Transferrin:
The Iron Carrier

Author

Simon Welch, Ph.D.
Department of Biochemistry
Queen Mary and Westfield College
University of London
London, England

CRC Press
Boca Raton   Ann Arbor   London   Tokyo

Library of Congress Cataloging-in-Publication Data

Welch, Simon.
    Transferrin: the iron carrier/author, Simon Welch.
      p.   cm.
    Includes bibliographical references and index.
    ISBN 0-8493-6793-X
    1. Transferrin. I. Title.
    QP552.T7W45   1992
    591.19'2454--dc20   91-39203
                                                                                  CIP

Direct all inquiries to CRC Press, Inc., 2000 Corporate Blvd., N.W., Boca Raton, Florida 33431.

© 1992 by CRC Press, Inc.

International Standard Book Number 0-8493-6793-X

Library of Congress Card Number 91-39203

Printed in the United States of America   1 2 3 4 5 6 7 8 9 0

Printed on acid-free paper

PREFACE

For all plants and animals, and for most microorganisms, iron is an essential nutritional requirement. Because of iron's subtle chemical properties, and possibly because of its abundance in the earth's crust, iron has been selected in molecular evolution to carry out a wide range of biological functions. This has not however been without a price. Iron is both insoluble and toxic. At the neutral pH and high oxygen tension of most physiological fluids, the predominant oxidation state of the transition metal iron is Fe^{3+} (ferric). In this form iron readily undergoes hydrolysis and polymerisation, resulting in a product of extreme insolubility. The toxicity of free iron is due principally to the ability of iron to catalyse the Fenton reaction, whereby the homolytic fission of hydrogen peroxide liberates the hydroxyl free radical (OH·). This highly reactive and aggressive free radical is capable of interacting with almost every type of molecule found in living cells, inflicting enormous damage on biological systems. Organisms have therefore been compelled to evolve specific molecules to store iron (ferritin) and to transport iron (transferrin) in a form that is both soluble and nontoxic whilst remaining readily available to biological systems.

Transferrin is a large glycoprotein molecule found in high concentration within the blood plasma of all vertebrates, as well as also being present in many other biological fluids. Whilst functioning principally as a vehicle for the transport of iron between the sites of absorption, storage and utilisation, transferrin also has an important role to play both as a growth promoter and as an antibacterial agent. In addition, the two high-affinity iron-binding sites of transferrin are also capable of binding as many as 29 other elements. Although most of these elements either have no known physiological role, or alternatively have their own independent transport proteins, there are four elements other than iron for which transferrin may act as a transport vehicle. These are the elements zinc, manganese, chromium, and vanadium.

Transferrin is but one member of a larger family of proteins known as the siderophilins. Other members include lactoferrin, ovotransferrin, and melanotransferrin. Whilst the biological roles of the other members of this family are somewhat different from the transport role of transferrin, all of the members of the siderophilin family are of a sufficiently similar structure, such that they are thought to have evolved from a common ancestral gene.

During recent years there have been many advances made in our understanding of transferrin structure, the mechanism by which the molecule binds iron, the process by which transferrin-bound iron enters cells, the structure and control of expression of the transferrin gene, and the inherited variability of the transferrin gene within human and other animal populations. These are the subjects of this book. It is hoped that the contents have been arranged in such a way as to appeal to a wide audience, including undergraduates in many fields of the biological sciences, as well as geneticists, physicians, and pathologists.

THE AUTHOR

Simon Welch, Ph.D., is Senior Lecturer in Biochemistry in the Faculty of Basic Medical Science at Queen Mary and Westfield College, University of London.

Dr. Welch graduated in Biochemistry in 1967 at The London Hospital Medical College, and obtained his Ph.D. in 1970. From 1970 to 1978 he served as Lecturer in Biochemistry at The London Hospital Medical College. In 1978, Dr. Welch was appointed as Senior Lecturer in Biochemistry — a post he held until 1990 — before assuming his present position at Queen Mary and Westfield College.

Dr. Welch's major research interests have been in the field of genetic variation of human and animal proteins, for which he has been the recipient of grants from the Medical Research Council and the Ministry of Overseas Development. In addition, he has researched and published on the subject of non-enzyme glycosylation of hemoglobin and its relationship to diabetic control, and on the mechanism of lactate transport across the hepatocyte membrane. His current research interest is the comparative structure and properties of human and animal transferrins.

TABLE OF CONTENTS

DEDICATION

Christine, Matthew, Jeremy, and Katherine

My family, without whose support, encouragement, and assistance the writing of this book would not have been possible.

Chapter 1

THE CHEMISTRY AND BIOLOGY OF IRON

I. INTRODUCTION

The element iron has been known since prehistoric times and it is probably true to say that no other element has played a more important role in the material progress of man. There is archeological evidence that iron was first smelted in Asia Minor by the Hittites about 3000 B.C. However, the secret of this process did not become more widely known until the fall of the Hittite empire 2000 years later, and with it the beginning of the "Iron Age". The name "iron" is Anglo-Saxon in origin (*iren*, cf. German *Eissen*). The symbol Fe and words such as "ferrous" originate from the Latin for iron — *ferrum*. Iron is an essential nutritional requirement for nearly every living organism. It is only in the case of a few microorganisms, such as *Lactobacillus,* that this element does not appear to be absolutely essential for survival. Iron would seem to have been selected during the process of molecular evolution to carry out a wide range of biological functions. In all probability this situation has arisen, not just as a result of the abundance of iron within the crust of the Earth, but also because of the rich and varied chemical properties exhibited by this transition element.

II. ATOMIC STRUCTURE

Iron has an atomic number of 26. Within the neutral atom, the 26 protons of the nucleus are surrounded by an electron cloud containing 26 electrons. The first two shells, K and L, are full, with two and eight electrons, respectively. The third shell, M, is incomplete, containing only 14 of the maximum 18 electrons permissible. The final outer N shell of iron contains two electrons. It is the incomplete filling of the penultimate M shell that characterises iron as a first series transition element. Within the M shell the s and p orbitals are full, with two and six electrons, respectively. The d orbital, which is gradually being filled with electrons as one progresses through the first series of the main transition elements from scandium, has only acquired six of the maximum ten possible electrons at the stage of iron. Since these six electrons, along with the two outer electrons of the N shell, have similar energy levels, the result is that iron has a total of eight valence electrons capable of participating in chemical bonding. It is this property that gives iron such a wide variety of chemical characteristics, including the formation of coloured ions, paramagnetism, catalytic activity, ready formation of stable coordination complexes, and the ability to exist in a wide range of oxidation states. Under certain circumstances iron can be found in oxidation states as high as $6+$ and as low as $2-$. However, in nature the most commonly encountered oxidation states for iron are Fe^{2+} (ferrous) and Fe^{3+} (ferric). Both of these oxidation states can exist as either high- or low-spin ions. The high-spin state has a larger atomic radius than the low-spin form. This difference in size is of great significance in the process of oxygenation of haemoglobin, since the reduction in size of the ferrous ion from high to low spin that occurs on oxygenation allows the smaller-diameter low-spin ion to slip into the plane of the porphyrin ring. This very small movement of the iron acts as the trigger that initiates much larger conformational changes within the globin polypeptide chain which are then transmitted to the adjoining three subunits of the haemoglobin tetramer. As a consequence, the binding of the first oxygen to haemoglobin increases the affinity of the remaining three binding sites for oxygen. This is the phenomenon of cooperativity.

In common with the other transition elements, iron exhibits a considerable propensity for forming coordination compounds with a wide range of ligands. Although coordination numbers from 3 to 8 are possible, the most common coordination number for complexes of iron is 6. An important biological example of such a 6-coordination complex is found within the molecule of haemoglobin. Within the haem group, four of the coordination sites are used to attach the iron to the four nitrogens of the porphyrin ring. The fifth coordination site is used to attach the haem group, via the iron, to an imidazole-nitrogen of one of the histidine residues of the globin polypeptide chain. The vacant sixth coordination site is free and available to bind oxygen during the process of oxygenation. Many further examples of iron-coordination complexes will be discussed in later chapters.

Naturally occurring iron has a relative atomic mass of 55.847 and is composed of a mixture of the four stable isotopes with mass numbers 54, 56, 57, and 58 (Table 1). In addition, a further six unstable and radioactive isotopes of the element iron can be produced. Some of these radioactive isotopes have been extensively used in studies of iron metabolism.

III. ORIGIN AND ABUNDANCE OF IRON IN THE SOLAR SYSTEM

Iron is an extremely abundant element. Taking the Earth as a whole, iron is second in abundance only to oxygen. Within the core of the Earth, however, iron is by far and away the most abundant element, making up some 90% of the mass of the core. Most of this is in the form of liquid iron, but at the very centre of the Earth (inner core), seismic studies suggest that solid iron is present. Even within the crust of the Earth, the layer of rocks forming the top few kilometres of the surface of our planet, iron is the fourth most abundant element behind oxygen, silicon, and aluminium. Nearly all the 30 elements that are essential to life, and this of course includes iron, are obtained from minerals within the crust. The chief iron-containing minerals found in the crust are haematite (Fe_2O_3), magnetite (Fe_3O_4), siderite ($FeCO_3$), and pyrite (FeS_2). Although the great abundance of iron within our environment does not of itself explain why the element has been selected to carry out such diverse biological roles, it is worth considering briefly how and why this situation has arisen. The combination of evidence from the sun and meteorites has allowed reasonably good estimates to be made of the abundances of all of the elements within the solar system as a whole. When these results are

TABLE 1
Iron, Electronic Configuration and Isotope Structures

IRON – Fe

Atomic number 26
Relative atomic mass 55.847

Electronic configuration:

Shell	K	L		M			N	
Orbital	s	s	p	s	p	d	s	
Number of electrons	2	2	6	2	6	6	2	Total: 26

					Isotope					
	Fe^{52}	Fe^{53}	Fe^{54}	Fe^{55}	Fe^{56}	Fe^{57}	Fe^{58}	Fe^{59}	Fe^{60}	Fe^{61}
Protons	26	26	26	26	26	26	26	26	26	26
Neutrons	26	27	28	29	30	31	32	33	34	35
Electrons	26	26	26	26	26	26	26	26	26	26
Mass no.	52	53	54	55	56	57	58	59	60	61
% Natural abundance	—	—	5.8	—	91.72	2.2	0.28	—	—	—
Half-life	8.2 h	8.5 m	—	2.6 y	—	—	—	45 d	3×10^5 y	6 d

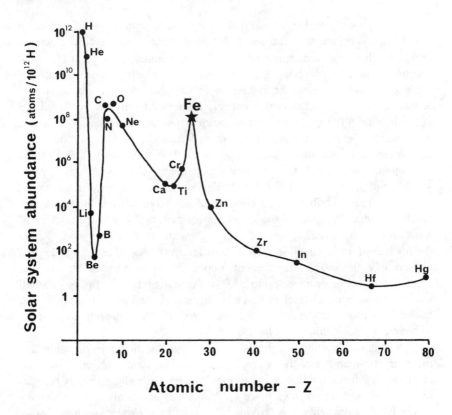

FIGURE 1. The abundance of the elements in the solar system in relation to their atomic numbers (Z), and the occurrence of the "Iron Peak" at Z = 26.

plotted against the atomic number (the number of protons within the nucleus of an atom), several interesting features can be seen (Figure 1). First, the very lightest elements hydrogen and helium make up a very high proportion of the total. Second, there is a general decline in the amount of an element in the solar system as the atomic number increases. The lighter elements predominate. Third, there is an obvious interruption in the relatively smooth curve that relates the decline in element abundance to increasing atomic number. This occurs when the number of protons has reached 26, and is known as the "Iron Peak".

To understand why iron is so abundant, it is necessary to consider how the individual elements are thought to have arisen since the birth of the universe 16 billion years ago, and in addition, why iron-56 has the most energetically stable nucleus of all of the elements.

The overall size of an atom is determined by the radius of the electron orbits, and whilst this is dependent upon the position of the element in the Periodic Table, it is generally of the order of 2×10^{-10} m. The nucleus of an atom, on the other hand, is very much smaller, with a diameter in the region of 1×10^{-14} m. This very large difference in size between the volume occupied by the nucleus of an atom and the volume occupied by the electron cloud helps to explain why the energy levels associated with nuclear reactions are so much greater than those of chemical reactions. In a typical chemical reaction, a process involving the redistribution of electrons between atoms, the energy involved is in the region of 700 kJ/mol. At this sort of energy level the nucleus of an atom is entirely stable and remains unaltered. In contrast, within the small volume of the nucleus, the nucleons (protons and neutrons) are very closely packed together. Therefore, the energy required to add or subtract nucleons in the process of nuclear reactions is many orders of magnitude higher than that required for chemical reactions. A typical value would be in the region of 100 GJ/mol. Yet despite this, atomic nuclei are not as entirely indestructible as had been originally thought by Dalton. Nuclear reactions, whereby the numbers of protons or neutrons within the nucleus of an atom can be altered, do indeed occur. These transmutation events change the nucleus of one element into either a different isotope of the same element or into an entirely different element, depending upon whether the nucleon change involves neutrons or protons. Processes involving the fusing of small nuclei, the addition of nucleons to existing nuclei, or the splitting of larger nuclei have provided the synthetic routes by which the elements are thought to have evolved within the solar system.[1]

The nucleon-binding energies associated with atomic nuclei are some 10^6 times greater than the energies associated with chemical reactions involving electrons. Synthetic nuclear reactions therefore have very large energy barriers to overcome and do not take place spontaneously, certainly at temperatures below 10^8 K, unless energy is provided by a nonthermal source such as cosmic rays or man-made particle accelerators. The temperature range in which nuclear reactions do become possible (10^9 to 10^{10} K) is similar to the temperatures thought to exist within the interior of stars. At temperatures above 10^{11} K, even the nuclei become unstable and dissociate into elementary particles. At the birth of the universe the temperature at the time of the big bang is thought to have been in the region of 10^{12} K. One second after the big bang, rapid expansion and cooling of the embryonic universe is likely to have reduced this temperature to 10^{11} K. In this environment stable atomic nuclei could not have existed, only the nuclear building blocks — electrons, protons, neutrons, photons, and other elementary particles. Further cooling of the universe resulted in temperatures that would have allowed these to combine by processes of fusion and neutron capture, resulting in the synthesis of the lightest elements, hydrogen and helium. The atomic ratio of hydrogen to helium within the sun is about 10 to 1, and together these two elements make up more than 99% of the mass of the sun. The sun alone contains more than 99% of the mass of the entire solar system. The continuing process of cooling and expansion within the interior of many of the stars, punctuated with episodes of explosive burning, sometimes resulting in the total disruption of the star, provided the environment in which further nuclear reactions would have occurred. This process resulted in the synthesis of many of the heavier elements. There is, however, a limit to which the processes of nuclear fusion leading to the production of ever heavier elements could have continued. It is in this connection that certain of the properties of the nucleus of the element iron assume significance.

When a nucleus is formed from smaller nuclei, energy is released. This is known as the binding energy, and gives a measure of the stability of that nucleus. The higher the binding energy, the more stable the nucleus. It is difficult to measure the binding energy directly in all but a few nuclear reactions. However, it is possible to obtain a good estimate of the value in a more subtle way. Accurate measurements of the mass of individual atoms have revealed that the mass of the nucleus is fractionally less than the sum of the masses of the component parts — protons and neutrons. Whilst this missing mass cannot be explained by the laws of classical physics, it is consistent with a prediction made by Einstein in his Special Theory of Relativity. Einstein's theory led to the famous equation that relates the mass of a body (m) to its energy (E) and the velocity of light (c):

$$E = mc^2$$

Since the velocity of light is known, and the mass loss of the nucleus can be measured, it is therefore possible to calculate the value of the nuclear binding energy (E) for each of the elements and their isotopes. If the nuclear binding energy is divided by the mass number, the result gives the binding energy per nucleon within an individual atomic nucleus. When the binding energy/nucleon is plotted against the mass number (Figure 2) it can be seen that the nuclear binding energy, and therefore the stability, rises rapidly with increasing mass number, reaches a peak at iron-56, and then decreases slowly as the nuclides become heavier. The nucleus of iron-56 is therefore the most energetically stable of all the atomic nuclei.

This experimental observation can only be explained by postulating the existence of an attractive force operating between nucleons strong enough to overcome the electrostatic repulsion between the positively charged protons within the nucleus. This force is known as the Strong Interaction. It differs from the electrostatic force in three ways. It is attractive, it operates over very short distances, and it operates equally between protons and neutrons. The binding force of the nucleus of any atom, and therefore its stability, will be dependent upon the balance between the electrostatic repulsion (long range) between protons and the Strong Interaction (short range) between nucleons. Within a small atomic nucleus the nucleons have space between themselves and are thought to be distributed mainly at the periphery of the nucleus. Long-range repulsive forces dominate, so the binding energies are low. As more protons and nucleons are added to the nucleus, and the mass number increases, the nucleons become more densely packed. The short-range attractive forces assume a greater importance and the binding energies increase. At iron-56, the optimum packing density of the nucleons has been reached and the

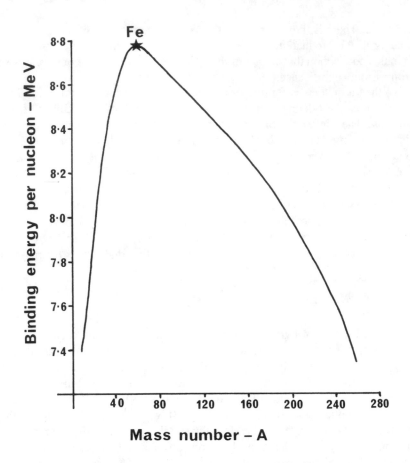

FIGURE 2.   The binding energy of the nucleons (protons and neutrons) in relation to the mass number (A) of the elements.

maximum advantage of the Strong Interaction occurs. As additional nucleons are added, and the mass number rises still further, the distance between the nucleons does not decrease any further. Therefore, whilst the short-range attractive force between nucleons does not increase in atomic nuclei beyond iron-56, the long-range electrostatic repulsive force between ever more distant protons continues to rise. The net effect is a gradual reduction in nucleon binding energy beyond iron-56. This explains why iron-56 has the most energetically stable of all the atomic nuclei.

During the synthesis of the elements within the stars, it remained energetically favourable to produce elements up to and including iron by processes involving the fusion of lighter nuclei. By far the greatest release of energy came from the initial reactions of this pathway generating the very light elements hydrogen and helium. As the sequence continued it would have been progressively more difficult to overcome the energy barriers and synthesise the heavier elements. Elements beyond iron could have been formed by these fusion reactions, but only by the addition of extra energy. It is also likely that a proportion of the heavier elements have been formed by the splitting of even heavier nuclei into smaller fragments — nuclear fission. However, the generally accepted route by which most of the heavier nuclides were formed is that they were the products of the major nuclear burning reactions of supernovae. At the exceptionally high temperatures involved during these explosive reactions, electrons were forced into such high transitional energy levels that it became favourable for them to combine with protons and form neutrons. Elements above iron could then have been formed by neutron capture. This is energetically favourable, since neutrons, unlike electrons, do not experience the Coulomb barrier, since they have no charge. During this synthetic process, as the mass of the isotope increases with the addition of successive neutrons, so the stability decreases. The unstable nucleus will undergo β-decay, ejecting an electron as a neutron is converted into a proton. This results in an increase in atomic number and the transmutation of the starting nuclide into a new element. In addition, some of the unstable heavy nuclides would have split into smaller fragments by the process of α-decay in which a helium nucleus (two protons and two neutrons) is ejected, resulting in a new element with an atomic number of two less than the starting nuclide. The difficulties associated with the synthesis of the elements heavier than iron may at least in part explain why their abundancies fall rapidly after the "iron peak".

However, the fact that nearly every living organism uses iron for a wide range of biological functions cannot be explained entirely on the basis of the abundance of iron within the crust of the Earth. For reasons already discussed, the stability of the iron-56 nucleus that may have indirectly led to the abundance of the element has no effect on the chemical reactivity of iron. It is only the configuration of the electrons of this transition metal that explains its rich and varied chemical properties. It is these very properties that have been exploited to the full by nearly every form of life on our planet.

IV. BIOLOGICAL ROLES OF IRON

Rather than having one single biological role, iron is found to participate in a very wide range of biochemical reactions. Since free iron is both insoluble and toxic, the form in which iron functions in living organisms is always in association with a suitably tailored protein environment, where iron assumes an irreplaceable role as a catalyst for many intracellular and extracellular reactions. The many and varied iron proteins and iron enzymes have been traditionally divided into three major categories:

1. The iron-tetrapyrrole complexes
2. The iron-sulphur proteins
3. The iron proteins

The brief account that follows is not intended to be an extensive and complete catalogue of every iron-containing protein found in living organisms. Instead, a few selected examples within each of the three categories will be described in order to demonstrate the versatility of iron within biological systems.

A. THE IRON-TETRAPYRROLE COMPLEXES

Members of this large group of iron-containing proteins are sometimes better known as the haem proteins, and they consist of two component parts, an iron porphyrin and a protein unit. Porphyrins are cyclic compounds formed by the linkage of four pyrrole rings. A characteristic property of the porphyrins is that they readily form complexes with metal ions. In the case of the iron porphyrins, the iron is situated at the centre of the porphyrin ring attached by four coordination links to the nitrogen atoms of the four pyrrole rings. A fifth coordination link attaches the iron directly to the protein, and this is most commonly to an imidazole nitrogen of a histidine residue. Finally, the sixth coordination link of the iron in many respects dictates the ultimate function of the haem protein. In molecules such as haemoglobin and myoglobin the ligand is water. This can then be displaced by oxygen when these molecules assume their intended biological roles as oxygen-binding proteins. In the case of other examples of haem proteins, the sixth coordination link is to the protein itself, the ligand usually being an imidazole nitrogen or the sulphur atom of either a cysteine or methionine residue. In this situation the molecule is then unable to function as an oxygen carrier, but instead is frequently found to participate in redox reactions in which the iron can reversibly alternate between the two common oxidation states Fe^{3+} and Fe^{2+}. The electron-carrying cytochromes belong to this group of haem proteins.

Examples of the iron-tetrapyrrole complexes include:

1. *Haemoglobin* — A family of haem proteins that function as oxygen-binding respiratory pigments. Haemoglobins are found not only in the red cells of vertebrates, but also in the tissues of a wide range of lower organisms including some bacteria, yeasts, moulds, root nodules of leguminous plants, molluscs, crustaceans, and insects. Whilst the haemoglobin of higher vertebrates consists of four polypeptide chains, each containing an iron group, the structure in lower organisms is more varied. In some invertebrates, haemoglobin contains up to 100 iron porphyrin groups in one giant molecule, whereas in other organisms the molecule consists of a single polypeptide chain with one haem group.
2. *Myoglobin* — A haem protein found in vertebrate muscle cells consisting of a single polypeptide chain with one iron porphyrin group. It functions as an oxygen-storage pigment.
3. *Cytochromes* — The cytochromes are a large family of haem proteins in which the iron functions as a redox couple. These electron carriers are found in both prokaryotes and eukaryotes. In higher organisms,

many of the cytochromes are an integral part of the structure of the inner mitochondrial membrane.

4. *Catalase* — An Fe^{3+} haem-containing enzyme that catalyses the reduction of one molecule of hydrogen peroxide with the simultaneous oxidation of a second molecule of hydrogen peroxide, the reaction products being water and oxygen.
5. *Peroxidase* — An Fe^{3+} haem enzyme that catalyses the reduction of a molecule of hydrogen peroxide to water, with the simultaneous oxidation of a second substrate (RH_2).

B. THE IRON-SULPHUR PROTEINS

This is a large and varied group of proteins with examples found in bacteria, plants, and higher organisms. The proteins contain iron complexed to the sulphydryl groups of cysteine residues in the polypeptide chain. In addition, many of the iron-sulphur proteins contain additional atoms of inorganic sulphur. Many of the more complex iron-sulphur proteins contain additional atoms and prosthetic groups including molybdenum, flavinoids, or haem. The number of atoms of iron present can range from one to as many as eight. Examples of iron-sulphur proteins include:

1. *Rubredoxins* — Small-molecular-weight bacterial proteins containing one or two atoms of iron bound to cysteine residues. No additional inorganic sulphur is present. Rubredoxins participate in redox reactions as well as being involved in the hydroxylation of alkanes and fatty acids.
2. *Ferrodoxins* — A large family of plant and bacterial proteins containing two, four, or eight atoms of iron and additional inorganic sulphur. In plants the ferrodoxins are involved in the electron-transport reactions associated with photosynthesis. In bacteria their functions are more numerous and include nitrate reduction, sulphate and sulphite reduction, nitrogen fixation, photosynthesis, and ATP synthesis.
3. *Adrenodoxin* — A mammalian ferrodoxin-like protein found in the mitochondria and microsomes of the liver, kidney, and adrenal gland. Adrenodoxins participate in the hydroxylation of steroid hormones and vitamin D in association with cytochrome P-450.
4. *Mitochondrial ferrodoxins* — This is a family of iron-sulphur proteins found in association with the respiratory complexes of mitochondria. They function as electron carriers within the electron-transport chain. An iron-sulphur protein component of respiratory complex III was originally termed Rieske's protein.
5. *Xanthine oxidase* — This enzyme, containing eight atoms of iron, catalyses the hydroxylation of purines and is present in liver, milk, and even some microorganisms.
6. *Aconitase* — A mitochondrial enzyme of the Krebs citric acid cycle. It is one of the few iron-sulphur proteins not involved in a redox reaction.

7.   *Amido phosphoribosyl transferase* — A mammalian and bacterial enzyme catalysing the first reaction in the *de novo* synthesis of purines.

C. THE IRON PROTEINS (NONHAEM; NONSULPHUR)

The third group of iron-containing proteins comprises a large family of molecules in which the iron atoms are not linked either to a porphyrin group or to the sulphur atoms of amino acid residues. This group is conveniently subdivided into (1) the iron oxygenases and (2) the binuclear oxo-bridged iron proteins.

The Iron Oxygenases

1.   *Dioxygenases* — Enzymes that catalyse the introduction of both atoms of molecular oxygen into the substrate. Examples of dioxygenases include homogentisic acid oxidase and proline hydroxylase.
2.   *Monoxygenases* — These enzymes are also known as mixed-function oxidases. They catalyse hydroxylation reactions in which one oxygen atom is attached to the substrate, whilst the second oxygen atom combines with hydrogen to form water. Examples include phenylalanine hydroxylase and a group of enzymes present in liver microsomes associated with the detoxification of drugs and other foreign substances.

The Binuclear Oxo-Bridged Iron Proteins

Binuclear oxo-bridged iron proteins contain two atoms of iron, each attached to three histidine residues of the protein. In addition, the iron atoms are linked to each other by an oxygen bridge. Four members of this family are worthy of mention:

1.   *Hemerythrin* — An oxygen-carrying protein present in the erythrocytes of various invertebrates, including annelid worms and brachiopods. The molecules are composed of eight identical polypeptide chains, each containing two atoms of iron (Fe^{2+}).
2.   *Ribonucleotide reductase* — An essential enzyme for all living organisms that catalyses the conversion of ribonucleotide diphosphates into the deoxyribonucleotides that are required for the synthesis of DNA. Those few organisms that do not require iron for growth, such as *Lactobacillus,* contain a ribonucleotide reductase enzyme that uses cobalt at the active site rather than iron.
3.   *Uteroferrin* — Otherwise known as the purple acid phosphatases, these mammalian enzymes have been isolated from the spleen and uterus. They catalyse the removal of protein-bound phosphates.
4.   *Methane oxygenase* — A bacterial enzyme that catalyses the oxidation of methane to methanol.

V. PROBLEMS ASSOCIATED WITH THE USE OF IRON BY LIVING ORGANISMS

A. SOLUBILITY OF IRON

Considering the abundance of iron within the crust of the earth and the rich and varied chemical properties of the element that have been so extensively exploited by most species, one might be led to imagine that an ideal and problem-free situation exists — organisms making use of the properties of iron and living in an environment where the element is in plentiful supply. This, however, is not the case. One of the very properties of this transition metal upon which cells have become so dependent, namely the redox couple Fe^{2+}/Fe^{3+}, has itself imposed severe problems for living organisms. This can be best appreciated by a brief consideration of the aqueous solution chemistry of iron.

The hydrated forms of the two most common oxidation states of iron, $Fe(H_2O)_6^{2+}$ and $Fe(H_2O)_6^{3+}$, are stable in acid solutions. However, as the pH is raised protons are lost, resulting in the formation of hydroxy-iron species in a process known as hydrolysis. These hydroxy-iron species have a tendency to polymerise, and as this proceeds, so the solubility of the iron decreases. There is, however, a significant difference between the ferrous and ferric ions in this respect.

In the case of the hydrated ferrous (Fe^{2+}) ion, hydrolysis does not begin to occur until the pH has risen to about 7. The result is that the solubility for Fe^{2+} is 10^{-1} M at pH 7 and has only reduced to about 10^{-3} M by pH 8.

On the other hand, $Fe(H_2O)_6^{3+}$ is far more acidic than its ferrous counterpart. In aqueous solution the process of hydrolysis starts at low pH, with the result that the solubility of Fe^{3+} is 10^{-2} M at pH 2, and by the time the pH has risen to 7 the solubility of the ferric ion is extremely low — 10^{-18} M!! This in effect means that ferric salts are intrinsically unstable in aqueous solution unless acid is added. For example, ferric chloride is readily soluble in water. If the solution is left to stand for even a short period of time, irreversible hydrolytic formation of insoluble hydroxy-Fe^{3+} polymers readily occurs. The particles have a fairly uniform size of 70 Å and each contains about 1200 iron atoms.

This insolubility of iron, particularly Fe^{3+}, due to the hydrolytic reactions, creates considerable problems for all organisms for which iron is an essential nutrient. There is no doubt that the problem is far greater with respect to the ferric ion than if living organisms could obtain and utilise the ferrous ion from their environment. At the beginning of chemical evolution before the appearance of life forms on Earth, the atmosphere was completely different from the contemporary one. Oxygen was missing, and the main constituents were H_2, N_2, CO, CO_2, and CH_4. Within this reducing environment, Fe^{2+} would have been the predominant iron species, and there is evidence to this effect in old rock formations. However, once oxygen appeared in the atmosphere the situation would have dramatically changed. The potential for the Fe^{3+}/Fe^{2+} couple (0.77 V) is such that molecular oxygen will rapidly convert Fe^{2+} into Fe^{3+}. As a result of the change to an oxidising environment in which Fe^{3+} is the predominant oxidation state for iron, present-day plants, bacteria, and higher organisms are faced with a series of problems relating to the acquisition, transport, and storage of iron.

B. TOXICITY OF IRON

Although iron is essential for a wide variety of metabolic processes, the element, particularly as the free ferrous or ferric ion, can also have several deleterious effects within an organism. It is for this reason, in addition to its insolubility, that iron in biological systems is tightly bound to proteins or small-molecular-weight chelators. Normally the "free-iron" pool is kept extremely small and only becomes significant in situations of iron overload.

The toxicity of free iron is due principally to the ability of Fe^{2+} to catalyse the Fenton reaction. This involves the homolytic fission of the O–O bond in hydrogen peroxide (H_2O_2):

$$Fe^{2+} + H_2O_2 \rightarrow Fe^{3+} + OH^- + OH\cdot \tag{1}$$

The products of the Fenton reaction, in addition to the ferric (Fe^{3+}) and hydroxyl (OH^-) ions, include the hydroxyl free radical $OH\cdot$. A broad definition of a free radical is a species capable of independent existence that contains one or more unpaired electrons.[2]

The $OH\cdot$ radical is a highly reactive species that is capable of interacting with almost every type of molecule found in living cells — including sugars, amino acids, membrane lipids, and nucleic acids. Frequently, the products of the reaction between $OH\cdot$ and these nonradical species are a range of new free radicals, usually less aggressive than $OH\cdot$. The extent of the damage that $OH\cdot$ radicals can inflict upon biological systems is enormous, ranging from membrane destruction to DNA mutation.

Equation 1 describes only part of the complex Fenton reaction. Other associated reactions include:

$$Fe^{3+} + H_2O_2 \rightarrow Fe^{2+} + O_2^- + H^+ \tag{2}$$

$$OH\cdot + H_2O_2 \rightarrow H_2O + H^+ + O_2^- \tag{3}$$

$$O_2^- + Fe^{3+} \rightarrow Fe^{2+} + O_2 \tag{4}$$

$$OH\cdot + Fe^{2+} \rightarrow Fe^{3+} + OH^- \tag{5}$$

A simple mixture of iron salts and H_2O_2 can therefore provoke a series of free-radical reactions, the overall result of which, assuming no other reaction is available to intercept the $OH\cdot$ radical, is an iron-catalysed decomposition of the hydrogen peroxide:

$$2H_2O_2 \xrightarrow{\text{Fe salt catalysis}} 2H_2O + O_2$$

For the catastrophic effects of the Fenton reaction to be significant in any biological situations, it is necessary for the two participating reactants to be present — hydrogen peroxide and free iron. Hydrogen peroxide is produced in normal cellular metabolism, much of it coming from the dismutation of the superoxide ion — O_2^-. Most aerobic cells form superoxide ions when the oxygen molecule (O_2) accepts a single electron. The presence of the highly active enzyme superoxide dismutase rapidly converts O_2^- into H_2O_2, thereby producing the necessary substrate for the Fenton reaction. All that is now required is the presence of a suitable Fenton catalyst such as free iron in order for the chain of events summarised in Equations 1 to 5 to be initiated. No doubt this is why organisms strive to keep the pool of free iron as small as possible by complexing the element with suitable proteins and small-molecular-weight chelators.

Some of the strategies that have been evolved in the animal, plant, and microbial kingdoms in order to overcome the problems associated with both the toxicity of free iron and the insolubility of the ferric ion at neutral pH will be discussed in the following brief review.

VI. EVOLUTION OF SYSTEMS WITHIN NATURE TO OVERCOME THE PROBLEMS OF IRON SOLUBILITY AND TOXICITY

A. MICROORGANISMS

With a few exceptions, such as *Lactobacillus,* all microorganisms including the fungi have an absolute requirement for iron,[3] with the minimal requirement for iron in their growth medium being in the range 0.4 to $4 \times 10^{-6} M$. Since the concentration of soluble ferric iron in the aqueous environments in which microorganisms live (soil, water, tissue fluids of host organisms, etc.) rarely exceeds $10^{-18} M$, bacteria have had to devise mechanisms to scavenge and solubilise iron in order to survive. This has been achieved by evolving a range of low-molecular-weight iron chelators exhibiting extremely high complex-formation constants. These molecules are known as the **siderophores**, a term proposed by Lankford in 1973.[4] Under conditions of iron deprivation, bacteria synthesise and secrete the siderophores into their external environment. With their high affinity for ferric iron, the siderophores chelate and solublise Fe^{3+} from minerals, organic substrates, and possibly even from the small amount of iron in solution. Although there is a great diversity in the structures of the siderophores, one common feature is that they all provide an octahedral coordination sphere for the iron, usually formed by six oxygen atoms (hexadentate). In some cases all six oxygen atoms are contributed by a single siderophore molecule, whereas in other examples as many as three separate siderophore molecules are necessary to provide the

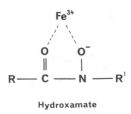

Hydroxamate

Catechol

FIGURE 3.   The basic structures of the two classes of siderophores — hydroxamates and catechols.

six oxygens that chelate a single Fe^{3+}. Most of the siderophores that have been isolated and characterised can be classified into one of two chemical categories, catechols or hydroxamates (Figure 3).

1.   *Catechols*: A good example of a catechol-phenolate siderophore is the molecule enterobactin, produced by many of the enteric bacteria, including *Escherichia coli*. This is a cyclic structure composed of three molecules of 2,3-dihydroxy-*N*-benzoyl serine (Figure 4). Further siderophores from this group include examples where the amino acid serine is replaced by either glycine or threonine. Other examples of catechol siderophores have linear rather than cyclic structures (pseudobactin).

2.   *Hydroxamates*: Members of this very large and variable group of siderophores are either cyclic or linear peptides containing various types of hydroxamic acids. Since there is no one model compound that describes all the characteristics of this group, a selection of examples are shown in Figure 5 — ferrichrome, ferrioxamine, and aerobactin.

Many other low-molecular-weight iron chelators have been isolated from microorganisms, and the molecules exhibit a range of novel structures that do not readily fit into either of the two main groups described.

Once the siderophores have chelated the Fe^{3+} from the external environment, the complex then has to be taken up by the cell, and this process involves specific receptors on the cell membrane. In some cases the iron-siderophore complex is transported into the cell, the iron is released, and the

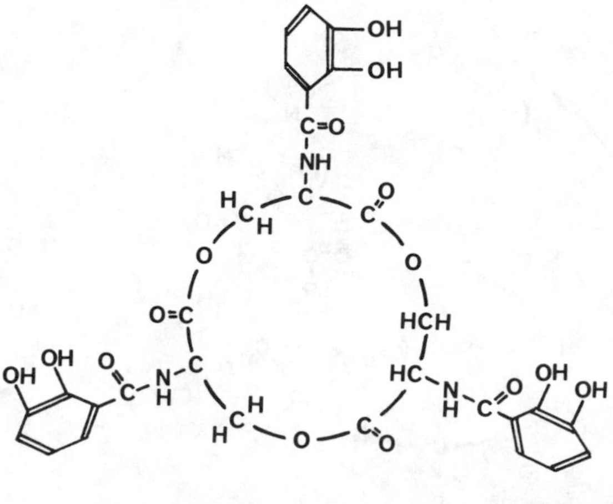

FIGURE 4. The structure of enterobactin — a cyclic catechol produced by *Escherichia coli*.

siderophore is either degraded or recycled for further use. In other examples only the ferric ion is transported across the membrane. The genetic control of siderophore, receptor, and transporter synthesis is extremely complex and there are examples of microorganisms that secrete more than one type of siderophore in situations of iron deprivation. Once inside the cell, the ferric ion has but a short journey in order to reach the sites of iron utilisation. Whether or not this process involves additional chelators is a matter of speculation, but there is no evidence that microorganisms use specific iron-transport proteins, unlike the higher organisms to be described later.

There seems no limit to the ingenuity demonstrated by microorganisms in their search for iron. It has recently been shown by Schryvers[5] that the pathogenic organism *Haemophilus influenzae* can use as a sole source of iron the Fe^{3+} transport protein of the vertebrate host, namely transferrin. Cell membranes of iron-deficient strains of this bacteria were found to contain a specific receptor for transferrin. A similar situation has been described in the Gram-negative bacteria *Neisseria meningitides* and *N. gonorrhoeae*. Neither of these organisms secrete siderophores, but instead synthesise and express cell membrane receptors specific for human transferrin and lactoferrin.[6-8] Another example of an organism that has evolved a means of obtaining iron from human transferrin is the malarial parasite. *Plasmodium falciparum*, whilst living within the human erythrocyte, apparently utilises none of the 20 mM intraerythrocytic haem for its iron supply. Instead, iron is obtained from human plasma transferrin. Since the mature erythrocyte has no transferrin receptors, the malarial parasite overcomes the problem by synthesising its own transferrin receptors, which are subsequently incorporated into the host red cell membrane, thereby enabling the parasite to acquire iron from human transferrin.[9,10]

As recently as 1978, it was generally considered that bacteria, unlike complex multicellular higher organisms, had neither the need to store iron,

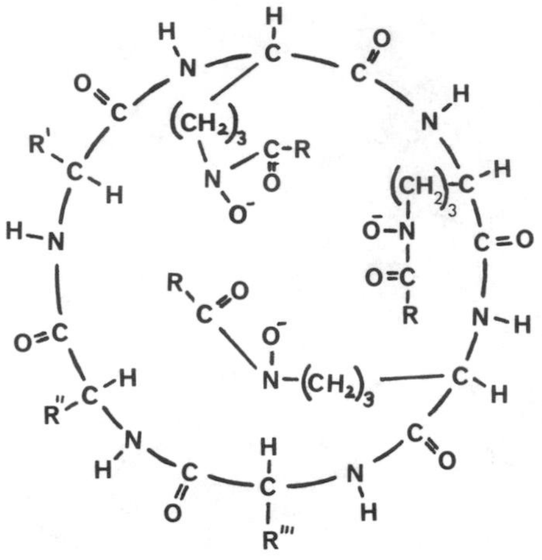

Ferrichrome

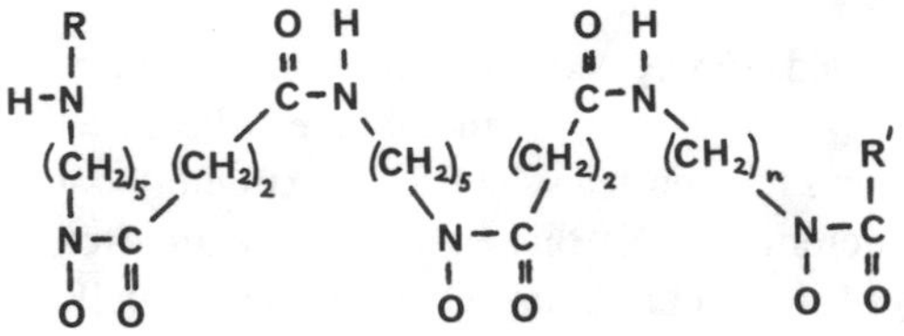

Ferrioxamine

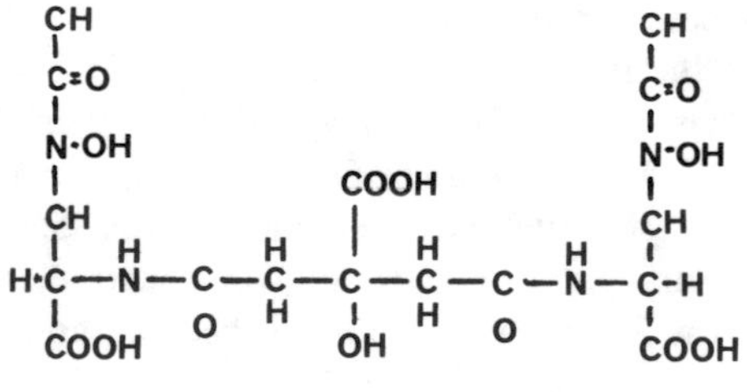

Aerobactin

FIGURE 5. Three examples of hydroxamate siderophores — ferrichrome, ferrioxamine, and aerobactin.

nor the mechanism to do so. This view has changed with the discovery of a class of bacterial iron-storage proteins known as the **bacterioferritins**.[11] Unlike the ferritin of higher organisms, bacterioferritins contain haem iron as well as nonhaem iron.

Harrison and Lilley[12] have suggested that these bacterial proteins may serve a dual function as both iron stores and *b*-type cytochromes. It has recently been possible to crystallise bacterioferritin free of the haem component. Whilst the bacterial protein has much in common with mammalian ferritin, namely

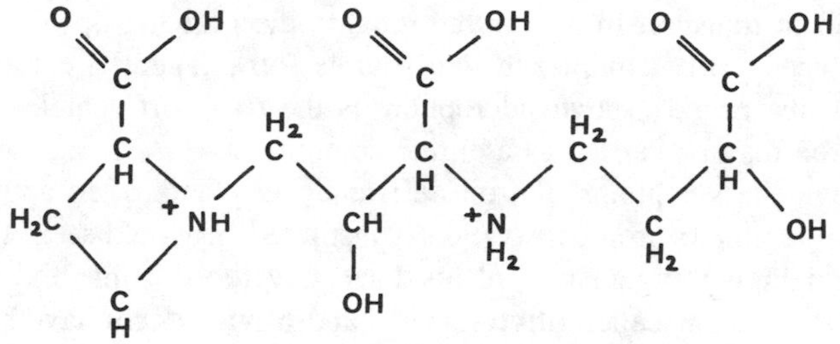

FIGURE 6. Mugineic acid — an example of a plant siderophore (phytosiderophore).

24 identical polypeptide subunits, the lack of sequence homology suggests that there is no direct evolutionary relationship between the two proteins.

B. PLANTS

In many respects, plants and soil-living microorganisms share a common problem in acquiring iron from an external environment where, although insoluble iron is often in abundance, the concentration of soluble and available Fe^{3+} is extremely low ($10^{-18} M$). The minimum concentration of iron required for normal plant growth is between 10^{-4} and $10^{-9} M$, depending upon the species and other environmental factors.[13] Iron deficiency is characterised by the appearance of chlorosis (a yellowing of the leaves). The problem for some plants is made even more acute if the soil contains large numbers of bacteria and fungi which compete for the iron with their high-efficiency siderophores.

Whereas microorganisms rely on a single method in order to obtain iron (siderophore secretion), plants have evolved a range of mechanisms in order to increase iron solubilisation from the soil. Four strategies have been characterised, occuring within the root tips: (a) secretion of acid into the soil, by means of an ATP-dependent proton pump; a decrease of one pH unit will increase the solubility of iron by a factor of 10^3; (b) secretion of reducing equivalents via either $NADH_2$ or $NADPH_2$, stimulating the release of iron from iron complexes by reducing Fe^{3+} to Fe^{2+}; (c) gross morphological changes in root structure; and (d) secretion of low-molecular-weight iron chelators into the soil. These **phytosiderophores**, such as mugineic acid (Figure 6), have far lower affinities for iron than the bacterial siderophores.

In addition to these four mechanisms, some crop plants, such as wheat and potatoes, have entered into a symbiotic relationship with a group of rhizobacteria — *Pseudomonas fluorescens*.[14] The rhizobacteria colonise the plant roots and secrete their own siderophore — pseudobactin. On the one hand this reduces the amount of iron available for other microorganisms, particularly the pathogenic fungi to which the plant would otherwise be susceptible. At the same time the plant roots have evolved a mechanism by which they can specifically absorb the Fe^{3+}-pseudobactin complex to use as their own supply of iron.

In order to transport iron from the roots to the growing tip of the plant, ferric iron needs to be complexed in a soluble form. There is evidence that in some plants the Fe^{3+}-phytosiderophore is the transport vehicle, whereas in others iron may be carried as a citrate complex.

Although the symptoms of iron deficiency in plants often appear very soon after a regime of iron deprivation is instituted, it would seem that, like bacteria and higher organisms, plants have developed a method for iron storage. Two proteins called **phytoferritin** and **phytosiderin** have been partially characterised. They strongly resemble the corresponding iron-storage proteins of higher organisms that will be described in the next section.

C. HIGHER ORGANISMS (e.g., VERTEBRATES)

Iron deficiency is generally regarded as the single most prevalent nutritional syndrome in man. It has been estimated that as many as 750 million people, one seventh of the population of the world, suffer from iron deficiency. Negative iron balance arises when the amount of iron required for growth plus the iron lost from the body is less than that absorbed. Whilst a far more detailed account of human iron metabolism will be given in Chapter 2, the very brief synopsis that follows is given in order to complete the comparison of the strategies employed by bacteria, plants, and higher organisms for the acquisition, transport, and storage of iron.

Higher organisms have developed complex digestive systems in order to deal with the wide range of food substances, of plant and animal origin, in their diet. Whilst vertebrates have little or no control over the amount of iron lost from their bodies, they can, to a limited extent, regulate the amount of iron absorbed from the diet in order to prevent the consequences of iron deficiency or iron overload. Nevertheless, the efficiency of iron absorption from an average diet is rather poor, and in the region of 10%. This figure is dependent upon the nature of the diet. Iron from plant sources has an absorption level of between 1 and 6%, compared with a value of between 10 and 20% for the iron of animal origin. Dietary iron comes principally from two pools. The first is the haem iron from molecules such as haemoglobin, myoglobin, and the cytochromes. The second is the nonhaem iron. As a general rule, haem iron is absorbed far better than nonhaem iron. Iron from mineral sources makes an insignificant contribution.

Many factors affect the bioavailability and absorption of iron by higher organisms, and only a few will be mentioned at this stage. In man, Fe^{2+} is absorbed far better than Fe^{3+}, explaining why the treatment of iron deficiency is usually achieved by the administration of ferrous salts. On the other hand, the efficiency of absorption of Fe^{2+} and Fe^{3+} is the same in animals such as dogs, rats, and guineapigs. Therefore in humans, factors that promote the reduction of iron will enhance absorption. These include vitamin C and gastric acidity. Inhibitors of iron absorption include many dietary proteins such as those found in milk and eggs. This explains why these two foods are poor suppliers of dietary iron. Other smaller-molecular-weight iron chelators, particularly those of plant origin such as oxalate, phosphate, and phytic acid, all reduce the availability of dietary iron.

In summary, vertebrates have no need to synthesise and secrete iron scavengers equivalent to the bacterial and plant siderophores. A mixed and varied diet will contain far more "soluble" and available iron than is present in the environment of bacteria and plants. Even when only 10% of dietary iron is absorbed, this is usually sufficient to supply the normal daily need of about 1 mg of iron that is needed to replace the equivalent amount that is irreversibly lost from the body during the same period. It is only when the body iron stores are exhausted and inadequate diet, disease, or accelerated iron loss occurs, that the symptoms of iron deficiency will appear.

Large and complex higher organisms are faced with an additional problem not experienced by bacteria, and possibly only to a limited extent by very large plants. This relates to how the organisms can move the potentially insoluble ferric ion around the body. Once iron has been absorbed from the gut it needs to be transported to, and between, the sites of utilisation and storage. The problems associated with the hydrolysis of the hydrated ferric ion have necessitated the evolution by higher organisms of a specific transport vehicle for iron. In vertebrates this role is carried out by a glycoprotein found in blood plasma and many other tissue fluids. The molecule is called **transferrin**. It is an extremely abundant plasma protein — evidence of its vital role — and has been detected within the blood of every vertebrate in which it has been sought. The structure, function, mechanisms of action, and genetic control of transferrin are the subject matter of this book.

Finally, mention should be made at this stage of the mechanism of iron storage by higher organisms. In humans, the body of an adult male contains about 4 g of iron. Of this iron, 70% is directly involved in cell structure and function, principally in the form of haemoglobin (2.3 g), myoglobin (0.3 g), and the other iron-containing proteins and enzymes (0.2 g). The remaining gram is stored in a soluble and available form. For an adult male this is sufficient to maintain body iron status for about 2 years, assuming no iron is taken in the diet and daily iron loss is in the normal range. The vital role played by the iron stores of higher organisms is therefore apparent.

Most of the iron stores are found in the liver and spleen, but because of the insoluble nature of the ferric ion, this store needs to be in a form that prevents the hydrolysis and precipitation of the iron, whilst still retaining the capacity to be readily mobilised. A specific and well-characterised protein has been evolved to carry out the function of iron storage. The molecule is called **ferritin**. The structure, function, mechanism of iron uptake and release, and genetic control of ferritin synthesis has been an area of intensive research over the last 30 years, and the subject of many recent reviews.[15-17] The following brief account summarises a few selected characteristics of ferritin.

Ferritin is a 24-subunit protein with a molecular weight in the region of 500,000. The structure of the molecule is organised such that the subunits are packed together, forming a spherical shell of 25-Å thickness. The interior of the iron-free molecule (apoferritin) can be accessed via specific channels in this shell. These channels provide a pathway by which iron can enter and leave the storage molecule. When loaded with iron, the core of ferritin is found to contain a mixture of ferric hydroxide (FeOOH) and ferric phosphate ($FeOOPO_3H_2$) of microcrystalline structure. The phosphate/iron ratio within the iron core of ferritin has been found to vary considerably between different preparations of iron-loaded ferritin (1:4.5 to 1:20). When fully loaded with iron, each ferritin molecule can accommodate as many as 4500 Fe^{3+} atoms.

In tissues, ferritin has been found to exist in multiple molecular forms (isoferritins). This heterogeneity can be partly explained by the existence of two structurally different polypeptide subunits — H and L. These are under independent genetic control and the proportions of the two different subunits in the 24-subunit final structure can vary between tissues. In addition, variations in the composition of the sugar chains attached to the subunits can be the source of further structural heterogeneity. The mechanisms for the *in vivo* uptake and release of iron by ferritin are only partly understood, and much of the information obtained from *in vitro* experiments may not be strictly relevant. Fe^{2+} is far more rapidly assimilated into ferritin than is Fe^{3+}. There is evidence that specific primary binding sites within ferritin catalyse the oxidation of bound Fe^{2+}, since it is Fe^{3+} that is the final storage form of the iron within the microcrystalline core. The reverse process of iron release requires the reduction of the ferric ion. In addition, small-molecular-weight Fe^{2+} iron chelators with access to the core may also be involved in the process of iron mobilisation from ferritin.

In addition to ferritin, there is a second iron-storage compound that can be detected within the cells of higher organisms. This is the molecule called **haemosiderin**. It represents a far more insoluble iron deposit than ferritin, and it accumulates within tissues in situations of iron overload. Haemosiderin forms intracellular iron-containing granules that are visible under the light microscope. The granules which often appear to be membrane enclosed are thought to be iron-laden secondary lysozymes, and have been termed "siderosomes". The iron within the haemosiderin granules is not readily available to the organism. However, since the iron-containing particles within haemosiderin share many structural similarities with the iron of the ferritin core, it now seems clear that haemosiderin originates from the partial degradation of ferritin.[18]

REFERENCES

1. **Cox, P. A.**, *The Elements. Their Origin, Abundance and Distribution*, Oxford University Press, New York, 1989.
2. **Halliwell, B. and Gutteridge, J. M. C.**, in *Free Radicals in Biology and Medicine*, Clarendon Press, Oxford, 1985.

3. **Weinberg, E. D.**, Iron and infection, *Microbiol. Rev.*, 42, 45, 1978.
4. **Lankford, C. E.**, Microbial iron metabolism, *Crit. Rev. Microbiol.*, 2, 273, 1973.
5. **Schryvers, A. B.**, Identification of the transferrin and lactoferrin binding proteins in *Haemophilus influenzae*, *J. Med. Microbiol.*, 29, 121, 1989.
6. **West, S. H. and Sparling, P. F.**, Response of *Neisseria gonorrhoeae* to iron limitation: alteration in expression of membrane proteins without apparent siderophore production, *Infect. Immun.*, 47, 388, 1985.
7. **Tsai, J., Dyer, D. W., and Sparling, P. F.**, Loss of transferrin receptor activity in *Neisseria meningitides* correlates with the inability to use transferrin as an iron source, *Infect. Immun.*, 50, 3132, 1988.
8. **Lee, B. C. and Schryvers, A. R.**, Specificity of the lactoferrin and transferrin receptor in *Neisseria gonorrhoeae*, *Mol. Microbiol.*, 2, 827, 1988.
9. **Pollack, S. and Fleming, J.**, *Plasmodium falciparum* takes up iron from transferrin, *Br. J. Haematol.*, 58, 289, 1984.
10. **Halder, K., Henderson, C. L., and Cross, G. A. M.**, Identification of the parasite transferrin receptor of *Plasmodium falciparum*-infected erythrocytes and its acylation via 1,2-diacyl-5n-glycerol, *Proc. Natl. Acad. Sci. U.S.A.*, 83, 8565, 1986.
11. **Yariv, J., Kalb, A. J., Sperling, E. R., Bauminger, E. R., Cohen, S. G., and Ofer, S.**, The composition and structure of bacterioferritin of *E.Coli*, *Biochem. J.*, 197, 171, 1980.
12. **Harrison, P. M. and Lilley, T. H.**, Ferritin, in *Iron Carriers and Iron Proteins*, T. M. Loehr, Ed., VCH Press, New York, 1989, chap. 2.
13. **Winkelmann, G., van der Helm, D., and Nielands, J. B., Eds.**, *Iron Transport in Microbes, Plants and Animals*, VCH Publishers, Weinheim, West Germany, 1987.
14. **Meyer, J.-M.**, Siderophores of *Pseudomonas* — biological properties, in *Iron Transport in Microbes, Plants and Animals*, VCH Publishers, Weinheim, West Germany, 1987, chap. 11.
15. **Harrison, P. M., Hoare, R. J., Hoy, T. G., and Macara, I. G.**, Ferritin and haemosiderin: structure and function, in *Iron in Biochemistry and Medicine*, A. Jacobs and M. Worwood, Eds., Academic Press, London, 1974, chap. 3.
16. **Harrison, P. M., White, J. L., Smith, J. M. A., Farrants, G. C., Ford, G. C., Rice, D., Addison, J. M., and Treffry, A.**, Comparative aspects of ferritin structure, in *Proteins of Iron Storage and Transport*, G. Spik, J. Montreuil, R. R. Crichton, and J. Mazurier, Eds., Elsevier, Oxford, 1985.
17. **Bezkorovainy, A.**, *Biochemistry of Nonheme Iron*, Plenum Press, New York, 1980, chap. 5.
18. **Andrews, S. C., Treffry, A., and Harrison, P. M.**, Siderosomal ferritin, the missing link between ferrtin and haemosiderin?, *Biochem. J.*, 245, 439, 1987.

Chapter 2

IRON METABOLISM IN MAN

I. INTRODUCTION

As long ago as 2735 B.C., iron was listed by the then emperor of China, Shen Nung, as a cure for "anaemia". For many centuries thereafter, iron was used as a remedy by ancient civilisations. The Greeks recognised that the muscular weakness experienced by injured soldiers improved after the administration of iron salts, no doubt as a result of correcting iron deficiency associated with blood loss. The first rational use of iron therapy was made by Thomas Syndenham (1624 to 1689), who administered iron preparations to treat chlorosis in young women. A further 200 years elapsed before it was demonstrated by Frodisch that chlorosis is associated with low levels of blood iron, and that this could be corrected by the administration of iron salts.

The involvement of the liver in human iron metabolism was first shown at the end of the 19th century with the demonstration that this organ contained Prussian blue positive granular and nongranular pigments. These we now recognise today as haemosiderin and ferritin, respectively. In 1825, Engelhardt determined the iron content of haemoglobin and found it to be 0.35%. During the next century the relationship between dietary iron and circulating haemoglobin was intensively studied. Nutritional iron deficiency anaemia was found to be particularly common in young infants and postpubertal women.

The foundations of our present day understanding of the relationship between dietary iron and body iron levels were laid by McCance and Widdowson[4] in 1937. They demonstated that amongst the 30 elements essential for normal growth and development, iron was unique in that the body had little or no ability to excrete iron, and therefore iron status was regulated almost entirely at the level of absorption in the gut. With the advent of the ready availability of radioisotopes in the period immediately following the Second World War, the methods used to study iron balance changed dramatically. It then became possible to study not only the fate of dietary iron, but also the movement and daily turnover of iron between tissues in the body.

II. BODY IRON AND ITS DISTRIBUTION

The body of a 70-kg male contains about 4 g of iron, equivalent to the mass of a 7-cm nail. Nutritionists conveniently divide the elemental composition of the body into the main elements, such, for example, as calcium and sodium, and the trace elements exemplified by copper and zinc. Since the usual definition of a trace element[1] is one that occurs at not more than 1 part in 20,000 in an organism and is concerned with enzymic activity, iron has been variously classified as both a main and a trace element (Table 1). Because ionized iron is toxic, body iron is always found in association with protein, and the approximate distribution of the iron within the body is shown in Table 2. Four different situations are illustrated, ranging from the newborn

TABLE 1
The Mass (Grams) of Some of the Elements in the Body of a 70-kg Man

	Grams	Parts per 20,000
Calcium	1500	430
Phosphorus	700	200
Sodium	80	23
Magnesium	25	7.2
Iron	**4**	**1.1**
Copper	0.150	0.043
Zinc	0.070	0.020
Cobalt	0.0001	0.00003

TABLE 2
The Distribution of Body Iron (mg)

	Newborn child	6-Month child	Adult male	Adult female
Body weight (kg)	3.4	7.6	70	55
Red cells (haemoglobin)	165 (64%)	210 (70%)	2500 (63%)	1700 (68%)
Tissues (myoglobin, enzymes, cytochromes, and bone marrow)	15 (6%)	45 (15%)	500 (12%)	450 (18%)
Plasma (transferrin)	0.25	0.4	4	3
Stores (liver and spleen — ferritin/haemosiderin)	80 (30%)	45 (15%)	1000 (25%)	350 (14%)
Total iron (mg)	260	300	4000	2500
Body iron (mg/kg body weight)	76	39	57	45

child to the adult. Such are the differences that a short discussion of each seems justified.

In an adult male, one quarter of the body iron (1 g) is found stored as ferritin, and to a lesser extent haemosiderin. The two principal sites of storage are the liver and the spleen. Since the average daily loss of iron from the body of an adult male is about 1 mg, this means that if iron was totally excluded from the diet, the body stores would be sufficient to last for between 2 to 3 years. Although nearly two thirds of the iron within the body of the adult male is found in the circulating red cell haemoglobin, most of this cannot be considered as a second iron store since a reduction in haemoglobin by as little as 20% will severely compromise oxygen delivery to the tissues. Most of the remaining iron (0.5 g) is distributed between muscle myoglobin and the iron-containing cytochromes and enzymes discussed in Chapter 1. Finally, it might initially appear from the data in Table 2 that the amount of iron carried in the blood plasma bound to transferrin is so small as to be insignificant. This is a good example of the situation where data relating to concentration alone can be misleading. It is only when one considers the dynamics of iron metabolism, and the daily turnover of iron between tissues and organs that the central role of plasma transferrin becomes apparent. These subjects will be considered in later sections of this chapter.

In the adult female, between the ages of puberty and the menopause, the total amount of body iron (2.5 g) is considerably less than in males. This can be partly explained by a smaller body size and blood volume. An additional and very significant contributing factor, however, is the much smaller amount of iron in the iron stores. The figure of 350 mg given in Table 2 is an average value. In a random survey of female college students, Scott and Pritchard[2] discovered that 25% of the women had no detectable iron stores, and as many as 65% of the women tested had iron stores less than 350 mg. Only 5% had iron stores approaching the levels found in men (1000 mg). The average daily iron loss experienced by women in their fertile years has been variously reported as between 2 and 3 mg. This is more than twice the loss experienced by males.

Menstrual blood loss is the principal factor accounting for this difference. It can be calculated that for a blood loss of 80 mL each period (normal range 5 to 200 mL), the daily intake of iron from the diet would need to be increased to 25 mg (since only 10% is absorbed) in order to prevent depletion of the iron stores. These 25 mg of iron are far more than is present in the average daily diet (10 mg). The adult female is therefore in a far more precarious position than the male in terms of iron balance. Even in those countries where neither malnutrition nor debilitating diseases are prevalent, the incidence of iron-deficiency anaemia amongst the adult female population can be as high as 20% (Cook et al.).[3] Women also experience a further burden on their iron stores as a result of pregnancy. About 300 mg of iron is lost to the foetus, with an additional loss of 150 mg in the placenta.

Of the four examples given in Table 2, the newborn child appears to have by far and away the best iron status (76 mg/kg body weight). For full-term infants, iron deficiency is extremely rare. During pregnancy the concentration of maternal plasma transferrin and the number of transferrin receptors on the placenta both increase (see later). This means that the placenta can compete very successfully with the maternal erythroid mass for transferrin-bound iron. This iron is rapidly passed to foetal transferrin to be finally deposited in the foetal tissues. From conception to birth a child will acquire 250 to 300 mg of iron. Since these requirements are considerably less than those of the maternal bone marrow over the same period, the placenta has no trouble in obtaining adequate iron for the developing foetus. This situation pertains even when the mother may be experiencing severe iron deficiency. The ferritin stores of the newborn child contain about 80 mg of iron, but, unlike the adult, there is an additonal useful iron store in the form of excess haemoglobin. At birth the haemoglobin levels (17 to 18 g per 100 mL) are higher than in adults (12 to 14 g), and during the first few postnatal weeks there is a rapid destruction of red cells coupled to a period of bone marrow hypoplasia. This provides a useful additional source of body iron. By 3 months the level of haemoglobin (10 to 11 g per 100 mL) is below the adult value. Therefore, iron stores during the first 2 months of life are proportionately higher than at any subsequent time.

By 6 months of age the situation is beginning to change dramatically (Table 2). Body weight has more than doubled, and as growth progresses the demands for iron become acute. This cannot be supplied by either human or cow's milk, since both have low concentrations of "available" iron. To provide sufficient iron for the child's daily needs, 10 pints of milk would be required. The amount of iron in the body stores at birth can usually satisfy the additional demands for iron during the first 6 months. At the end of this period the iron stores are severely depleted (Table 2). For the next 6 months of life the growing infant needs to absorb at least 1 mg of iron per day. It has been estimated that a substantial proportion of the children in this age group in the English population do not receive a diet containing this amount of absorbable iron.

Iron deficiency anaemia is therefore a fairly common problem during at least two periods of life — infancy, and the child-bearing age in women.

III. IRON ABSORPTION, BALANCE, AND TURNOVER

In the previous section, the description of the major sites where body iron is located only presented a static picture. In order to appreciate the central role of plasma transferrin (the iron-carrying protein) in iron metabolism, we need to consider the dynamics of iron turnover. A number of questions need to be answered:

1. How much iron is absorbed from the diet and what factors affect the efficiency of iron absorption? What are the mechanisms of iron absorption by the mucosal cells of the intestine and how is the process controlled?
2. How much iron is lost from the body each day and by what routes? Can body iron loss be controlled?
3. How much iron moves around the body in a day and from what sources, other than dietary, is this iron derived? Which tissues contribute iron into, and which tissues remove iron from the plasma iron pool?

A. DIETARY IRON AND ITS ABSORPTION

In man, only 5 to 15% of orally ingested dietary iron is usually absorbed. For an adult, a normal daily mixed diet contains between 10 and 15 mg of iron. This means that about 1 mg of iron is absorbed by the intestinal mucosa, and the remaining 9 to 14 mg is excreted, unabsorbed, in the faeces. In situations where the body demands for iron are raised, such, for example, as increased red cell production, the amount af iron absorbed daily at the mucosa can be increased from 1 mg to as much as 3 mg. Conversely, in situations of iron overload the intestinal mucosa can reduce the amount of dietary iron that it absorbs to values as low as 0.5 mg. Our knowledge of the mechanism and control of food-iron absorption in man has progressed considerably since the proposal in 1937 by McCance and Widdowson[4] that body iron status must be regulated by controlled iron absorption as no mechanisms appeared to exist to regulate iron excretion from the body. Recent advances in the field of iron absorption have been the subject of many review articles (Cook,[5] Lynch,[6] Bothwell et al.[7]) and only a brief summary of these findings will be presented.

Dietary iron absorption takes place in the duodenum and the jejunum. Most of the iron present in a normal mixed diet is in one of two forms. It is either as haem iron (haemoglobin, myoglobin, and cytochromes) or as non-haem iron (ferritin, haemosiderin, other nonhaem iron proteins, and low-molecular-weight iron chelates).

Although probably less than 10% of the dietary iron is **haem**, because the efficiency of absorption of this form of iron is five- to tenfold higher than nonhaem iron, it can supply as much as one third, or 0.4 mg, of the normal daily iron requirements of an adult male. Haem is released from its protein anchor by the acid present in the stomach. The haem then enters the mucosal cell of the duodenum, via haem receptors, with the porphyrin ring intact. There is no exchange of this iron with the nonhaem iron component of the diet. Once within the mucosal cell, the haem group is catabolised by the enzyme haem oxygenase and the ferric iron is released. The concentration of this enzyme is high in the duodenum, where iron is absorbed, and its activity is increased during iron deficiency. The released ferric iron either enters the blood bound to transferrin, or is stored as ferritin within the mucosal cell. This can only be a temporary store, however, since the life-span of the mucosal cells is short (3 to 4 days). Once these cells are shed into the intestine, the iron is effectively lost from the body, as no mechanisms exist for the retrieval of the iron further down the intestine. This process represents one of the nonregulated routes by which iron is lost from the body each day (see later).

The world supply of food iron is predominantly in the form of **nonhaem** iron. In most countries cereals and cereal products (bread) alone contribute nearly half of the iron in the diet. However, the efficiency of absorption of this nonhaem iron is low compared with haem iron. In addition, unlike haem iron the absorption of nonhaem iron is considerably affected by other factors in the diet. Finally, the mechanisms of absorption of this nonhaem iron by the mucosal cell are not only separate and distinct from those responsible for haem iron, but they appear able to be regulated by the iron requirements of the body.

Gastric and other digestive secretions bring about the reduction and release of nonhaem iron from its conjugated forms within the diet. Since Fe^{2+} is far more soluble than Fe^{3+}, any additional factor, such as vitamin C, that helps to maintain iron in the reduced form will enhance absorption. It was established many years ago that ferrous iron is absorbed by man far more readily than ferric iron. In addition to gastric acidity and vitamin C, many other

TABLE 3
Some of the Many Factors that Have Been
Shown Experimentally to Affect the
Efficiency of Absorption of Nonhaem Iron

Increase	Decrease
Gastric acidity	Oxalates
Vitamin C	Phosphates
Cysteine and histidine	Carbonates
Animal protein	Phytic acid
Haem iron	Calcium
Fructose	Phosphoproteins (eggs)
	Tannins (tea)
	Milk proteins

factors that may be present within a normal diet have been found to influence the efficiency of absorption of nonhaem iron (Table 3). Most of these observations were made in the course of animal experiments, and it is by no means clear to what extent these results can be extrapolated to the *in vivo* situation in humans. What is clear, however, is that none of these dietary factors can be considered as being part of the normal physiological mechanism by which the body can regulate the intake of iron at the mucosal cell.

The way in which nonhaem iron is absorbed by the mucosal cell has been the subject of intense research during the last 40 years. As each new and often contradictory experimental observation has been reported, so different pathways for the absorption of nonhaem iron have been proposed. Each mechanism proposed has required in addition an explanation as to how the process might be regulated at the cellular level. The fact that nonhaem iron absorption can be regulated is universally accepted. One constant observation is that conditions that stimulate erythropoiesis or deplete iron stores, such as haemorrhage, pregnancy, and iron deficiency, increase the absorption of dietary iron. On the other hand, in situations associated with ample iron stores or reduced erythropoiesis, such as iron overload and radiation damage, the mucosal cell can respond by reducing the amount of iron absorbed from the diet. The list of physiological factors that have, at some time or another, been suggested as possible signals involved in the regulation of iron absorption is extensive (Table 4). However, attempts to construct a complete picture of both the mechanism and control of iron absorption at the mucosal cell are not yet possible.

The ultimate fate of the Fe^{2+} iron is to be absorbed into the mucosal cell. Two mechanisms have been suggested. One is via a saturable transport system within the membrane of the mucosal cell, and the other, possibly only operating at high iron concentrations, is by a passive diffusion process with apparently unlimited capacity.[8] Even for the receptor-mediated uptake of iron, two different routes have been proposed. One involves a specific ferrous iron receptor site located in the brush border of the mucosal cell,[9] whereas an

TABLE 4
Some of the Physiological Factors that Have Been Proposed as Possible Signals Involved in the Regulation of Iron Absorption by the Mucosal Cell

Hypoxia
Erythropoietin
Mucosal cell ferritin
Plasma ferritin
A protein factor in gastric juice
An unidentified factor in pancreatic secretions
Biliary-derived transferrin
Plasma transferrin concentration
Plasma transferrin iron saturation
Mobilferrin in the duodenal cells

alternative mechanism involves a transferrin receptor on the mucosal cell membrane. Transferrin has been detected in the lumen of the intestine.[10] The precise origin of mucosal transferrin is not yet known, but it has been suggested that biliary secretions might be the source. Very recently, a newly identified iron-binding protein has been discovered in the duodenal mucosa of rats. The molecule has a molecular weight of 56,000 and does not contain any significant amounts of carbohydrate. The protein has been called **mobilferrin**[11] and is capable of binding one atom of iron. Mobilferrin is located in the apical cytoplasm of the duodenal cells of the rat intestine, and has not been found in any other tissue. The molecular size, electrophoretic mobility, and amino acid composition distinguish mobilferrin from any of the other iron-binding proteins (transferrin, lactoferrin, and ferritin). Although the precise function of mobilferrin has yet to be elucidated, its localisation in cells known to be involved in iron absorption, as well as its ability to reversibly bind iron, suggest that it may have a role to play in iron transport across the mucosal cells of the intestine. Although the amount of dietary iron that is available for absorption at the mucosal cell surface can be profoundly influenced by a number of different substances that might be present in the diet (Table 3), these cannot be considered as being part of a normal physiological mechanism for the regulation of body iron status. However, there have been a number of reports of two factors, one secreted by the gastric mucosa and the other by the pancreas, that inhibit iron uptake. Since the concentration of both factors is reduced in iron deficiency, thereby stimulating iron uptake from the diet, these molecules may have a role to play in the maintenance of iron homeostasis.

Once within the cell, the initial fate of the nonhaem iron appears to follow a route which is quite separate from that of the haem iron. This has been clearly established from experiments using two different isotopes of iron, and the results from such experiments indicate the existence of two separate pools

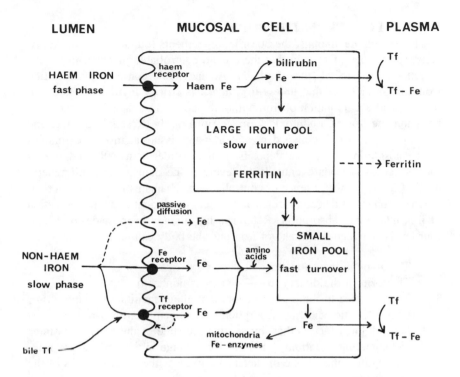

FIGURE 1. Possible routes for the absorption of haem iron and nonhaem iron by the mucosal cells of the small intestine.

of iron within the mucosal cell — haem iron and nonhaem iron. Soon after a meal, nonhaem iron is found within the mucosal cell bound to a number of different ligands. These include ferritin, transferrin, amino acids, and a second transferrinlike protein. Amino acids possibly participate in the initial binding of the iron once it has entered the cell. At this stage the absorbed iron is thought to follow one of two routes. A proportion is rapidly attached to a transferrinlike protein for transfer across to the serosal surface of the cell. Once there, the iron is released, moves across the serosal membrane, and becomes attached to plasma transferrin for transport to other sites in the body. Most of the remainder of the amino acid-bound iron is delivered to mucosal cell ferritin. Clearly, a mechanism that can regulate iron intake and match this to the iron demands of the body has to be able to alter the proportion of the iron that follows these two routes. Although the ferritin iron is available for mobilisation, it only remains so for the short life-span of the mucosal cell. Within 2 to 3 days this iron would be lost from the body when the cell dies and is shed into the intestine.

Figure 1 is an attempt to summarise the possible mechanisms by which both haem and nonhaem iron are absorbed by the mucosal cell. Many of the suggestions contained within this diagram are speculative.

B. IRON LOSS FROM THE BODY

Iron is unique amongst the 30 or more elements found within the fluids, cells, and tissues of man in that there is no controllable mechanism for the secretion of the metal from the body. An inevitable consequence resulting from this situation is that unless iron intake is strictly regulated, there will be a gradual accumulation of iron within the body. The capacity of the adult body to store iron in a nontoxic form (ferritin) rarely exceeds 2 g. Over and above this level iron becomes deposited in many tissues as insoluble granules of haemosiderin. Excessive deposits of haemosiderin in cells and tissues (haemosiderosis) leads eventually to severe tissue damage and, ultimately, death. Clearly, in the absence of controllable mechanisms for iron excretion, the maintenance of a healthy iron status is very dependent upon the regulation of iron intake and absorption. Reference has already been made to at least four levels at which the intake of iron into the body can be modified:

1.   The amount of iron in the diet
2.   The form of the dietary iron — haem or nonhaem
3.   The presence in the diet of factors that either facilitate (vitamin C) or inhibit (phytic acid) the absorption of nonhaem iron in particular
4.   Physiological factors that, by sensing the state of the body iron stores and signaling situations where there is change in the demand for iron, can regulate the uptake of dietary iron across the mucosal cells of the duodenum

Lack of a regulatory mechanism for iron excretion is not the same as the absence of iron loss from the body. If during the course of 24 hours humans did not lose any iron from the body, iron would not need to be an essential component of the diet, except in situations of growth and repair of iron-containing tissues. The reason that an adult absorbs about 1 mg of iron a day in order to remain in iron balance is because this amount of iron matches the normal iron loss from the body during the same period.

The figure of 1 mg a day is the average value for iron loss in adult males. The greatest proportion of this iron (0.8 mg) is lost from the gut via the faeces. This includes a small amount in the bile and the large iron content (ferritin) of the mucosal cells shed into the intestine. A further 0.1 mg of iron is present in the normal daily urine output. Finally, approximately 0.1 mg of iron is lost each day via the skin and its appendages (dead skin cells, sweat, hair, and nails). Whilst 0.8 mg of iron is "lost" from the body in the faeces, this does not represent the total iron content of faecal material. The faeces will also contain that proportion (85 to 95%) of the dietary iron that was never absorbed during its passage through the intestine. This can amount to between 10 and 15 mg of iron from a normal diet.

The normal routes of iron loss are ones over which the body has very little control. It is true that in situations of iron deficiency the daily iron loss can be reduced by about 50% (0.5 mg/day), but this is accounted for by the reduced ferritin content of the dead mucosal cells shed into the intestine.

Similarly, in situations of iron overload where the daily loss of iron via the faeces can be seen to increase (3 to 5 mg/day), this has been shown to be principally due to the increased ferritin-iron content of the mucosal cells and the intestinal macrophages.[12]

C. DAILY MOVEMENT OF IRON BETWEEN THE TISSUES OF THE BODY

For an adult male in iron balance, the daily loss of 1 mg of iron from the body is matched by the uptake of an equivalent amount of iron from the diet. In an earlier section of this chapter, the approximate distribution of the 4000 mg of iron within the body of an adult male was described (Table 2). Yet neither of these two pieces of information gives any indication of the daily turnover of iron within the body.

The earliest attempts to study this subject (ferrokinetics) were reported by Hahn et al.[13] in 1939, using radioactive iron to follow the fate of the iron in a mammalian organism. This was rapidly followed by numerous investigations in the post-World War II period as radioactive isotopes became more readily available. The pioneering work by Huff et al.[14] in the early 1950s, followed by technical refinements introduced by Pollycove and Mortimer[15] (1961) led to the subject of ferrokinetics being treated in a detailed mathematical fashion. The outcome was that a number of different models were proposed to explain iron turnover within the body. A detailed description of these models, including such concepts as stable and labile iron pools, plasma iron clearance kinetics, and multiple body-iron compartments, will not be attempted. These subjects have been reviewed by Cavill and Ricketts[16] and by Bezkorovainy.[8] The purpose of the following brief account is to attempt to answer the questions: Which tissues remove iron from or add iron to the blood plasma? How much iron is involved in these individual transfers each day? What is the turnover time (days) of iron within the tissues and body fluids?

Only by appreciating the answers to these questions will it be possible to understand the vital role played by plasma transferrin as the vehicle for iron transport between tissues.

1. Iron Uptake

Whilst all human tissues have a requirement for iron and have developed methods to acquire the iron from the transferrin circulating in the blood plasma, the majority of daily iron uptake is into one of the following four tissues — developing red cells in the bone marrow, liver, spleen, and muscle.

Bone marrow — During a period of 24 hours the bone marrow of an adult male removes about 30 mg of iron from the blood. From 20 to 22 mg of this iron has a short turnover time (1 day) and soon appears in the haemoglobin of red cells released into the circulation. This is the largest uptake of iron by any tissue in the body and is necessary in order to compensate for the daily destruction of the oldest population of red cells in the circulation, when these cells reach the end of their 120-day life-span. It has been estimated that an individual reticulocyte takes up about 90,000 atoms of iron per minute, and that for the even more immature normoblast this value increases to 500,000.[17] Since for an adult male, the total amount of iron within the circulating red cell mass is about 2500 mg, it can be calculated that the amount of iron removed from the circulation each day is 20 to 22 mg. To maintain the haemoglobin level, an equivalent amount of iron has to appear each day in the newly synthesised red cells. The remaining 8 mg of iron taken up by the bone marrow each day is temporarily stored as ferritin with a turnover time of about 6 days.

Liver — The liver removes between 2.5 and 4.5 mg of iron from the plasma each day, and most of this iron is destined for the ferritin iron stores. The turnover time for liver iron has been estimated as 6 days.

Spleen — The reticuloendothelial cells of the spleen are responsible for the initial removal of the dying red cells at the end of their 120-day life-span. The majority of the iron released from the haemoglobin of these red cells is not stored within the spleen, but is returned via the plasma transferrin to the bone marrow. The spleen cells themselves take up about 8 mg of iron a day and this, as in the liver, is stored as ferritin. The turnover time of ferritin iron within the spleen can be very slow, and this tissue represents the most stable of all the iron stores.

Muscle — Of all the remaining body tissues that remove iron from the blood plasma, skeletal muscle makes the largest contribution, taking about 1 mg of iron from the circulation each day. This is by virtue of the high concentration of myoglobin within the muscle cells. However, since myoglobin is such a stable molecule, the turnover of iron within muscle tissue is in the region of 150 days.

By combining together the figures for each of these four tissues, one can arrive at a value of about 40 mg as representing the total amount of iron removed from the blood plasma each day. Since the total concentration of iron in the blood plasma of an adult male is about 4 mg, this means that the turnover time for the plasma iron carried almost exclusively by transferrin is extremely rapid — 3 to 4 hours.

The factors that regulate the uptake of iron by the tissues include the concentration of iron within the plasma and the number of transferrin receptors expressed by the cells. The concentration of plasma transferrin rarely falls outside the range 2×10^{-5} to 9×10^{-5} M, and since the dissociation constant (Kd) for most cellular transferrin receptors is approximately 10^{-8} M, receptor-saturating concentrations of transferrin are always likely to exist.

The structure and regulation of expression of the specific transferrin membrane receptor will be discussed in Chapter 7.

2. Iron Release

In contrast to the large amount of information that is now known concerning the mechanism and control of iron uptake by cells, knowledge of the

TABLE 5
The Turnover Times of Iron Within Different Body Tissues

Plasma	3 hours
Spleen (labile pool)	1 day
Bone marrow (labile pool)	1 day
Gut mucosa	3 days
Bone marrow (stable pool)	6 days
Liver	6 days
Red cells	120 days
Muscle	150 days
Spleen (stable pool)	Long-term store

method and regulation of iron release from tissues is comparatively sparse. In a healthy adult where the amount of iron taken up by tissues is in the region of 40 mg per day, in order to maintain internal iron balance, this has to be matched by the release of an equivalent amount of iron into the plasma during the same period. The principal tissues that contribute to this figure are the red cells, the spleen, the bone marrow, the liver, the gut mucosa, and the muscle.

Spleen and red cells — About 75% (30 mg) of the iron turned over in the plasma during the course of a day has passed through the erythrophagocytosing cells of the reticuloendothelial system (RES). The organ primarily responsible for removing effete red cells from the circulation is the spleen. The flux of iron across the reticuloendothelial cell membrane is more than ten times that of even the most avidly iron-seeking erythropoietic cell. For an adult male with a blood volume of 5 L, it can be calculated that the number of red cells at the end of their 120-day life-span that are removed from the circulation each day by the spleen is in the region of 25×10^{10}. The total amount of iron released from these cells will be in the order of 30 mg per day. There is evidence that within the RES cells of the spleen there exists both an "early release" and a "late release" iron pool.[17] Most of the iron recovered from the effete red cells (20 to 25 mg) passes rapidly through the early-release iron pool and soon appears in the plasma bound to transferrin. With such a fast turnover, it is likely that this iron has never been incorporated into ferritin within the spleen. The remaining 5 mg of the iron released from red cell breakdown enters the ferritin stores of the spleen. Whilst the turnover time of this stable iron store is extremely slow, the iron released from the splenic stores each day amounts to about 5 mg in order to maintain internal iron balance.

Liver — The two principal sites of iron storage within the body are the liver and the spleen. Whilst the iron stored within the spleen is stable and has a very slow turnover (Table 5), iron stored as ferritin within the liver hepatocyte has a turnover time of about 6 days. In addition, the liver iron stores are particularly susceptible to iron overloading when the body burden of iron increases. The total amount of iron released from the liver during a period of 24 hours is in the region of 5 mg. The process of iron release from the hepatocyte cell, as well as being facilitated by iron chelators and by apotransferrin (iron-free transferrin), has also been shown to be temperature dependent and to be disrupted by metabolic inhibitors.[18] These observations suggest that there is an energy requirement for the process of iron release.

Bone marrow — The bone marrow of an adult removes about 30 mg of iron from the plasma each day. Much of this iron enters a labile bone marrow iron pool (turnover time 1 day), and soon appears in the newly synthesised haemoglobin. The remainder of the iron (6 to 8 mg) that is not required for haemoglobin synthesis enters a more stable iron pool within the bone marrow and is stored as ferritin. Within 6 days most of this iron has been released into the plasma.

Gut mucosa — The intestinal mucosal cells, particularly in the region of the duodenum, are responsible for the uptake of dietary iron. Over a period of 24 hours, approximately 1 mg of iron is released from these cells into the plasma.

In this brief review of human iron metabolism, the figures given for the amount of iron in an individual tissue or the quantity of iron released or taken up by a particular tissue during the course of a day are only approximations. They have been obtained from a large number of scientific publications, some of which were found to contain conflicting results. In Figure 2 an attempt has been made to summarise these results and represent in a schematic form not only the turnover of iron within the body, but the fate of ingested iron in an adult man.

IV. THE ROLE OF PLASMA TRANSFERRIN — A PREVIEW

During the course of 24 hours, approximately 45 mg of iron enters the blood plasma and 40 mg leaves the circulation. The function of plasma transferrin, in this respect, is to collect the iron from the tissues as it is released and to transport iron, in a nontoxic and soluble form, to those tissues that have a continual requirement for this element. The vital role played by plasma transferrin is best demonstrated by those very rare instances where an organism is born with an inherited deficiency of transferrin. A complete absence of plasma transferrin is not compatible with life.[19]

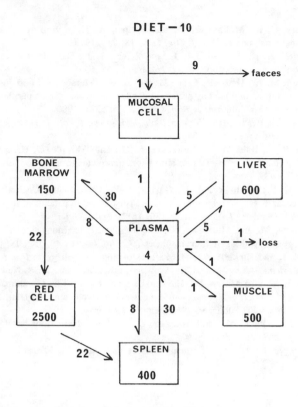

FIGURE 2. The daily turnover (mg) and tissues iron stores (mg) of an adult man.

REFERENCES

1. **Davidson, S. and Passmore, P.,** *Human Nutrition and Dietetics,* 2nd ed., Churchill Livingstone, London, 1963, chap. 12.
2. **Scott, D. E. and Pritchard, J. A.,** Iron deficiency in healthy college women, *J. Am. Med. Assoc.,* 199, 897, 1967.
3. **Cook, J. D., Finch, C. A., and Smith, N. J.,** Evaluation of the iron status of a population, *Blood,* 38, 449, 1976.
4. **McCance, R. A. and Widdowson, E. M.,** Absorption and excretion of iron, *Lancet,* 2, 680, 1937.
5. **Cook, J. D.,** Absorption of food iron, *Fed. Proc., Fed. Am. Soc. Exp. Biol.,* 36, 2028, 1977.
6. **Lynch, S. R.,** in *Current Topics in Nutrition and Disease ,* Vol. 12, N. W. Solomons and I. H. Rosenberg, Eds., Alan R. Liss, 1984, 89.
7. **Bothwell, T. H., Charlton, R. W., Cook, J. D., and Finch, C. A.,** in *Iron Metabolism in Man,* Blackwell Scientific, Oxford, 1979.
8. **Bezkorovainy, A.,** in *Biochemistry of Nonheme Iron,* Plenum Press, New York, 1980, chap. 3.

9. **Kimber, C. L., Mukherjee, T., and Weller, W. J.,** In vitro iron attachment to the intestinal brush border, *Am. J. Dig. Dis.,* 18, 781, 1973.
10. **Osterloh, K. R., Simpson, R. J., and Peters, T. J.,** The role of mucosal transferrin in intestinal iron absorption, *Br. J. Haematol.,* 65, 1, 1987.
11. **Conrad, M. E., Umbreit, J. N., Moore, E. G., Peterson, R., and Jones, M. B.,** A newly identified iron binding protein in duodenal mucosae of rats; purification and characterisation of mobilferrin, *J. Biol. Chem.,* 265, 5273, 1990.
12. **Hughes, E. R.,** in *Metal Ions in Biological Systems,* Vol. 7, H. Sigel, Ed., Marcel Dekker, New York, 1978, chap. 9.
13. **Hahn, P. F., Bale, W. F., Lawrence, E. O., and Whipple, G. H.,** Radioactive iron and its metabolism in anaemia; its absorption, transportation and utilisation, *J. Exp. Med.,* 69, 739, 1939.
14. **Huff, R. F., Elmlinger, P. J., Garcia, J. F., Oda, J. M., Cockrell, M. C., and Lawrence, J. H.,** Ferrokinetics in normal persons and in patients having various erythropoietic disorders, *J. Clin. Invest.,* 30, 1512, 1951.
15. **Pollycove, M. and Mortimer, R.,** The quantitative determinants of iron kinetics and haemoglobin synthesis in human subjects, *J. Clin. Invest.,* 40, 753, 1961.
16. **Cavill, I. and Ricketts, C.,** The kinetics of iron metabolism, in *Iron in Biochemistry and Medicine,* A. Jacobs and M. Worwood, Eds., Academic Press, New York, 1974.
17. **Theil, E. C. and Ainsen, P.,** The storage and transport of iron in animal cells, in *Iron Transport in Microbes, Plants and Animals,* G. Winkelmann, D. Helm, and J. B. Neilands, Eds., VCH Publishers, Weinheim, West Germany, 1987.
18. **Baker, E., Page, M., and Morgan, E. H.,** Iron release from hepatocytes, *Am. J. Physiol.,* 248, 993, 1985.
19. **Heilmeyer, L.,** Die atransferrinamien, *Acta Haematol.,* 36, 40, 1966.

Chapter 3

THE SIDEROPHILIN FAMILY

I. INTRODUCTION

The siderophilins are a family of monomeric, iron-binding glycoproteins, widely distributed in the animal kingdom. The name siderophilin, derived from the Greek and meaning "iron-loving", was first used in 1944 by Schade[1] to describe an iron-binding protein isolated and partially purified from hen egg white. This molecule is now called ovotransferrin. Most of the members of the siderophilin family are large proteins with molecular weights in the region of 80,000, each having two specific iron-binding sites. The binding of the ferric iron (Fe^{3+}) is only possible when a synergistic anion, usually bicarbonate (HCO_3^-), is also attached at the iron-binding sites. The function of the anion is to act as a bridging ligand between the iron and the protein, rendering the sixth coordination site of the ferric ion unavailable to water,[2] so preventing the hydrolysis of Fe^{3+} and the formation of insoluble polynuclear iron complexes. A distinctive characteristic of most of the siderophilins is that upon the binding of iron, the proteins take on a salmon-red colour with a visible absorbance maximum at 465 nm. In addition to the more well-known examples of siderophilins, including transferrin, lactoferrin, and ovotransferrin, other members of the family include proteins with molecular weights ranging from 150,000 (crab transferrin) to 40,000 (transferrin from the prochordate *Pyura stolonifera*). Some very recent possible additions to the family have included a number of low-molecular-weight (8000) protein products of tumour-transforming genes (human Burkitt's lymphoma-transforming gene HuBlym-1).

The nomenclature and classification of these iron-binding proteins have undergone frequent changes over the last 40 years, with a result that the present situation within the literature is complex, confusing, and controversial. The archetypal member of the family has always been considered to be transferrin, the iron-transport protein of vertebrates and some invertebrates. Once the amino acid sequence of transferrin had been determined in 1982,[3] it became apparent that the protein was composed of two halves, or domains, of approximately equal size. Within the monomeric protein these two domains, each possessing an iron-binding site, are joined by a short sequence of amino acid residues in an α-helix. Such is the amino acid sequence homology between the two domains that the suggestion was made that the human transferrin gene was the product of a gene duplication that had occurred at a much earlier stage in the process of evolution. This was later confirmed when the nucleotide sequence of the human transferrin gene was elucidated.[4,5] The determination of the amino acid and nucleotide sequences of other members of the family soon followed — lactoferrin,[6,7] melanotransferrin,[8] and ovotransferrin.[9,10] Once again, the evidence from these three proteins indicated a two-domain structure, with extensive sequence homolgy between the domains. In addition, it then became possible to compare the amino acid and nucleotide sequences of these four members of the siderophilin family. The

TABLE 1
The Siderophilin Family

Name	Alternative names that have been used to describe the same molecule
Transferrin	Serotransferrin, siderophilin, metal-binding β-globulin
Ovotransferrin	Conalbumin, siderophilin
Lactoferrin	Lactotransferrin, milk "red protein", ekkrinosiderophilin
Melanotransferrin	Melanoma-associated antigen, p97 antigen
Sertoli transferrin	Testicular transferrin
Neurotransferrin	Brain transferrin, sciatin
Mucosal transferrin	Biliary transferrin
ChBlym-1	Chicken lymphoma transforming factor
HuBlym-1	Human Burkitt's lymphoma transforming factor
T β G41	

results strongly indicated that all four proteins had most likely evolved from a common ancestral gene.[11]

Since the functional, structural, and genetic comparisons were made using transferrin as the model example, this ever expanding group of high-affinity iron-binding proteins were classified as members of the "transferrin family".[2,11-14] Recently, Williams[15] has suggested reverting to use of the older term — siderophilin — to describe this family of structurally related proteins. This seems far more appropriate. First, it allows the name transferrin to be used only to describe the iron-transport serum protein. Second, it permits the inclusion, within the same protein family, of molecules such as melanotransferrin, which, whilst clearly being related to the other members from an evolutionary point of view, has no role to play in the transport of iron between tissues, since it is a cell membrane component. The number of reported examples of siderophilins has increased, particularly over the last 10 years, and Table 1 is an attempt to list all those that have been cited in the literature.

A member of the family, and therefore by definition a siderophilin, is any unique protein or polypeptide with one or more of the following characteristics:

1.　A monomeric glycoprotein with (usually) two high-affinity iron-binding sites, e.g., **serum transferrin**. This definition does not therefore exclude proteins half the size of transferrin and with a single iron-binding site that may prove to be the product of the putative, nonduplicated, ancestral transferrin gene. One such example is the transferrinlike protein isolated from the primitive prochordate *P. stolonifera*.[16] Whilst most siderophilins are likely to be soluble globular proteins, an exception has been found in the case of the membrane protein **melanotransferrin**.[8] Within a single organism, different siderophilins may either be the product of an alternative gene locus, e.g., **lactoferrin**, or products of the same gene locus that have subsequently undergone significantly different posttranslational modifications that have resulted in distinct and stable structural forms. Under this definition, hen **ovotransferrin** is clearly distinguishable from hen serum transferrin. The two glyco-proteins differ not only in their tissue distribution, but also in the nature of the glycan chains attached to the polypeptide backbones. In mammals, the existence of tissue-specific, but structurally distinct transferrins is less well established. Although the gene coding for serum transferrin is expressed in many different tissues, it remains to be confirmed whether or not such examples as **mucosal transferrin**,[17] **neurotransferrin**,[18] or **Sertoli cell transferrin**[19] can justifiably be cited as separate sider-ophilins.

2.   A second and quite separate group of molecules, that have been ten-tatively classified as siderophilins, are a number of small-molecular-weight proteins that have been found to exhibit sufficient amino acid or gene nucleotide sequence homology with part of serum transferrin to suggest that they have evolved from a common ancestral gene. These transferrin-like proteins include **ChBlym-1** and **HuBlym-1**, factors re-sponsible for the transformation of chicken B-cell lymphomas[20] and human Burkitt's lymphomas.[21] A third example is **TG41**, a repeated DNA sequence in the human Kpnl family associated with the β-globin gene cluster.[22] None of these molecules are likely to be involved in iron binding, but it was Williams[15] in 1985 who suggested that sequence homology and not just affinity for iron should be used as the qualification for membership of the siderophilin family.

II. THE DISCOVERY OF THE MAJOR SIDEROPHILINS

A. OVOTRANSFERRIN

In 1900, during a study of the chemical composition of hen egg white, Osborne and Campbell[23] identified and partially purified a new protein com-ponent that exhibited similar physical properties to the major egg-white pro-tein, ovalbumin. Since the two proteins were precipitated together in the same ammonium sulphate fraction, it was suggested that the new protein should be called conalbumin. For the next 45 years, the iron-binding properties of conalbumin remained undiscovered. Towards the end of the Second World War, Schade and Caroline[24] were investigating means of stabilising bacteri-ophage isolates that were therapeutically active against *Shigella dysenteriae*. In order to protect the bacteriophage lysates from desiccation, a great variety of substances were added prior to freeze drying. One such additive was hen egg white. When these samples were reconstituted and tested against the *Shigella* bacteria, it was discovered from the results of control experiments that hen egg white alone strongly inhibited bacterial growth. Attempts to reverse the growth inhibition of *S. dysenteriae* by hen egg white were partially successful when either meat or yeast extracts were added. The factor present in both of these extracts that was responsible for the abolition of the growth-inhibiting properties of egg white was soon identified. It was iron. Schade concluded that egg white contained a material with potent antimicrobial properties, and since these properties could be abolished by the addition of iron, it seemed reasonable to conclude that the antimicrobial component of egg white functioned by binding iron and depleting the bacteria of this essential growth factor. Alderton,[25] two years later, identified the bacteria-inhibiting, iron-binding component of egg white as conalbumin. The conalbumin, which accounts for at least 10% of all egg white protein, was for a short period of time renamed siderophilin. Both terms have now been replaced by the name ovotransferrin.

B. TRANSFERRIN

Some of the earliest definitive work on plasma iron was carried out in 1925 by Fontes and Thivolle.[26] They discovered that the small but significant concentration of iron in blood plasma was decreased in experimental anaemia. Later, Barkan and Schales,[27] by demonstrating that the iron in plasma was nondialysable, suggested that iron was protein bound within the plasma. Most of this iron was found to be associated with the globulin fraction[28] to which it was firmly bound over the pH range 5 to 10, but could be released when the pH was reduced to 4. The isolation and partial characterisation in 1946 of a unique iron-binding protein in blood plasma can be attributed to two independent groups. In America, Schade and Caroline[29] detected the protein in human plasma, not by accident as had been the case with the discovery of ovotransferrin, but on the contrary as the result of a deliberate search for the protein amongst the various Cohn fractions of human plasma. Cohn fraction IV-3,4 was found, like the conalbumin of egg white, to possess antibacterial properties and to bind iron. Schade et al.[30] later reported that the iron-binding protein, which they called siderophilin, had a molecular weight of 90,000 and was capable of binding two atoms of iron. Upon the binding of iron, which required the presence of bicarbonate, the protein was seen to acquire a salmon-pink colour. Independent of the American group, the Swedish researchers Laurell and Ingelman,[31] using as a starting material pig plasma because of its high iron-binding capacity, identified and isolated an iron-binding protein with a molecular weight of 88,000. The term transferrin was suggested as an appropriate name for the protein, in order to signify a possible biological role for the molecule.

C. LACTOFERRIN

For many years, researchers working on the protein content of milk had noticed the presence of a red-coloured protein in many of their preparations.[32] It was not, however, until the end of the 1950s that this protein was isolated and characterised. Johansson[33] was the first to report the isolation of an iron-binding protein from human milk, as a by-product of his lactalbumin purification procedure. The fraction contained a small amount of iron and exhibited an absorbance maximum at 465 nm, accounting for the red colour. Johansson commented at the time that the iron was not easily removed from the protein. By 1960, several reports had appeared of an iron-binding protein isolated from both human[34,35] and bovine milk.[36] These initial studies revealed that the protein, variously called lactosiderophilin, lactotransferrin, or lactoferrin, had many characteristics in common with both transferrin and ovotransferrin. It was shown to be a glycoprotein of molecular weight 80,000, capable of binding two atoms of iron, but only in the presence of bicarbonate. Naturally, the question arose as to whether or not the lactoferrin of milk and the transferrin of plasma were the same protein. By the use of immunological techniques, Montreuil et al.[35] showed that the two molecules were not immunochemically related. An additional significant difference between the two molecules was that lactoferrin was found to bind the iron far more avidly than transferrin, and a pH as low as 2 was required to release the iron from the protein. The most definitive evidence that lactoferrin and transferrin from the same species were indeed different proteins came with the elucidation of their respective amino acid sequences. Whilst the sequence homology between the two human proteins has been shown to be as high as 59%,[6] clearly they must be the product of two different gene loci. In humans, these two genes have both been found to be present on chromosome 3, closely linked on the long arm of this chromosome.[7]

Within the siderophilin family, the relationship between human transferrin and human lactoferrin is quite different to the one that exists between hen transferrin and hen ovotransferrin. The transferrin/lactoferrin pair are distinct siderophilins and the products of different genes. On the other hand, in birds, transferrin and ovotransferrin are the products of the same gene locus and the structural differences that exist between the two are the result of posttranslational modifications.

D. MELANOTRANSFERRIN

In 1980, during the course of a study of the membrane proteins of human melanoma tumour cells, a range of cell-surface glycoproteins antigens were identified using monoclonal antibodies.[37-39] Amongst the many antigens detected was one with a molecular weight of 97,000, and this was called the p97 antigen. It was studied extensively with regard to its expression in normal and neoplastic tissues and found to be present in the cell membranes of most human melanoma cells, certain foetal tissues, and in trace amounts in normal adult tissues. The glycoprotein antigen p97 was isolated, purified, and the sequence of the first 12 amino acids was determined by Brown et al.[40] in 1982. A computer search of an amino acid sequence library revealed that the first 12 amino acid residues of human p97 showed considerable sequence homology with the first 12 residues of both human transferrin (58%) and human lactoferrin (50%). Brown et al. further demonstrated that a polyvalent antiserum obtained by immunising rabbits with denatured p97 melanoma-associated antigen crossreacted with human transferrin. In addition, p97 antigen, when part of the melanoma cell membrane, had the ability to bind iron.

The complete amino acid sequence of the p97 melanoma-associated antigen, now known as simply melanotransferrin, was elucidated by Rose et al.[8] from the cloned mRNA nucleotide sequence. The protein, with a molecular weight of 80,196, was found to exhibit extensive sequence homology with human transferrin (40%). In addition, there was found to be an extra sequence of 25 hydrophobic amino acids at the C-terminal end of the protein that were thought to be responsible for anchoring the molecule to the cell membrane.

III. A BRIEF COMPARISON OF THE STRUCTURES, FUNCTIONS, AND PROPERTIES OF THE MAJOR SIDEROPHILINS

The remaining chapters of this book are devoted almost entirely to an account of the structure, function, and properties of the iron-transport protein transferrin, with particular emphasis being paid to the human protein. Much of this information has come, either directly or indirectly, from research on the structure and properties of other members of the siderophilin family, particularly ovotransferrin and lactoferrin. It therefore seems appropriate at this stage to very briefly summarise and compare the structural and functional characteristics of all the major siderophilins, including transferrin, before embarking upon a detailed description of the latter.

A. TRANSFERRIN

Human transferrin is a single polypeptide glycoprotein containing 679 amino acid residues and two N-linked glycan chains, resulting in a calculated molecular mass of 79,570 Da. In solution, the iron-free protein behaves like a prolate ellipsoid of revolution, with an axial ratio of 1:3. Upon binding of two atoms of iron (Fe^{3+}), transferrin becomes more compact or spherical in shape, and this conformational change results in the iron-laden protein becoming more resistant to denaturation than the apotransferrin. On the basis of its amino acid sequence, transferrin can be divided into two homologous regions, the N-terminal domain (residues 1 to 336) and the C-terminal domain (residues 337 to 679). X-ray crystallography indicates that these domains form two separate globular lobes within the molecule, connected by a short helical section. Of the amino acids in the N-domain, 42% have identical counterparts in the C-domain. It is because of this homology of amino acid sequence between the two domains, subsequently confirmed by base sequence analysis of transferrin DNA, that it has been suggested that the present day transferrin gene has arisen by a process of intragenic gene duplication. Each of the two domains within the transferrin molecule contains a metal-binding site. The concomitant binding of an anion at each site, which in the physiological situation is a bicarbonate ion (HCO_3^-), is essential for iron binding.

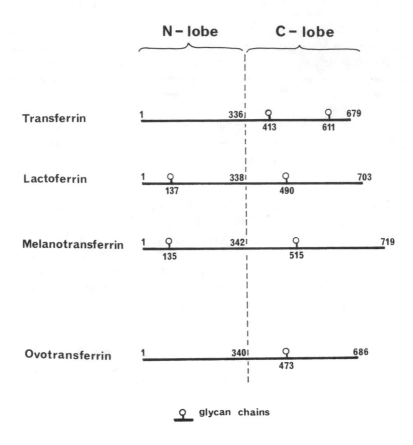

FIGURE 1.   The general structures of human transferrin, lactoferrin, melanotransferrin, and chicken ovotransferrin, showing the location of the glycan chains.

The two iron-binding sites have similar, but not identical, affinities for iron, and it is still a matter of considerable debate as to whether or not these small differences have any biological significance.

The C-terminal domain of human transferrin carries two glycan chains, attached to asparagine residues at positions 413 and 611, respectively (Figure 1). Each of the oligosaccharide chains is of a complex type exhibiting considerable variation in both the degree of branching and the nature of the sugar residues at the outermost ends of the branches. Biantennary, triantennary, and tetra-antennary structures have been shown to exist (Figure 2), and each of the branches has the possibility of ending with a negatively charged sialic acid residue. As a result of this potential microheterogeneity, nine different structural varieties of human serum transferrin are possible, ranging from a molecule with no sialic acid residues to a transferrin with eight sialic acids per molecule. Whilst all of these nine varieties have been shown to exist in biological fluids, the most predominant species in human plasma is a transferrin molecule with two biantennary glycan chains, with each of the four branches ending with a sialic acid residue.

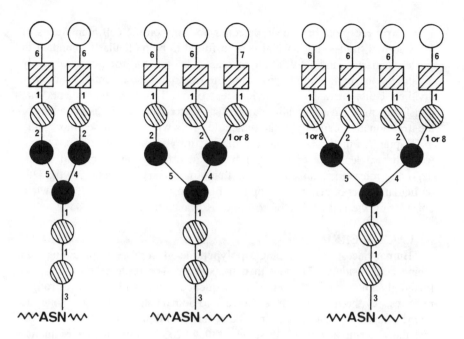

FIGURE 2. The three different types of glycan chains (biantennary, triantennary, and tetraantennary) of human serum transferrin. Each molecular of transferrin contains two glycan chains, which can be the same or different structures, attached to asparagine residues at positions 413 and 611. Further heterogeneity arises from the possible absence of the sialic acid residues at the ends of the branches. Key to symbols: ○, sialic acid; ◉, *N*-acetyl glucosamine; ▨, galactose; ●, mannose; **ASN**, asparagine residue; ∿, polypeptide chain; **1**, β1–4; **2**, β1–2; **3**, β1–N; **4**, α1–3; **5**, α1–6; **6**, α2–6; **7**, α2–3; and **8**, β1–6.

Transferrin has been detected in the blood of all vertebrates, including mammals, birds, fish, amphibia, and reptiles. As well as being a major protein of blood plasma (2.5 g/L), transferrin has been detected in a variety of other biological fluids including lymph, bile, cerebrospinal fluid, milk, and amniotic fluid. Like most plasma proteins, transferrin is synthesised primarily in the liver. However, important extrahepatic sites of transferrin synthesis include nervous tissue, testis, ovary, placenta, mammary gland, thymus, and lymphocytes. The synthesis of transferrin by some of these nonhepatic tissues may be important in those situations where cells are separated by blood barriers from the transferrin in plasma. Additional sites where very low levels of transferrin synthesis have been demonstrated using Tf cDNA probes include muscle, kidney, lung, spleen, heart, and intestine.

The major function of serum transferrin is to transport iron from the intestine, liver, and reticuloendothelial cells to tissues requiring iron for normal growth and development. The cellular uptake of transferrin-bound iron occurs by means of a transferrin-specific cell membrane receptor protein.

Transferrin receptors have been detected not only on the cell membranes of most normal tissues, but have also been found to be particularly abundant in cancerous tissues, indicative of the increased demand for iron by these rapidly dividing cells. In addition to providing the iron that is so essential for rapidly dividing cells, there is some evidence from cell culture experiments that transferrin may have an additional growth factor role that is independent of the iron-donating capacity of the molecule. This will be discussed more fully in Chapter 7. Finally, by acting as a high-affinity iron-binding protein, transferrin has at least the potential of being an effective antimicrobial agent, depriving microorganisms of the iron that is necessary for their growth. This particular aspect of general siderophilin function becomes more relevant when considering the roles of lactoferrin and ovotransferrin.

B. LACTOFERRIN

Human lactoferrin is a single polypeptide glycoprotein containing 703 amino acid residues, 24 more than transferrin. The protein carries two N-linked glycan chains. The amino acid sequence of human lactoferrin strongly indicates that the molecule has a similar two-domain structure as was found to be the case for human transferrin. The N-terminal domain (residues 1 to 338) and the C-terminal domain (residues 339 to 703) exhibit a 37% sequence homology corresponding to 125 amino acid residues in identical positions. In addition to this internal sequence homology, 59% of the amino acid residues of lactoferrin are in the same positions as they are in the molecule of transferrin. This observation has been taken to indicate that although lactoferrin and transferrin are the products of two distinct gene loci, these two loci have evolved from a common ancestral gene. Unlike transferrin, where the two glycan chains are both attached to asparagine residues in the C-domain, the two glycan chains of the lactoferrin molecule are located one in each domain, at asparagine residues 137 and 490, respectively (Figure 1). These glycans differ from those found in human transferrin. The methyl pentose sugar fucose is present, and the sialic acid content is substantially reduced. There is also considerable heterogeneity of the glycan chains, and some of the oligosaccharide structures that have been identified in human lactoferrin are shown in Figure 3. For the purposes of comparison, Figure 2 also includes the structures of the principal glycan chains of human transferrin. The lactoferrin glycans from species other than man have often been found to have quite different structures. For example, the glycans of bovine lactoferrin are composed of nine mannose residues and two molecules of *N*-acetyl glucosamine.

Although the molecule of human lactoferrin is structurally similar to that of human transferrin, particularly in respect to its amino acid sequence and X-ray diffraction pattern, there are some significant differences in their properties. The two molecules are immunolocally distinct. Polyclonal antibodies raised against transferrin do not react with lactoferrin. The affinity of lactoferrin for iron is 300 times greater than that of transferrin, and in addition,

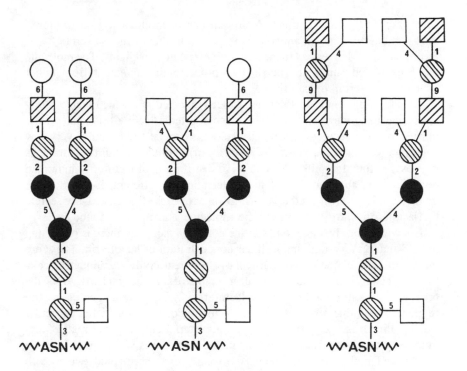

FIGURE 3. The three different types of glycan chains of human lactoferrin. Each molecule of lactoferrin contains two glycan chains, which can be the same or different structures, attached to asparagine residues at positions 137 and 490. Key to symbols: ○, sialic acid; □, fucose; ◉, N-acetyl glucosamine; ▨, galactose; ●, mannose; **ASN**, asparagine residue; ∿, polypeptide chain; **1**, β1–4; **2**, β1–2; **3**, β1–N; **4**, α1–3; **5**, α1–6; **6**, α2–6; and **9**, β1–3.

lactoferrin holds on to the two atoms of bound iron (Fe^{3+}) at low acid pH where transferrin iron would have been released.

Lactoferrin was first detected in milk. In human milk lactoferrin is a major component (1 to 3 g/L), accounting for as much as 30% of the total protein content of this fluid. In other animals the lactoferrin content of their milk is often much lower. For example, cow's milk contains less than 10% of the lactoferrin found in human milk. It has been suggested that lactoferrin may be a vehicle whereby young children in particular can acquire dietary iron. Specific receptors for lactoferrin have been identified on the brush-border membranes of the mucosal cells lining the intestine.[41] The lower lactoferrin content of bovine milk probably accounts for the observation that the frequency of iron deficiency amongst breast-fed babies is far less than that found in babies fed on cow's milk alone. The lactoferrin content of human breast milk is highest at the start of the lactation period (5 g/L). Rabbit milk contains little, if any, lactoferrin. However, what is present is a siderophilin that cross-reacts immunologically with rabbit serum transferrin. A similar situation has been described in the mouse.[42] A protein has been characterised in mouse milk that has an identical amino acid sequence to that of mouse serum transferrin, but differs in respect to the structure of the glycan chains. The molecule has been called "milk transferrin" in order to distinguish it from either lactoferrin or serum transferrin.

In addition to milk, lactoferrin has been detected in a wide range of body fluids and exocrine secretions. These include tears, saliva, bile, pancreatic juice, bronchial secretions, seminal plasma, synovial fluid, and at very low concentrations in blood plasma. The lactoferrin content of human tears is as high as that found in milk. The extensive distribution of lactoferrin in human body fluids is an indication of the wide range of different tissues that are involved in lactoferrin synthesis. Whilst most of these tissues actively secrete the lactoferrin into fluids, where the molecule is frequently found in association with either IgA antibodies or the enzyme lysozyme, there is one group of cells that retain a high intracellular concentration of lactoferrin. These are the white cells of the blood, particularly the neutrophil granulocytes, cells that are actively involved in the destruction of microorganisms. It is the presence of the iron-binding protein lactoferrin in many serous secretions and in granulocytes that provides the clue to the major function of this particular siderophilin. It is one of the principal antibacterial agents of the body, functioning by depriving microorganisms of the iron that is so essential for their growth and multiplication. There is a wealth of experimental evidence to support the role of lactoferrin as an important bacteriostatic agent. The locations of many of the fluids with a high lactoferrin content, such as tears, bronchial secretions, and saliva, are the very sites for potential bacterial invasion. The neutrophil granulocytes represent a more specialised form of defence mechanism. The granules within the mature granulocytes contain large amounts of iron-free lactoferrin which is subsequently released during the phagocytosis of pathogenic organisms by these cells. Lactoferrin, with its very high iron affinity, has been shown to be capable of removing the iron bound to serum transferrin. The iron-laden lactoferrin is very rapidly cleared by the liver, such that the half-life of plasma lactoferrin is measured in minutes, whereas that for plasma transferrin is comparatively long (5 to 7 days). It is therefore likely that this course of events accounts for the significant decrease in the serum iron level that is a typical secondary clinical finding in infections.[43]

The bacteriostatic growth-inhibiting role of lactoferrin is attributable to its high affinity for iron, thereby decreasing the availability of this essential element to the invading microorganisms. In addition, there is some evidence that lactoferrin might act as a more direct bactericidal agent, particularly against *Streptococcus mutans* and *Vibrio cholerae*. It has been suggested that the rapid killing of these pathogenic organisms may result from the formation of toxic hydroxyl radicals by the iron bound to the lactoferrin.[43]

Since the concentration of lactoferrin within the plasma of healthy individuals is extremely low (2 mg/L) in comparison with the levels of transferrin

(2500 mg/L), it is likely that plasma transferrin acts as the initial bacteriostatic agent. Only at a later stage in the course of an infection when lactoferrin has been released by the granulocytes will the bacteriostatic role of plasma lactoferrin become significant. Sawatzki[43] has calculated that the amount of lactoferrin released into the circulation each day increases from 0.5 g to as much as 30 g during the course of a bacterial infection.

In those body fluids and serous secretions where the concentration of lactoferrin is high, even in healthy individuals (tears, milk, bronchial secretions, and saliva), the molecule plays a vital role in the first line of defence against invading pathogens. In many of these fluids the bacteriostatic action of lactoferrin is augmented by the antibacterial effect of the secretory IgA antibodies that are present. Infants fed on breast milk will normally receive daily between 0.5 and 2.5 g of IgA and between 0.8 and 1.2 g of lactoferrin. Since neither of these two proteins are particularly well digested, together they provide a significant protective shield within the intestine against the invading pathogens.

It has recently been demonstrated that some pathogens have made attempts to avoid a body defence mechanism based upon the iron-sequestering action of lactoferrin and transferrin. *Haemophilus influenzae* and *Neisseria meningitidis* have evolved specific lactoferrin- and transferrin-binding proteins located on their cell membranes.[44] Membrane-associated transferrin-binding proteins have also been detected in a number of unicellular parasitic organisms that infect humans. These include *Trypanosoma cruzi*,[52] *Plasmodium falciparum*,[53] and *Leishmania donovani*.[54] In the case of some of these organisms, the transferrin-binding proteins are only present at certain stages in their life cycles, possibly reflecting differences in the demands for iron.

C. MELANOTRANSFERRIN

Human melanotransferrin, previously known as human melanoma-associated antigen p97, is a single polypeptide glycoprotein containing 719 amino acid residues (Figure 1). It is a cell membrane component of human melanomas, but has also been found in trace amounts in normal adult tissues.[8,37,38,40,45] From the amino acid sequence that has been deduced from the nucleotide sequence of the cDNA, it would appear that the protein is organised into three domains. The extracellular N-domain (residues 1 to 342) and C-domain (residues 343 to 694) each contain an iron-binding site. The remaining 25 residues (695 to 719) comprise a region of predominantly uncharged and hydrophobic amino acids, and are thought to be involved in the anchoring of the molecule in the cell membrane. The extracellular N- and C-domains show an interdomain sequence homology (46%) that is even more striking than that found in either transferrin (42%) or lactoferrin (37%). Two potential sites for the attachment of glycan chains have been identified at asparagine residues 135 and 515. Until sufficient of the protein has been isolated and purified from human melanoma cells, it remains to be established, firstly, whether or not these putative glycosylation sites are correct, and secondly, what is the structure of the glycan chains.

The function of melanotransferrin in either normal or malignant cells can only be speculated at the present time. The structural similarities with other members of the siderophilin family and the ability of the extracellular portion of the molecule to bind iron[40] support the proposal that melanotransferrin has a role to play in transmembrane iron transport,[45] particularly in rapidly dividing melanoma cells. Human melanotransferrin is a good example of a situation where the modern techniques of biotechnology have resulted in the complete amino acid sequence of a protein being deduced well in advance of establishing a biological role for the molecule.

D. OVOTRANSFERRIN

Ovotransferrin is a single polypeptide glycoprotein and a major component of the egg white of birds and reptiles. Chicken ovotransferrin contains 686 amino acid residues, and the amino acid sequence suggests a two-domain structure (Figure 1). The N-terminal domain (residues 1 to 340) and C-terminal domain (residues 341 to 686) share extensive internal sequence homology (37%). The total sequence homology between chicken ovotransferrin and human serum transferrin is even greater (51%), suggesting that the gene duplication resulting in a bilobar two-iron sited siderophilin preceded the evolutionary divergence of birds and mammals.

For a while it was thought that chicken ovotransferrin and chicken serum transferrin were two structurally and genetically distinct proteins, sharing the common characteristic of binding two atoms of iron. However, in 1962, Williams[46] demonstrated by chemical and immunological techniques that the two molecules differed only in the nature of their respective carbohydrate chains. It has now been confirmed that within the same species, ovotransferrin and transferrin are the products of the same gene locus. As a result of different pathways of glycosylation, occuring principally in the liver and oviduct, respectively, the single glycan chain attached to the N-domain of both proteins at asparagine 473 differs significantly in structure between the two siderophilins (Figure 4). The chicken ovotransferrin glycan chain contains no fucose, galactose, or sialic acid.

Ovotransferrin was initially discovered by virtue of its ability to suppress bacterial growth. The bacteriostatic properties of ovotransferrin are, like lactoferrin, attributable to the high affinity the molecule has for ferric iron. Whilst this is probably the major biological role for ovotransferrin within the egg white, the possibility that ovotransferrin acts as an iron store for the developing bird cannot be excluded.

E. OTHER TISSUE-SPECIFIC TRANSFERRINS

Although the majority of the transferrin that is present in the blood plasma has been synthesised in the liver, mention has already been made of the many other tissues in which transferrin mRNA has been detected and transferrin synthesis has been confirmed. For many of these extrahepatic sites, the molecule is secreted into the extracellular fluid from where it has access to the

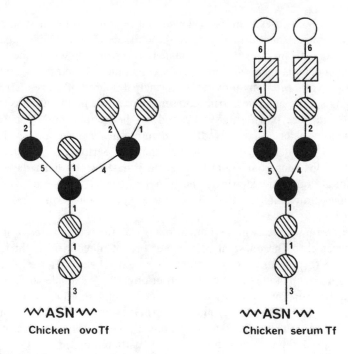

FIGURE 4. The glycan chains of chicken ovotransferrin and chicken serum transferrin. In each case the single glycan chain is attached to asparagine residue 473. Key to symbols: ○, sialic acid; ◕, N-acetyl glucosamine; ▨, galactose; ●, mannose; ASN, asparagine residue; ∿, polypeptide chain; **1**, β1–4; **2**, β1–2; **3**, β1–N; **4**, α1–3; **5**, α1–6; and **6**, α2–6.

bloodstream via the lymphatic system. There is as yet no evidence that the transferrin synthesised in tissues such as the heart, the lung, the kidney, and the intestine is in any way structurally different from the molecule made in the liver. The situation with regard to the mammary gland may be an exception. Levels of transferrin in the mammary glands of virgin mice are significantly lower than in the glands of pregnant or lactating animals. Transferrin synthesis in the mammary glands of lactating rabbits has been reported to be extremely high, three times that of the liver.[47] In mice the mammary gland epithelium synthesises transferrin which is secreted into the milk, constituting a major milk protein in this species. Mention has already been made of the fact that mouse "milk transferrin" is distinct from either mouse lactoferrin (different amino acid sequence) or mouse serum transferrin (additional fucose residue on the glycan chain).[42] Human milk contains lactoferrin and transferrin. It has always been assumed that all of the transferrin present in human milk has an identical structure to that found in the serum. It has not yet been confirmed whether or not this is actually the case.

Of the remaining nonhepatic tissues where transferrin synthesis has been shown to occur, two sites warrant special mention. These are the brain and the testis. In both cases there is evidence that *in situ* transferrin synthesis is particularly important to the cells, since these tissues are effectively separated from the bloodstream, preventing adequate transferrin supply from the serum.

Tight junctions between Sertoli cells constitute a blood-testis barrier.[48] The Sertoli cell secretions provide the principal source of nutrients for the developing sperm, and transferrin represents one of the major proteins of this nutrient fluid. The transferrin synthesised by the Sertoli cells of the testes functions to transfer iron, received from serum transferrin, to the developing germ cells. Whilst there is no evidence that the Sertoli cell transferrin is structurally different from serum transferrin, it has recently been shown that factors that stimulate transferrin synthesis in Sertoli cells (testosterone, insulin, and follicle-stimulating hormone) have little effect on transferrin synthesis by the liver.[19]

Transferrin synthesis in the human brain was first demonstrated in 1978 by Levin et al.[49] The question of whether or not transferrin might have a special role to play in nervous tissue has recently been reviewed.[18] It has been established that the blood-brain barrier effectively excludes much of the serum transferrin from reaching the nerve cells, although there is some evidence that a small amount of serum transferrin may cross the barrier by means of a specific receptor-mediated transport mechanism.[50] The existence of local transferrin gene expression within the brain, particularly in the oligodendrocytes and the choroid plexus, suggests a special requirement by these cells or possibly an alternative function for the locally synthesised transferrin. In addition to transferrin synthesis occurring within the central nervous system, it has now been thought that transferrin has an important role to play in the peripheral nervous system, particularly in the region of the motor end plates in muscle tissue. There is evidence to suggest that a specific transferrin is produced locally, either by the motor neuron itself or by the adjacent Schwann cells. It has been demonstrated, using monoclonal antibodies, that the transferrin produced at these sites is structurally different from serum transferrin in that it possibly expresses an embryonic epitope by way of an altered glycan chain structure.[51] It has been suggested very recently that transferrin may function as a neurotransmitter or neuromodulator in the developing vertebrate nervous system.[55]

The function and control of transferrin synthesis by these and other non-hepatic tissues will be considered in more detail in Chapter 6.

REFERENCES

1. **Schade, A. J.,** Conalbumin and siderophilin as iron-binding proteins: a review of their discovery, in *Proteins of Iron Storage and Transport,* G. Spik, J. Montreuil, R. R. Crichton, and J. Mazurier, Eds., Elsevier, Amsterdam, 1985, 3.
2. **Heubers, H. A. and Finch, C. A.,** The physiology of transferrin and transferrin receptors, *Physiol. Rev.,* 67, 520, 1987.

3. **MacGillivray, R. T. A., Mendez, E., Sinha, S. K., Sutton, M. R., Lineback-Zins, J., and Brew, K.,** The complete amino acid sequence of human transferrin, *Proc. Natl. Acad. Sci. U.S.A.,* 79, 2504, 1982.

4. **Yang, F. J., Lunn, J. B., McGill, J. R., Moore, C. M., Naylor, S. C., Van Bragt, P., Baldwin, B. H., and Bowman, B. H.,** Human transferrin gene: cDNA characterisation and chromosomal localisation, *Proc. Natl. Acad. Sci. U.S.A.,* 81, 2752, 1984.

5. **Uzan, B., Frain, M., Park, I., Besmond, C., Massen, G., Trepat, J. S., Zakin, M. M., and Kahn, A.,** Molecular cloning and sequence analysis of cDNA for human transferrin, *Biochem. Biophys. Res. Commun.,* 119, 273, 1984.

6. **Metz-Boutigue, M., Jolles, J., Mazurier, J., Schoentgen, F., Legrand, D., Spik, G., Montreuil, J., and Jolles, P.,** Human lactoferrin: amino acid sequence and comparison with other transferrins, *Eur. J. Biochem.,* 145, 659, 1984.

7. **McCombs, J. L., Teng, C. T., Pentecost, B. T., Magnuson, V. L., Moore, C. M., and McGill, J. R.,** Chromosomal localization of human lactoferrin gene, *Cytogenet. Cell Genet.,* 47, 16, 1988.

8. **Rose, T. M., Plowman, G. D., Teplow, D. B., Dreyer, W. J., Hellstrom, K. E., and Brown, J. P.,** Primary structure of human melanoma-associated antigen p97 (melanotransferrin) deduced from the mRNA sequence, *Proc. Natl. Acad. Sci. U.S.A.,* 83, 1261, 1986.

9. **Williams, J., Elleman, T. C., Kingston, I. B., Wilkins, A. G., and Kuhn, K. A.,** The primary structure of hen ovotransferrin, *Eur. J. Biochem.,* 122, 297, 1982.

10. **Jeltsch, J-M. and Chambon, P.,** The complete nucleotide sequence of the chicken ovotransferrin mRNA, *Eur. J. Biochem.,* 122, 291, 1982.

11. **Bowman, B. H., Yang, F., and Adrian, G. S.,** Transferrin: evolution and genetic regulation of expression, *Adv. Genet.,* 25, 1, 1988.

12. **Ainsen, P. and Listowsky, I.,** Iron transport and storage proteins, *Annu. Rev. Biochem.,* 49, 357, 1980.

13. **Chasteen, N. D.,** Transferrin: a perspective, *Adv. Inorg. Biochem.,* 5, 201, 1983.

14. **Morgan, E. H.,** Transferrin biochemistry, physiology and clinical significance, in *Molecular Aspects of Medicine,* Pergamon Press, Oxford, 1981, 1.

15. **Williams, J.,** The structure of transferrin, in *Proteins of Iron Storage and Transport,* G. Spik, J. Montreuil, R. R. Crichton, and J. Mazurier, Eds., Elsevier, Amsterdam, 1985, 13.

16. **Martin, A. W., Heubers, E., Heubers, H., Webb, J., and Finch, C. A.,** A monosited transferrin from a representative deuterostome, *Blood,* 64, 1048, 1984.

17. **Osterloh, K. H., Simpson, R. J., and Peters, T. J.,** The role of mucosal transferrin in intestinal iron absorption, *Br. J. Haematol.,* 65, 1, 1987.

18. **Espinosa de los Monteros, A., Pena, L. A., and Vellis, J.,** Does transferrin have a specific role to play in the nervous system?, *J. Neurosci. Res.,* 24, 125, 1989.

19. **Huggenvik, J. I., Izerda, R. L., Haywood, L., Lee, D. C., McKnight, G. S., and Griswold, M. D.,** Transferrin messenger ribonucleic acid: molecular cloning and hormonal regulation in rat Sertoli cells, *Endocrinology,* 120, 332, 1987.

20. **Goubin, G., Goldman, D. S., Luce, J., Neiman, P. E., and Cooper, G. M.,** Molecular cloning and nucleotide sequence of a transforming gene deleted by transfection of chicken B-cell lymphoma and DNA, *Nature,* 302, 114, 1983.

21. **Diamond, A., Cooper, G. M., Ritz, J., and Lane M-A.,** Identification and molecular cloning of the human Burkitts Lymphoma transforming gene, *Nature,* 305, 112, 1983.

22. **Hattori, M., Hidaka, S., and Sakaki, Y.,** Sequence analysis of a Kbeta n1 family member near the 3' end of human β-globin gene, *Nucleic Acids Res.,* 13, 7813, 1985.

23. **Osborne, T. B. and Campbell, G. F.,** The protein components of egg white, *J. Am. Chem. Soc.,* 22, 422, 1900.

24. **Schade, A. L. and Caroline, L.,** Raw hen egg white and the role of iron in growth inhibition of *Shigella dysenteriae, Science,* 100, 14, 1944.

25. **Alderton, G., Ward, W. H., and Fevold, H. L.,** Identification of the bacteria-inhibiting, iron-binding protein of egg white as conalbumin, *Arch. Biochem. Biophys.,* 11, 9, 1946.
26. **Fontes, G. and Thivolle, L.,** The presence of non-haemoglobin iron in serum, and its reduction in experimental anaemia, *C.R. Seances Soc. Biol. Paris,* 93, 687, 1925.
27. **Barkan, G. and Schales, O.,** Chemischer Aufban und physiologische Bedeutung des "leicht abspaltbaven" Bluteisens, *Hoppe-Seylers Z. Physiol. Chem.,* 248, 96, 1937.
28. **Vahlquist, B. C. S.,** Serum iron, *Acta Paediatr. Suppl.,* 5, 28, 1941.
29. **Schade, A. L. and Caroline, L.,** An iron-binding component in human blood plasma, *Science,* 104, 340, 1946.
30. **Schade, A. L., Reinhart, R. W., and Levy, H.,** Carbon dioxide and oxygen complex formation with iron and siderophilin, the iron-binding component of human plasma, *Arch. Biochem. Biophys.,* 20, 170, 1949.
31. **Laurell, C. B. and Ingelman, B.,** The iron-binding protein of swine serum, *Acta Chem. Scand.,* 1, 770, 1947.
32. **Sorensen, M. and Sorensen, S. P. L.,** A red protein present in bovine milk, *C.R. Trav. Lab. Carlsberg,* 23, 55, 1939.
33. **Johansson, B. G.,** Chromatographic separation of lactalbumin from human milk whey on calcium phosphate columns, *Nature,* 181, 996, 1958.
34. **Johansson, B. G.,** Isolation of an iron-containing red protein from human milk, *Acta Chem. Scand.,* 14, 510, 1960.
35. **Montreuil, J., Tonnelat, J., and Mullet, S.,** Preparation and properties of lactosiderophilin from human milk, *Biochim. Biophys. Acta,* 45, 413, 1960.
36. **Groves, M. L.,** The isolation of a red protein from milk, *J. Am. Chem. Soc.,* 82, 3345, 1960.
37. **Woodbury, R. G., Brown, J. P., Yeh, M., Hellstrom, I., and Hellstrom, K. E.,** Identification of a cell surface protein, p97, in human melanoma and certain other neoplasms, *Proc. Natl. Acad. Sci. U.S.A.,* 77, 2183, 1980.
38. **Brown, J. P., Wright, P. W., Hart, C. E., Woodbury, R. G., Hellstrom, K. E., and Hellstrom, I.,** Protein antigens of normal and malignant human cells identified by immunoprecipitation with monoclonal antibodies, *J. Biol. Chem.,* 255, 4980, 1980.
39. **Dippold, W. G., Lloyd, K. O., Li, L. T., Ikeda, H., Oettgen, H. F., and Old, L. J.,** Cell surface antigens of human malignant melanoma: definition of six antigenic systems with mouse monoclonal antibodies, *Proc. Natl. Acad. Sci. U.S.A.,* 77, 6114, 1980.
40. **Brown, J. P., Hewick, R. M., Hellstrom, I., Hellstrom, K. E., Doolittle, R. F., and Dryer, W. J.,** Human melanoma-associated antigen p97 is structurally and functionally related to transferrin, *Nature,* 296, 171, 1982.
41. **Cox, T., Mazurier, J., Spik, G., Montreuil, J., and Peters, T.,** Human lactoferrin receptors on the membranes of enterocytes, *Biochim. Biophys. Acta,* 588, 120, 1979.
42. **LeClerq, Y., Sawatzki, G., Wieruszeski, J-M., Montreuil, J., and Spik, G.,** Primary structure of the glycans from mouse serum and milk transferrins, *Biochem. J.,* 247, 571, 1987.
43. **Sawatzki, G.,** The role of iron binding proteins in bacterial infections, in *Iron Transport in Microbes, Plants and Animals,* G. Winkelmann, D. Van der Helm, and J. B. Neilands, Eds., VCH Publishers, Weinheim, West Germany, 1987, chap. 25.
44. **Schryvers, A. B.,** Identification of the transferrin- and lactoferrin-binding proteins in *Haemophilus influenzae, J. Med. Microbiol.,* 29, 121, 1989.
45. **Brown, J. P., Rose, T. M., and Plowman, G. D.,** Human melanoma antigen p97, a membrane-associated transferrin homologue, in *Proteins of Iron Storage and Transport,* G. Spik, J. Montreuil, R. R. Crichton, and J. Mazurier, Eds., Elsevier, Amsterdam, 1985, 39.
46. **Williams, J.,** A comparison of conalbumin and transferrin in the domestic fowl, *Biochem. J.,* 83, 355, 1962.

47. **Jordan, S. M. and Morgan, E. H.,** Plasma protein metabolism during lactation in the rabbit, *Am. J. Physiol.,* 219, 1549, 1970.

48. **Fawcett, D. W.,** Ultrastructure and function of the Sertoli cell, in *Handbook of Physiology: Male Reproductive System,* Vol. 5, D. W. Hamilton, and R. D. Grup, Eds., American Physiological Society, Bethesda, MD, 1975, 21.

49. **Levin, M. J., Tuil, D., Uzan, G., Dreyfus, J-C., and Kahn, A.,** Expression of the transferrin gene during the development of non-hepatic tissues: high levels of transferrin mRNA in fetal muscle and adult brain, *Biochem. Biophys. Res. Commun.,* 122, 212, 1984.

50. **Jeffries, W. A., Brandon, M. R., Hunt, S., Williams, A. F., Gatter, K. C., and Mason, D. Y.,** Transferrin receptor on the endothelium of brain capillaries, *Nature,* 312, 162, 1984.

51. **Festoff, B. W., Munoz, P. A., Patel, M. K. N., Harris, M., and Beach, R. L.,** Monoclonal antibodies detect embryonic epitope specific for nerve derived transferrin, *J. Neurosci. Res.,* 22, 425, 1989.

52. **Lima, M. F. and Villalta, F.,** A transferrin-binding protein associated with the membrane of *Trypanosoma cruzi, Mol. Biochem. Parasitol.,* 38, 245, 1990.

53. **Rodriguez, M. H. and Jungery, M.,** A protein on *Plasmodiun falciparum*-infected erythrocytes functions as a transferrin receptor, *Nature,* 324, 388, 1986.

54. **Voyaitzaki, C. S. and Soteriadou, K. P.,** Evidence of transferrin binding sites on the surface of *Leishmania* promastigotes, *J. Biol. Chem.,* 265, 22380, 1990.

55. **Hyndman, A. G., Hockberger, P. E., Zeevalk, G. D., and Connor, J. A.,** Transferrin can alter physiological properties of retinal neurons, *Brain Res.,* 561, 318, 1991.

Chapter 4

TRANSFERRIN STRUCTURE AND IRON BINDING

I. THE OCCURRENCE OF TRANSFERRINS WITHIN THE ANIMAL KINGDOM

The need for a vehicle to transport iron in a nontoxic form between tissues is clearly demonstrated by the presence of transferrin in the blood of the more complex organisms of the animal kingdom. If the use of the term transferrin is restricted to those plasma glycoproteins with a molecular weight in the region of 80,000 that are able to reversibly bind two atoms of ferric iron in the obligatory presence of bicarbonate, then it is true to say that such molecules have been detected in the blood from representatives of all the major classes of the superclass Gnathostomata, subphylum Vertebrata, phylum Chordata. This includes mammals, birds, reptiles, amphibians, bony fish, and cartilaginous fish. However, if one is prepared to accept a more flexible definition of a transferrin as being a protein, with or without carbohydrate chains, capable of reversibly binding at least one atom of iron, with or without the need for the bicarbonate anion, and with any acceptable molecular weight, then the presence of transferrins throughout the animal kingdom is far more widespread (Figure 1).

Of the many phyla within the animal kingdom, five have been examined for the presence of iron-binding proteins. In the case of representative examples from the phyla Nematoda, Annelida, and Mollusca, no iron-binding proteins were detected in a study carried out by Palmour and Sutton.[1] From the phylum Arthropoda, which includes the insects and crustacea, a number of putative transferrins have been reported. Iron-binding proteins have been identified in three species of moths, although no details were given of either the size of the proteins or the number of iron atoms bound.[2] During the course of a study of the metabolism of iron in the tarantula spider, *Dugesiella hentzi*, Lee et al.[2] identified an iron-binding plasma protein with a molecular weight of 90,000. Iron-binding proteins have been detected in three species of crabs. In two early reports,[3,4] a brief reference was made to a protein in the blood from *Callinectes sapidus* and *Macropipus puber* that was able to reversibly bind ^{59}Fe. In neither of these reports was the protein further characterised. More recently, Heubers et al.[5] have isolated and characterised an iron-binding protein from the blood of the crab *Cancer magister*. The molecule is a single polypeptide chain with a molecular weight of 150,000. In the presence of bicarbonate ions the protein was shown to bind two atoms of iron and exhibited an absorbance spectrum very similar to that of mammalian transferrin. Furthermore, the crab transferrin was shown to be capable of delivering iron to rat erythroid and nonerythroid tissues. Apart from the significantly larger size of the crab transferrin in comparison with its mammalian counterpart, the two proteins have many common structural and functional characteristics. This would appear to negate a previously held view that transferrin is a newcomer to the evolutionary scene, confined to the phylum Chordata.

The situation regarding the iron-binding proteins present in crab haemolymph has become more complicated as a result of two recent findings.

Phylum ARTHROPODA

Phylum CHORDATA :

    Subphylum UROCHORDATA

    Subphylum VERTEBRATA :

        Superclass AGNATHA :

            Class CYCLOSTOMASTA

        Superclass GNATHOSTOMATA :

            Class ELASMOBRANCHII

            Class ACTINOPTERIGYII

            Class AMPHIBIA

            Class REPTILIA

            Class AVES

            Class MAMMALIA

FIGURE 1. The phyla, subphyla, superclasses, and classes of the animal kingdom in which transferrinlike molecules have been discovered.

Topham et al.[6] have reported that the haemolymph of the horseshoe crab, *Limulus polyphenus,* contains a very large iron-binding protein (M.W. 282,000). The molecule is composed of ten identical subunits, each capable of binding two atoms of iron. The same authors have recently characterised an iron-binding protein from the haemolymph of the blue crab, *Callinectes sapidus.*[7] This protein has a molecular weight of 155,000 and is composed of a single polypeptide chain, with the capacity to bind ten atoms of iron. Clearly, such are the differences in structure between the iron-binding proteins present in the haemolymph of these three species of crab, that it is difficult to imagine how the three crab proteins are in any way analogous either to each other, or to the transferrin from higher organisms.

The phylum Chordata is divided into two subphyla, Urochordata and Vertebrata. Urochordates are small marine organisms possessing a notochord only during the larval stage of their development. The group is an ancient one, separated by millions of years of separate evolution from the members of the vertebrate line. Many of the Urochordates accumulate metal ions as seawater is drawn through their feeding syphons. For example, some species have been shown to have the ability to bind vanadium in their blood plasma and to concentrate this metal up to 10^6 times in blood cells called vanadocytes.[8] An iron-binding protein from the blood of a representative Urochordate, the ascidian *Pyura stolonifera,* has been isolated and characterised.[8] The protein was found to have a molecular weight of 41,000 and to bind just one atom of iron in the presence of bicarbonate. Confirmation that the molecule was a true monosited transferrin came with the demonstration that it was able to bind to the transferrin receptor on rat reticulocytes, and furthermore was subsequently internalised within these cells. The Pyura protein is the only substantiated example that has so far been found of a monosited transferrin, half the size of the vertebrate protein. Yet the existence of such a molecule was postulated well before its discovery. The extensive amino acid sequence homology between the two domains of all the vertebrate transferrins that have so far been characterised strongly suggested that the mammalian transferrin was the product of gene duplication of a primitive ancestral monosited protein with a molecular weight of about 40,000.

The large subphylum Vertebrata is subdivided into two superclasses. Cyclostomes are the most primitive living vertebrates, appearing anatomically to be a connecting link between invertebrates and vertebrates.[9] Together with the now extinct Ostracoderms they form the superclass Agnatha (without jaws), which has followed an independent evolution since the earliest vertebrate origins. The only living representatives today are the hagfish (marine) and lampreys (marine and/or freshwater). In 1971, Palmour and Sutton,[1] whilst carrying out a study of the transferrins from a large range of vertebrates, reported on an iron-binding protein from the serum of the Californian hagfish *Eptatretus stouitii*. The protein appeared to have a molecular weight of 45,000 and a single iron-binding site. Not unnaturally, the authors suggested that this was the much sought after ancestral precursor of modern transferrins. However, within a year, Ainsen et al.,[10] using the same source of hagfish as Palmour and Sutton, failed to confirm this finding. In a more detailed analysis, and using a range of procedures to measure molecular weight, they showed conclusively that the hagfish transferrin was a single polypeptide chain (M.W. 77,000) with two iron-binding sites. Lampreys are close relatives of the hagfish. The sea lamprey *Petromyzon marinus* has been shown to possess a plasma transferrin with a molecular weight of 79,000 and two iron-binding sites.[11] Interestingly, the molecule contains no sialic acid, nor does it appear to contain the amino acid arginine. By comparison, the plasma iron-binding proteins from another lamprey, *Geotria australis,* demonstrate a more complex situation.[12] The larval stage of this species spends a number of years lying dormant in the mud deposits of rivers and streams. The plasma iron levels are extremely high (20 mg/100 mL) compared to the iron levels found in human plasma (0.1 mg/100 mL). The iron is associated with a large protein (M.W. 354,000) that appears to be analogous to mammalian ferritin. However, in the adult of this species, which by now has migrated to the sea, plasma iron levels are considerably reduced (0.03 mg/100 mL). The major iron-binding plasma protein is a tetrameric structure (M.W. 296,000) which readily dissociates into four identical subunits (M.W. 78,000). Each subunit reversibly binds two atoms of iron and therefore appears to be analogous to mammalian transferrin.

TABLE 1
The Concentration of
Human Transferrin in
Different Body Fluids

	mg/L
Plasma	2500
Lymph	2200
Amniotic fluid	300
Tears	100
Milk	25
Seminal fluid	22
Cerebrospinal fluid	18
Bile	16

Most of the present day vertebrates belong to the superclass Gnathostomata (with jaws). Of the seven principal classes, only one has not been examined for the presence of transferrin within the plasma. These are the lungfish belonging to the class Crossopterygii. In all the other vertebrate classes — Elasmobranchii (cartilaginous fish), Actinopterygii (bony fish), Amphibia, Reptilia, Aves, and Mammalia — evidence for the presence of a plasma transferrin (M.W. 75,000 to 85,000; two iron-binding sites) has been forthcoming on every occasion that it has been sought. Whilst interclass and interspecies differences have been shown to exist, these only relate to amino acid sequences and glycan structures. The basic model of a large-molecular-weight, single polypeptide, with a bilobar structure and two iron-binding sites, has remained remarkably consistent throughout the vertebrates.

For the remainder of this chapter, during which the chemical and physical properties of transferrin will be considered, human serum transferrin will be taken as the archetypal example. Reference to the structure of other animal transferrins will only be made where a comparison seems appropriate and relevant.

II. HUMAN SERUM TRANSFERRIN

A. PLASMA CONCENTRATION AND ELECTROPHORETIC MOBILITY

The body of an adult contains about 14 g of transferrin, of which approximately half is found in the blood plasma. The remainder is distributed amongst a wide variety of body fluids, including lymph, tears, cerebrospinal fluid, bile, amniotic fluid, milk, saliva, aqueous humour, and seminal fluid (Table 1). Plasma transferrin (2.5 g/L) accounts for about 4% of the protein content of this fluid and is the fourth most abundant plasma protein.

An extensive range of techniques are available in order to measure plasma transferrin concentration. Most of the original procedures were based on the capacity of this plasma protein to bind iron, but these methods are now being progressively replaced by more direct immunological procedures using anti-bodies specific for human transferrin.

The iron-binding techniques are based on the assumption that when plasma is deliberately saturated with iron, and the excess unbound iron is then removed, the remaining protein-bound iron is attached exclusively to transferrin. Since it is known that one molecule of transferrin (M.W. 79,570) has the capacity to bind a maximum of two atoms of iron (atomic mass 55.847), if the protein-bound iron is removed and its concentration measured colorimetrically, it is then possible to calculate the original transferrin concentration in the plasma sample (1 g of transferrin binds a maximum of 1.403 mg of iron). The iron that is released from the proteins of iron-saturated plasma gives a result that is referred to as the total iron-binding capacity (TIBC). From a separate measurement of the protein-bound iron that was present in the plasma before excess iron had been added to achieve saturation (serum iron concentration), it can be calculated that the iron-binding plasma protein fraction, and therefore by inference transferrin, is about 30% saturated with iron in a healthy individual. As has already been mentioned, to calculate the transferrin concentration in plasma from the TIBC result, two basic assumptions are made:

1.   The addition of excess iron to a sample of plasma results in a rapid and complete saturation of the iron-binding sites of the transferrin.
2.   Iron added to plasma only binds to the protein transferrin.

There is evidence to suggest that neither of these assumptions are any longer fully justified. The kinetics and mechanism of iron uptake by apotransferrin is very much influenced by the nature of the iron donor used in the experiments. The reaction of transferrin with either ferric chloride or ferric citrate, the iron donors used in many of the clinical assays of TIBC, is slow and never reaches completion.[13] Rapid (10 s) and complete saturation of transferrin is, however, achieved using monomeric complexes such as Fe^{3+}-nitrilotri-acetic acid (FENTA).[13] In addition, it has been clearly demonstrated that TIBC methods using either ferric chloride or ferric citrate result in about 20% of the protein-bound iron becoming attached to plasma proteins other than transferrin.[14]

These observations explain why plasma transferrin concentrations calculated from the TIBC value consistently give results that are higher than those obtained by using the more direct immunological methods. A wide range of immunological techniques are now available in order to measure plasma transferrin concentration including immunodiffusion, immunoelectrophoresis, immunoturbidometry, enzyme-linked immunoassay, and radioimmunoassay. In addition to providing a more accurate measure of the plasma transferrin concentration, these methods have proved to be extremely useful for measuring the low levels of transferrin that are often associated with other biological fluids (Table 1).

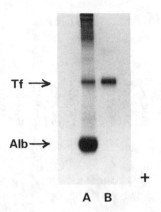

FIGURE 2. Polyacrylamide gel electrophoresis of human serum and pure human transferrin at pH 8.8. A, Human serum; B, pure human transferrin.

Transferrin migrates electrophoretically with the β_1-globulin fraction of human plasma. The concentration of transferrin in human serum is sufficiently high, such that the position to which the protein has migrated during electrophoresis can be readily identified using one of the nonspecific protein stains, for example, Coomassie Blue, Amido Black, or Ponceau S (Figure 2). If in doubt, the identity of transferrin can be confirmed using a more specific technique — Nitroso R (an iron stain),[15] ^{59}Fe autoradiography,[16] or immunofixation.[17] The initial electrophoretic identification of transferrin from other animal sera is often not as simple as is the case with the human protein (Figure 3), and in these situations one of the more specific staining techniques has to be employed.[18]

In nondenaturing buffer systems the isoelectric point of transferrin, and therefore its electrophoretic mobility, is influenced by at least two factors. The first is the degree of iron saturation. Under normal physiological conditions serum transferrin is about 30% saturated with iron. Consequently, in fresh serum four different forms of transferrin with respect to iron content can be distinguished: apotransferrin (Tf); monoferric transferrin with a single iron atom attached to the N-domain binding site (Fe_NTf); monoferric transferrin with a single iron atom attached to the C-domain binding site ($TfFe_C$); and diferric transferrin (Fe_2Tf). The binding of iron to apotransferrin is associated with the release of three protons. In addition, the molecule undergoes a conformational change, resulting in a more spherical shape and an alteration in the positions of the N-glycan chains relative to the polypeptide. As a result, at alkaline pH diferric transferrin (pI 5.5) has a slightly greater negative charge than apotransferrin (pI 5.9). Using the more commonly employed techniques of plasma protein electrophoresis at pH 8.9 (cellulose acetate, starch, and acrylamide gel), these small differences in net negative charge cannot readily be distinguished, and transferrin (30% iron saturated) migrates as a single broad band. It is only when a more discriminatory electrophoretic technique

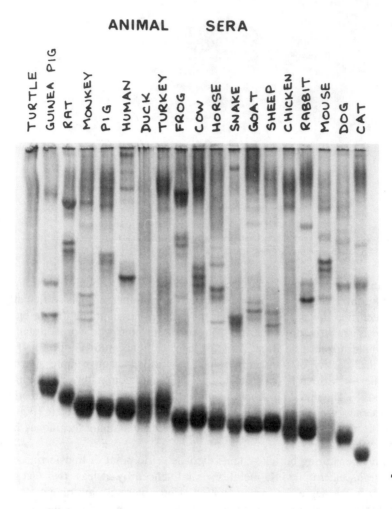

FIGURE 3.   Polyacrylamide gel electrophoresis of a variety of animal sera at pH 8.8.

such as isoelectric focussing is used that these four isotransferrins can be separated.

The second factor that increases the potential heterogeneity of serum transferrin concerns the structure, degree of branching, and sialic acid content of the two glycan chains. The cause and extent of this heterogeneity will be discussed in a later section. It is, however, worth mentioning at this stage that it has recently been calculated that the potential number of structurally different forms of human transferrin that can result from differences in iron and sialic acid content is 36.[19] Isoelectric focussing in a narrow pH range (5 to 6.5) has the potential to resolve these complex mixtures.[19] It is usually the case that only a proportion of these isotransferrins exists at any one time in a sample of fresh plasma. Nevertheless, in order to reduce the microheterogeneity of transferrin and convert all the forms into a single molecular species, it is necessary to first saturate the plasma with iron, and then to remove all of the sialic acid residues with the enzyme neuraminidase.[19] If, as a result of such treatment, human serum still appears to contain more than one transferrin protein, the cause is likely to be due to genetic polymorphism. Inherited variation at the transferrin gene locus will be discussed in Chapters 8 and 9.

B. PURIFICATION OF TRANSFERRIN

The concentration of transferrin in human plasma is at a sufficiently high level (2.5 g/L), such that there are very few technical problems associated with the extraction of the protein in a pure and homogeneous state. Over the years a wide variety of purification procedures have been published[20-24] in which the most frequently employed practical methods have included some of the following:

1. Ammonium sulphate precipitation
2. Rivanol precipitation of nontransferrin plasma proteins
3. Ion-exchange chromatography
4. Gel-filtration chromatography
5. Preparative isoelectric focussing
6. Immunoaffinity chromatography
7. Preparative starch block electrophoresis
8. Phenyl-boronate affinity chromatography (for glycoproteins)
9. Fast protein liquid chromatography

An example of a purification protocol that has proved very successful in this laboratory is shown in Figure 4. The entire procedure takes 4 days to complete, and between 50 and 60 mg of pure transferrin can be recovered from 25 mL of plasma.

C. PHYSICAL AND CHEMICAL PROPERTIES
1. Size, Shape, and Quaternary Structure

Some of the earliest measurements on the hydrodynamic properties of transferrin were made 45 years ago.[25] These initial experiments estimated the molecular weight of human serum transferrin as being close to 90,000, and from this data the dimensions of the molecule were calculated to be 19 × 3.7 nm. These values have been subsequently modified as the methods for the isolation and purification of transferrin have improved. In addition, the physical methods for measuring the molecular weights of proteins have become more precise. In a detailed study of the molecular weight and sedimentation properties of human transferrin in 1966, Roberts et al.[26] reported a value of 74,000 for the molecular weight of the polypeptide chain. The physical methods that were used to obtain this result would not have taken into account the carbohydrate component of the glycoprotein. It is now known that transferrin contains two glycan chains which together contribute an additional 4400 Da to the gross molecular weight. On this basis, the measured

25 ml plasma + 50 μmole bicarbonate
+ 20 μmole Fe^{3+} - nitrilotriacetate

↓

Dialyse for 24 hr against 10mM Tris/20mM NaCl pH 8.3

↓

DEAE Sephacel column : 10mM Tris/20mM NaCl pH 8.3
to
10mM Tris/150mM NaCl pH 8.3

Collect and pool Tf fractions (A_{470})

↓

DEAE Sephacel column : 10mM Tris/55mM NaCl pH 8.3
to
10mM Tris/110mM NaCl pH 8.3

Collect and pool Tf fractions (A_{470})

↓

SEPHADEX G-200 column : 0.1M Tris/0.2M NaCl pH 8.0

Collect and pool Tf fractions (A_{470})

Dialyse Tf for 24 hr against 0.02M sodium citrate pH 5.0
This removes the bound iron and the Tf changes from
salmon-pink to colourless

↓

SP SEPHADEX C-50 column :

1. 0.02M Na citrate pH 5.0 - discard eluate

2. 0.02M Na citrate pH 5.55 - collect and pool
Tf fractions (A_{280})

↓

PURE TRANSFERRIN $A_{280} \div A_{470} < 22.0$

FIGURE 4.   An example of a protocol for the purification of transferrin from human serum.

molecular weight of human transferrin would now be increased to 78,400.
This turns out to be remarkably close to the true molecular-weight value which
it has recently been possible to calculate from a knowledge of the complete
amino acid sequence of the polypeptide chain.

Human transferrin contains 697 amino acid residues. From the amino
acid sequence, a molecular weight for the polypeptide chain can be calculated:
75,095. This value is for the apotransferrin, devoid of iron and bicarbonate,

and assumes that all 38 cysteine residues are involved in disulphide bridges. The glycan chains of transferrin are known to have the potential of exhibiting considerable heterogeneity with respect to both sugar composition and sequence. If, however, the assumption is made that both of the glycan chains are of the most common configuration — biantennary and fully sialylated — this will add a further 4412 Da to the weight of the molecule. The final calculated molecular weight of human serum apotransferrin comes to a value of 79,469.

The shape of the apotransferrin molecule in solution is that of a prolate ellipsoid. The ratio of major to minor axes is between 2.5:1 and 3:1.[27] Upon binding two atoms of iron, the molecule becomes more compact or spherical, and the axial ratio of diferric transferrin is approximately 2:1.[28] Iron-saturated transferrin is more resistant to thermal and chemical denaturation or proteolytic attack compared with apotransferrin.

For a short period of time some 25 years ago, the quaternary (subunit) structure of transferrin was unresolved. Since the molecule was known by then to be capable of binding a maximum of two atoms of iron, it was suggested that the protein might consist of two identical polypeptide subunits. In 1967, Jeppson[29] reported that he had been able to split transferrin into two identical subunits by either reduction-alkylation or by performic acid oxidation. However, later in the same year, Bezkorovainy and Grohlich[30] found that the molecular weight of transferrin did not change when the protein was exposed to a range of physical conditions that might have been expected to disrupt quaternary structure. The controversy was finally resolved in 1970 by Mann et al.[31] when it was conclusively shown that the molecular weight of transferrin in both the native and the reduced alkylated form remained constant at 78,000. Transferrin therefore has no quaternary structure. Only under special and exceptional circumstances can the covalent structure of the protein be split chemically into two portions, each with a molecular weight of about 40,000. Indeed, it would be a considerable disadvantage to higher organisms if the molecule of transferrin were to be reduced to a molecular weight of 40,000. At this relatively small size the molecule could escape from the circulation into the glomerular filtrate at the kidneys. The protein, and more importantly its bound iron, would be irreversibly lost from the body in the urine. This scenario has recently been shown experimentally by Williams et al.[32] and probably provides the best evidence to support the evolutionary advantage that accrued from the gene duplication that is thought to have given rise to the modern transferrin gene.

2. Primary Structure

The isolation and subsequent purification of a protein that is present in human plasma at a concentration of 2.5 g/L, and alone comprises 4% of the total protein content of this fluid, should not have been a major problem for the protein chemist. This has certainly been true in the case of human transferrin. Over the last 25 years, sufficient quantities of pure human transferrin

TABLE 2
The Amino Acid Composition of Human Serum Transferrin

	Data from known sequence	Ref.										
		33	34	35	36	37	31	38	39	40	41	42
Lysine	58	58	61	60	61	64	51	64	60	51	59	54
Histidine	19	18	20	19	22	17	19	20	20	18	18	18
Arginine	25	27	27	27	25	28	24	24	27	24	24	25
Threonine	30	31	30	30	26	29	30	28	28	26	30	30
Serine	41	42	40	38	39	39	40	37	39	37	38	41
Proline	32	35	32	34	35	31	30	25	31	38	39	30
Alanine	58	57	57	58	57	57	59	53	56	53	59	56
Aspartic	42 } 79	79	80	80	81	81	81	64	79	74	80	79
Asparagine	37 }											
Glutamic	43 } 59	60	64	58	63	61	58	58	63	55	57	64
Glutamine	16 }											
Cysteine	38	39	40	35	24	35	35	38	39	31	37	37
Valine	45	46	44	43	47	38	43	42	43	42	41	42
Methionine	9	10	8	8	24	9	4	8	8	7	8	8
Isoleucine	15	15	15	15	14	15	14	13	15	15	14	15
Leucine	59	58	59	62	58	62	57	57	57	54	58	59
Tyrosine	26	25	23	26	18	25	24	41	22	25	29	25
Phenylalanine	28	27	28	29	30	39	38	38	38	38	32	28
Tryptophan	8	8	9	8[a]	22	8	9	10	8[a]	8[a]	8[a]	8
Total	679	684	686	681	700	678	660	637	671	634	679	669

Note: The number of amino acid residues has been recalculated from the original reported values[31-42] on the basis of a polypeptide chain, molecular weight of 75,095, and a gross molecular weight of 79,469.

[a] Eight tryptophan residues have been assigned to those reports where no value for tryptophan was given.

have been isolated by many research groups such as to allow the amino acid composition of the molecule to be elucidated and, more recently, the complete amino acid sequence to be determined. Since 1962, there have been many reports in the literature of the amino acid composition of human transferrin,[31,33-42] and the results of many of these studies are given in Table 2. In order to allow a more valid comparison, much of the original data has been recalculated on the basis of what is now known to be the true molecular weight of the whole glycoprotein (79,469) or the polypeptide chain alone (75,095). It is quite clear from the results shown in Table 2 that even in the absence of a known amino acid sequence, there has been a remarkably consistent agreement as to the amino acid composition of the protein. Once the amino acid sequence of human transferrin had been finally established with the cloning and sequencing of the transferrin gene,[43] the amino acid composition of the protein was confirmed.

The complete sequence of the 679 amino acid residues in human transferrin has been established as a result of the combined efforts of the protein chemists and the molecular biologists. The first attempts at sequence analysis were carried out in the early 1970s. It was soon realised that for such a large protein with so many arginine and lysine residues, the conventional approach of initially cleaving the polypeptide chain into tryptic peptides would yield far too many fragments for sequence and overlap analysis. However, since it was already known at the time that transferrin contained only nine methionine residues, cleavage with cyanogen bromide was selected as the method of choice, in order to produce a small number (ten) of large peptides. In 1973, six cyanogen bromide fragments were reported[44] with a combined molecular weight of 76,000. Seven fragments were isolated[45] one year later, and once again the combined molecular weight of these seven fragments accounted for most, if not all, of the entire transferrin polypeptide. Since a total of ten cyanogen bromide fragments would be expected, clearly, in both of these experiments either some of the methionine bonds had not been broken, or a few of the peptides were of such a small size that they had been lost during the purification procedures. The situation was finally clarified in 1982 by MacGillivray et al.,[46] who showed that by combining cyanogen bromide cleavage with disulphide bond reduction and alkylation, a full complement of ten peptides could be isolated. These ranged in molecular weights from as large as 26,000 to as small as 340. These peptides, along with subsequent ones generated by the proteolytic enzymes trypsin, chymotrypsin, thermolysin, and *Staphylococcus aureus* protease, were sequenced. After position of overlap had been determined, the complete amino acid sequence of human transferrin was reported. The molecule was found to contain 678 residues, and within the polypeptide chain, two domains with considerable sequence homology were identified — residues 1 to 336 and residues 337 to 678. The extent of sequence homology between the two halves of the polypeptide chain was taken as evidence to support the hypothesis that the structural gene for human transferrin had arisen during the course of evolution by the contiguous duplication of an ancestral gene for an iron-binding transferrin containing about 340 amino acid residues.[47]

A year after the first publication of an amino acid sequence by MacGillivray et al.,[46] the same group reported a second and slightly modified sequence, based upon results obtained using an automated sequence analysis procedure.[48] The most significant change was an increase in the number of amino acid residues from 678 to 679. Other revisions included alterations in amide assignments and a small number of sequence inversions.

It was at this stage that the intervention by the molecular biologists provided the final confirmation of amino acid sequence. In 1984, Yang et al.[43] isolated and sequenced human transferrin cDNA from a cDNA library constructed from human liver messenger RNA. The complete 2324-base sequence of the cDNA was found to contain a single reading frame from which the amino acid sequence of the polypeptide coded by transferrin mRNA was deduced. The initial translation product of liver transferrin mRNA was found to be a polypeptide containing 698 amino acid residues, which is 19 amino acids longer than the molecule isolated from human plasma.[48] These extra residues are accounted for by a leader sequence or signal peptide which is essential for the secretion of the protein from the liver cell, but is subsequently cleaved from the amino-terminal end of the polypeptide. The amino acid sequence of transferrin as deduced from the cDNA base sequence was found to agree almost exactly with the sequence determined by the protein chemists. The small number of changes related mainly to those of amide assignments. What is now generally accepted as being the definitive amino acid sequence of human transferrin is shown in Figure 5. An identical sequence has recently been confirmed as a result of the analysis of the complete structure of the human transferrin gene. Schaeffer et al.[49] isolated the gene from human foetal liver and human leukocyte genomic libraries. The gene has a total length of 33,500 bases, and is organised into 17 coding exons which are separated by 16 intron sequences ranging in size from 675 to 5300 bases. This means that the total coding region, divided amongst the 17 exons, accounts for less than 7% of the entire transferrin gene. The structure, organisation, and control of expression of the transferrin gene will be discussed more fully in Chapter 6.

A particularly striking feature of the amino acid sequence of human transferrin is the similarity between the N-terminal and C-terminal halves of the protein. The data shown in Figure 5 have been arranged, with appropriate gaps in the sequence, in order to emphasise this homology. Of the amino acids in the N-terminal domain (residues 1 to 336), 42% have identical counterparts in the C-terminal domain (residues 337 to 679). It is difficult to imagine that any evolutionary process, other than a gene duplication, could have resulted in such a structure.

The amino acid sequences of two additional members of the human siderophilin family, namely lactoferrin (Lf) and melanotransferrin (Mf), have also been determined.[50,51] In both cases a similar degree of internal sequence homology between the N-terminal and C-terminal domains has been discovered. In addition, the sequence homology between these three proteins (Tf:Lf, 59%; Tf:Mf, 40%) suggests, although it is known that the proteins are coded for by three separate gene loci, that the genes must have evolved from a common ancestor. This same gene is thought to have been the ancestor of the structural gene for transferrin in all other animal species. Evidence to support this view has come from the amino acid sequence analysis of transferrin from three widely different animal species — pig,[52] chicken,[53] and toad.[54] The sequence homology between the protein from these three species and human transferrin is 70, 51, and 46%, respectively.

3. Secondary Structure

In the absence of the data that would have been provided by high-resolution X-ray diffraction studies, it has only been possible to predict the secondary structure of human transferrin from more indirect methods of analysis. Optical rotatory dispersion and circular dichroism studies have indicated that the molecule has a low α-helix content and a substantial β-pleated sheet

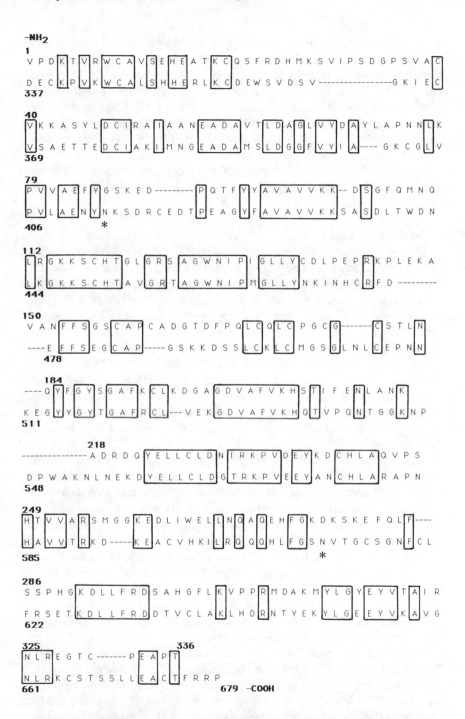

FIGURE 5. The primary sequence of human serum transferrin. The upper sequence corresponds to the N-terminal domain (1–336), and the lower sequence to the C-terminal domain (337–679). The boxed segments indicate the regions of sequence homology between the two domains. The asterisks (*) show the positions of attachment of the two glycan chains at asparagine residues 413 and 611. The one-letter amino acid abbreviations are as follows: A, alanine; C, cysteine; D, aspartic acid; E, glutamic acid; F, phenylalanine; G, glycine; H, histidine; I, isoleucine; K, lysine; L, leucine; M, methionine; N, asparagine; P, proline; Q, glutamine; R, arginine; S, serine; T, threonine; V, valine; W, tryptophan; and Y, tyrosine.

component. In a study carried out in 1976 by Mazurier et al.,[55] the distribution of secondary structure within the polypeptide chain of iron-free human transferrin was suggested as being 17% α-helix, 68% β-sheet, and 15% random coil. In addition, it was found that the secondary structure did not change significantly upon the binding of iron. Predictions of secondary structure by computer analysis of the amino acid sequence also suggested a low (17%) content of α-helix.[46] However, this same procedure predicted a very low (10%) β-structure content, with the majority of the molecule being composed of a random coil. Clearly, the details of the secondary structure of human transferrin will only finally be resolved when suitable X-ray diffraction data becomes available.

4. Tertiary Structure

Human transferrin has yet to be subjected to the high-resolution X-ray diffraction analysis that is necessary to provide detailed information on the secondary and tertiary structure and the topographical folding of the polypeptide chain. Although the analytical techniques are available, the problem is one of producing stable crystals with appropriate heavy atom replacements. Fortunately, this situation does not apply for two closely related siderophilins — human lactoferrin and rabbit transferrin. X-ray crystallographic stuctures of both human lactoferrin and rabbit transferrin have been determined to a resolution of 3.3 Å,[56,57] and the three-dimensional structures of these two proteins have been shown to be remarkably similar. Since human serum transferrin shares both functional and sequence homology with these two closely related siderophilins, it is unlikely to differ significantly in terms of its tertiary structure.

In the period between 1970 and 1978, preliminary crystallographic data were reported on four siderophilins — pig transferrin,[58] rabbit transferrin,[59] human lactoferrin,[60] and human transferrin.[61] In each case, crystals were grown and subjected to X-ray diffraction analysis at a resolution of 6 Å. Attempts to produce heavy atom replacement derivatives were unsuccessful, and as a result the diffraction patterns could only be interpreted in terms of the crystal space groups and unit cell dimensions. In 1979, Gorinsky et al.[62] reported for the first time X-ray analysis results on rabbit transferrin for which heavy atom derivatives had been produced, using mercury, platinum, and uranium.[62] A 6-Å resolution electron density map was calculated, and from these results a crude model of the protein was constructed. This model clearly showed that transferrin, the iron-transport protein, consisted of two lobes of approximately equal size. Each lobe was seen to exhibit a pronounced cleft. Since it had already been established that transferrin was a single polypeptide chain,[31] and therefore had no quaternary structure, the two lobes must have been formed by folding at each end of the protein and remain connected by a central part of the polypeptide chain. Gorinsky et al. suggested that the two lobes might correspond to the two domains of the transferrin molecule, each containing an iron-binding site, possibly within the cleft in each lobe.

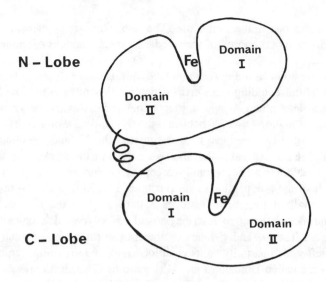

FIGURE 6. A diagrammatic representation of the structure of human transferrin, showing the two lobes and the two domains within each lobe (separated by the iron-binding site).

However, since the maximum resolution of these studies was at the 6-Å level, it was not possible to identify the iron-binding sites or the arrangement of amino acids within the polypeptide chain.

A further 8 years elapsed before, in 1987, the diffraction pattern of a member of the siderophilin family was determined at a sufficiently high level of resolution (3.2 Å) such as to divulge not only the topography of the polypeptide chain folding, but also the nature and location of the iron-binding sites. The molecule in question was human lactoferrin,[56] for which the amino acid sequence had already been determined.[50]

A year later, Bailey et al.[57] reported the first X-ray analysis of a transferrin at a resolution of 3.3 Å. This was for the diferric serum transferrin from the rabbit. The structure was solved using a combination of multiple isomorphous replacement (mercury, gold, and uranium) and solvent-flattening techniques. The interpretation of the electron density maps of rabbit transferrin by Bailey's group was greatly assisted by access to the data of Anderson et al.[56] on human lactoferrin prior to its publication. Nevertheless, one major problem remained. Only a fragment of the primary structure of rabbit transferrin was known at the time, so in order to build a molecular structure for the molecule from the electron density maps, Bailey et al.[57] used the established amino acid sequence for human transferrin. The overall organisation of the molecule is shown diagrammatically in Figure 6. The polypeptide chain is folded into two globular lobes joined by a short connecting sequence of amino acids. The N-lobe, comprising the N-terminal half of the protein, contains the first 330 amino acid residues, and the C-lobe, comprising the C-terminal half of the molecule contains the last 330 residues. Each lobe is a prolate ellipsoid (21 × 25 × 35 Å) and contains one iron-binding site. The two lobes are connected by a short, three-turn helix composed of the middle 15 to 20 residues of the polypeptide chain.

At this point in the description, mention should be made of a change in nomenclature regarding transferrin structure. When the amino acid sequence had been determined, it was apparent that there was extensive amino acid sequence homology (42%) between the N- and C-terminal halves of the protein. These two regions were designated the N- and C-domains. X-ray analysis has now revealed that the two halves of the protein are folded into two distinct lobes. The currently accepted nomenclature is to describe the first half of the polypeptide chain (residues 1 to 330) as the N-lobe, and the terminal half of the chain (residues 350 to 679) as the C-lobe. The term domain is now reserved to describe parts of the polypeptide architecture within each lobe. The N- and C-lobes of the transferrin molecule each contain a deep cleft which partially splits each lobe into two dissimilar regions. These regions are called Domains I and II (Figure 6). The cleft between these two domains contains the amino acid residues whose side chains comprise the iron-binding sites within each lobe.

The N- and C-lobes of transferrin have very similar tertiary structures, a fact that supports the suggestion that the transferrin gene of higher organisms has arisen from the duplication of an ancestral gene that coded for a one-iron-binding protein with a molecular weight of about 40,000. The folding patterns of the polypeptide chain within the N- and C-lobes can be super-imposed by a rotation of 167° and a translation of 23 Å. Both lobes, and indeed both domains within each lobe, consist of a mixture of sections of right-handed β-sheet connected by lengths of α-helix and nonhelical loops and bends. Figure 7 is a schematic drawing of the secondary structural elements within the N-lobe of transferrin.

Domain I is composed of two separate regions of the primary structure, residues 1 to 96 and residues 246 to 330, whereas Domain II comprises a continuous sequence of the primary structure from residues 97 to 245. The polypeptide chain in the N-lobe starts in Domain I with four segments of parrallel β-sheet (a, b, c, and d), each pointing towards Domain II and connected by three helices. The chain then crosses and enters Domain II at residue 97 as a long segment of β-sheet (e). It continues within this domain as four further sections of β-sheet (f, g, h, and i), each orientated towards Domain I and connected by helices. At residue 246 the chain leaves Domain II and reenters Domain I, where it forms two further segments of β-sheet (j and k), both of which run antiparallel to the β-sheets a, b, c, and d. The polypeptide chain in Domain II finishes with two helical sections, after which it leaves the N-lobe in order to enter the C-lobe via a short connecting helical peptide (residues 331 to 349).

The topography of the polypeptide chain of transferrin is very similar to that described by Anderson et al.[56] for the molecule of human lactoferrin. In addition, Anderson et al. also noted that there was an unexpected similarity

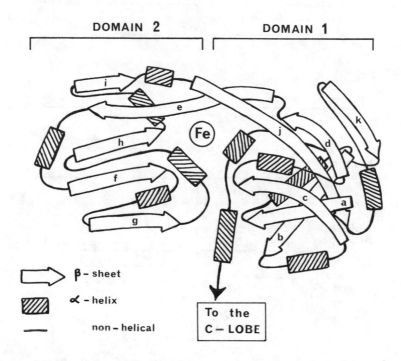

FIGURE 7. Secondary structures within the N-lobe of transferrin.

between the tertiary structure of lactoferrin and that of a number of other binding proteins functionally unrelated to any of the siderophilins. The most striking example is the case of the sulphate-binding protein of *Salmonella typhimurium*,[63] which has precisely the same sheet topography as lactoferrin, with many additional matching features in the helical regions.

5. Disulphide Bridges

The 38 cysteine residues of human transferrin are all involved in the formation of disulphide bridges, giving a total of 19 sulphur bridges which contribute significantly to the maintenance of the tertiary structure of this bilobar protein. The distribution of the disulphide bridges is shown in Figure 8. Whilst some of the bridges in both the N- and the C-lobes covalently cross link between residues in Domains I and II, there are no sulphur bridges connecting the two lobes. This fact may explain why it has been possible to split some of the transferrins into two separate 40,000-M.W. fragments by proteolytic enzymes without the need to reduce the disulphide bridges.

The position of the bridges is known, not only for transferrin, but also for two closely related siderophilins — lactoferrin and ovotransferrin. What is quite apparent is that their distribution in these three molecules is not

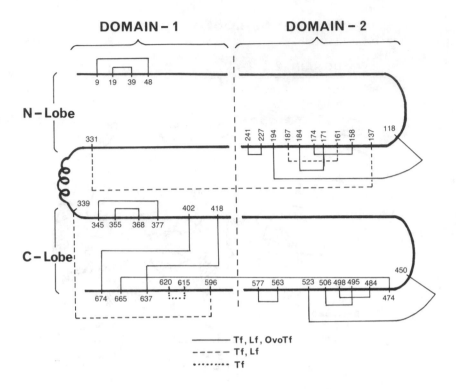

FIGURE 8. A diagram showing the positions of the sulphur bridges within transferrin, lactoferrin, and ovotransferrin.

random. In transferrin, 15 of the disulphide bridges (6 in the N-lobe and 9 in the C-lobe) are found in homologous positions in both lactoferrin and ovotransferrin. One further bridge is found only in transferrin and lactoferrin, whilst the remaining three are unique to transferrin. Williams[47] has suggested that this conservative distribution of disulphide bridges strongly supports the argument that siderophilins are the product of a gene duplication. The three conserved bridges of the C-lobe that do not have counterparts in the N-lobe are thought therefore to have evolved after the gene-duplication event. This implies that the ancestral gene, prior to its duplication to give rise to the precursor from which all present-day transferrins have evolved, coded for a 40,000-M.W. protein analogous to the N-lobe of transferrin.

6. Glycan Chains

Human transferrin is a glycoprotein with two N-linked oligosaccharide chains attached to asparagine residues 413 and 611 in the C-lobe. The structure of these glycan chains can exhibit a wide range of variability. This phenomenon has been called microheterogeneity and is a logical consequence of the mechanism of protein glycosylation in eukaryote cells. The synthesis of glycoprotein glycan chains is neither the result of a random assembly of sugar units, nor is it a precise, template-directed mechanism like protein synthesis. The synthesis of N-linked oligosaccharide chains is a sequential process of enzyme-catalysed addition and loss of sugar residues as the protein passes through the rough endoplasmic reticulum and Golgi system, *en route* to its final destination.[64] A range of highly specific enzymes are involved, including glycosyl transferases that add sugar residues, and glycosidases that remove them. The compartmentalisation of these enzymes and their substrates throughout the rough endoplasmic reticulum and Golgi region can profoundly affect the glycan structure of the end product. The microheterogeneity of transferrin is compounded by the fact that the glycoprotein is internalised by iron-requiring cells before it is recycled back to the plasma to pick up more iron. During the intracellular iron cycle, the glycan chains are subject to degradation and structural modification.

Transferrin invariably carries two "complex-type" glycan chains, and much of the microheterogeneity exhibited by transferrin isolated from fresh human plasma is due to differences in the degree of branching of the glycans and to the nature of the sugar residue at the outermost end of the branches.[65] The most frequently encountered structure is a biantennary chain with a residue of sialic acid at the end of each of the two branches. However, tri- and tetraantennary structures have been shown to exist, and in addition the negatively charged sialic acid residues can be missing from the ends of the branches. The stuctures of the glycan chains most commonly found attached to human transferrin have been described in Chapter 3 (see Figure 2 in that chapter). Chapter 3 also includes a brief description of the glycan chains of the two related siderophilins, lactoferrin and ovotransferrin.

As many as nine different isotransferrins, resulting from variable sialic acid content, have been identified in human plasma. The significance of this microheterogeneity in respect to differential transferrin uptake by tissues will be considered in Chapter 6. In addition, it has been known for a number of years that the proportions of the nine isotransferrins in human plasma can be significantly altered in a number of situations, including pregnancy and alcoholism. These aspects will be discussed further in Chapter 10.

D. IRON BINDING
1. Absorption Spectrum

Apotransferrin is a colourless protein. In the ultraviolet region of the spectrum, the molecule has an intense absorption peak at 280 nm (Figure 9), a characteristic of most proteins and due to the presence of the aromatic amino acids tryptophan, tyrosine, and, to a lesser extent, phenylalanine. When tyrosine looses the phenolic proton, the absorption at 295 and 245 nm increases dramatically. This change in the ultraviolet region of the spectrum is also seen when apotransferrin binds iron (Figure 9), and has been taken to indicate

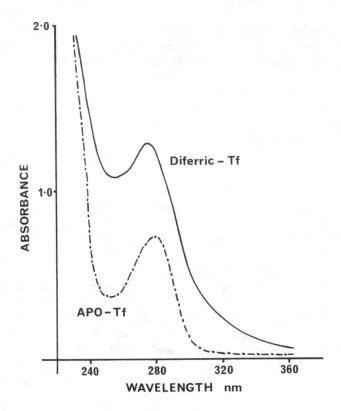

FIGURE 9. The ultraviolet spectrum of human apotransferrin and diferric transferrin. Both solutions are at a concentration of 1 mg/mL.

the involvement of one or more tyrosine residues in the process of iron binding by transferrin.

Diferric transferrin has as very distinctive salmon-pink colour. This property not only contributed to the original discovery of the siderophilins, but it also allows the presence of transferrin to be easily detected in chromatographic fractions during the course of the purification of the protein. In the visible region of the spectrum the absorption maximum of diferric transferrin is between 465 and 470 nm (Figure 10). An absorbance ratio (280/470) of 22.5 is indicative of pure human diferric transferrin.

2. Anion Requirements

In 1949, Schade et al.[66] demonstrated that CO_2 was required for the development of the characteristic salmon-pink colour of the iron-transferrin complex. Since the enzyme carbonic anhydrase was later shown to accelerate this process, it was concluded that bicarbonate (HCO_3^-), rather than carbon dioxide, was involved in the process of iron binding by transferrin. The cooperativity between Fe^{3+} and bicarbonate binding is very strong and is one

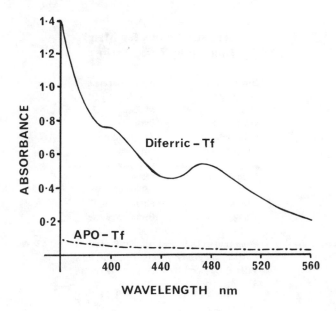

FIGURE 10. Part of the visible spectrum of human apotransferrin and diferric transferrin. Both solutions are at a concentration of 10 mg/mL.

of the most striking examples of site-site interaction in biochemistry. Despite the tightness of the iron-protein "bond" under normal physiological conditions, binding of iron at the two specific iron sites on the transferrin molecule does not occur unless the anion-binding requirements have been satisfied. The involvement of bicarbonate in the process of iron binding by transferrin was confirmed by Van Snick et al.,[67] who demonstrated that transferrin coupled to Sepharose was able to bind iron ($^{59}Fe^{3+}$) only after the addition of bicarbonate, indicating that the bicarbonate anion does not merely cause the formation of the pink colour of the iron-transferrin complex but is essential for the formation of the complex. However, these experiments and many that followed were unable to distinguish between the following two possibilities. Under physiological conditions, is the true synergistic anion bicarbonate (HCO_3^-) or carbonate (CO_3^{2-})? Despite extensive studies, this question remains unanswered.

The binding of a ferric ion (Fe^{3+}) to each of the two iron-binding sites of transferrin is associated with the release of three protons and an increase in the negative charge of the protein:

$$Fe^{3+} + ApoTf^Z + HCO_3^- \rightarrow [Fe^{3+}\text{--}Tf\text{--}bicarbonate]^{Z-1} + 3H^+$$

From proton-titration experiments it has been concluded that if the bound anion is carbonate rather than bicarbonate, then the extra proton released must remain bound to transferrin, since the three protons that are released are all

TABLE 3
Synergistic Anions for Metal
Binding by Transferrin

Bicarbonate	Nitrilotriacetate
Oxalate	EDTA
Malonate	Maleate
Glyoxalate	Pyruvate
α-Ketoglutarate	Ketomalonate
Acetoacetate	Glycolate
Lactate	Phenyllactate
Phenyllactate	Malate
Gluconate	Salicylate
Glycine	Phenylalanine
Thioglycolate	Bromopyruvate

From Harris, D. C. and Ainsen, P., in *Iron Carriers and Iron Proteins*, T. Loehr, Ed., VCH Publishers, New York, 1989, chap. 3. With permission.

derived from the side groups of the amino acid residues of transferrin, and not from the anion.

In fully iron-saturated transferrin, two molecules of bicarbonate (or carbonate) are bound per molecule of protein, one for each of the two iron atoms. When a solution of diferric transferrin labelled with $H^{14}CO_3^-$ is in contact with the air, the bound HCO_3^- slowly exchanges first with the HCO_3^- in the solvent, and then with atmospheric CO_2. At physiological pH and ambient CO_2 pressure, the half-life for this exchange is about 20 days, indicating that HCO_3^- is firmly bound in the iron-transferrin-anion complex. The process of bicarbonate exchange can, however, be accelerated by the presence of a variety of alternative anions.[68] This observation led to the discovery that whilst bicarbonate (or carbonate) acts as the true physiological anion, a range of other carboxylate anions can fulfill this function under appropriate experimental conditions.

The common feature of all the synergistic anions was first described by Schlabach and Bates,[69] who noted that each anion (some examples of which are listed in Table 3) contains an electron-withdrawing Lewis base near to the carboxylate group (Figure 11). Whilst it is unlikely that any of these synergistic anions, other than of course bicarbonate, has a true physiological role, an examination of the size and shape of these molecules has allowed certain predictions to be made regarding the geometry of the iron-binding site of transferrin. It has been proposed that the role of the anion is to form a bridge between the protein and the metal ion (Figure 12). In this simple model, the Lewis base is attached to one of the six coordination sites on the ferric ion, whilst the carboxylate group forms a salt bridge with the protein, possibly via a specific arginine amino acid residue. A more detailed discussion of the specific iron- and anion-binding sites of transferrin will be considered

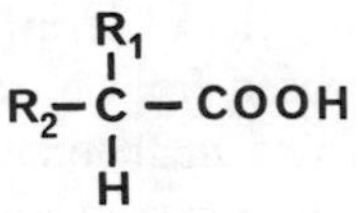

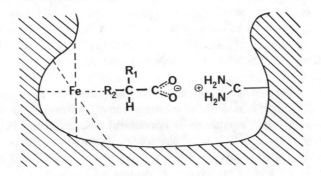

FIGURE 11. The basic structure of the synergistic anion.

FIGURE 12. The role of the synergistic anion in stabilising the metal complex in transferrin.

in Section D.7 in this chapter. What is clear from the list of synergistic anions in Table 3 is that one side of the iron-binding site must be open and spacious in order to accommodate molecules with large R_1 side groups, such as Xylenol Orange (M.W. 500). On the other hand, the space available for the R_2 group must be very small, since, whilst lactate is a synergistic anion, methyl lactate is not.[70]

Despite some early reports to the contrary, it is now generally accepted that in the absence of synergistic anions the affinity of the **specific** metal-binding sites of transferrin for Fe^{3+} is so low as to not compete favourably with either hydrolytic polymerisation of the ferric ion, or **nonspecific** binding effects. It is very likely that in many of these early reports claiming to show iron binding in the absence of bicarbonate, the transferrin preparations were never entirely bicarbonate free. It is technically very difficult to totally exclude bicarbonate from the system. On the other hand, the ability of transferrin to bind some metals other than iron (see Chapter 5) is not entirely abolished in the absence of bicarbonate. At high pH, and in the absence of bicarbonate, human transferrin is capable of binding a single copper ion (Cu^{2+}) at one of the two iron-binding sites. This may reflect the greater resistance of Cu^{2+} than Fe^{3+} to hydrolysis.[70]

3. The Reaction of Transferrin with Iron Salts and a Variety of Iron Chelates

The form or forms in which iron is presented to apotransferrin *in vivo* is as yet unknown. The major sources of the iron atoms that eventually become attached to the two iron-binding sites of serum transferrin are the intracellular stores of ferritin, the iron released from haemoglobin breakdown, and to a much lesser extent the haem and nonhaem iron from the diet. The major biological role of transferrin is to transport iron between tissues in a nontoxic and soluble form, since free iron becomes rapidly oxidised, hydrolysed, and polymerised into insoluble polynuclear complexes. Therefore, iron released from the ferritin stores or haemoglobin breakdown needs to be kept in a soluble form as it passes through the cytoplasm of the cell on its way to the plasma membrane to be eventually bound to transferrin. It is assumed that small-molecular-weight intracellular iron chelators are involved in this phase of iron transport. The identity of these physiological chelators remains to be determined.

From *in vitro* studies it appears that both ferrous (Fe^{2+}) and ferric (Fe^{3+}) iron can each serve as a source of transferrin iron. However, since the former is likely to be rapidly oxidised, it is doubtful whether or not Fe^{2+} is ever bound to transferrin under normal physiological conditions. Attempts to measure the binding constants for Fe^{2+} by direct means have always been hampered by the difficulties involved in preventing the oxidation of Fe^{2+} to Fe^{3+}. An indirect approach has been to extrapolate from the results obtained using an alternative divalent metal, namely zinc (Zn^{2+}). Using this approach, Harris[71] has estimated that the two thermodynamic binding constants for Fe^{2+} would be $8 \times 10^6 \ M^{-1}$ (K_1) and $3 \times 10^5 \ M^{-1}$ (K_2). These values indicate that the binding of Fe^{2+} by apotransferrin, even if it were able to occur physiologically, would be very weak when compared with Fe^{3+} where the binding constants are very much higher, at values of $7 \times 10^{22} \ M^{-1}$ (K_1) and $3 \times 10^{21} \ M^{-1}$ (K_2).[70]

A study of the reaction between apotransferrin and Fe^{3+}, in the presence of the synergistic anion bicarbonate, is central to an understanding of how transferrin functions within the body. It is relatively easy to purify human transferrin, to convert the protein to apotransferrin by removing any bound iron by reducing the pH to below 4.5, and then to follow the subsequent binding of added iron by monitoring the increase in absorbance at 470 nm. The most difficult problem is to decide in which soluble form to offer the ferric iron to the apotransferrin molecule in order to study the mechanism of iron binding. Over the last 25 years, extensive studies have been carried out in order to more fully understand how transferrin functions as an iron-transport protein. Many questions have been asked and these have included:

1. How many atoms of iron are bound by transferrin?
2. What is the structure and chemistry of the iron-binding site(s)?
3. Are the two iron-binding sites independent of each other?
4. Are the two iron-binding sites functionally different?
5. What are the values of the iron-binding constants?
6. How is iron distributed between the two sites when, under normal circumstances, human plasma transferrin is only 30% iron-saturated? Is the site selection random or nonrandom?

7. What physiological factors affect the binding of Fe^{3+} at the two separate iron-binding sites?
8. How stable is the iron bound at the two sites, and what factors promote iron release?

These questions and many others have been the subject of a number of excellent reviews,[70,72-74] and only a brief summary will be presented in this chapter.

Schade et al.[66] had reported as early as 1949 that the protein transferrin bound two iron atoms per molecule. By 1973 it had become apparent that the reaction between apotransferrin and simple iron salts such as ferric chloride was difficult to control primarily to the rapid hydrolysis and subsequent polymerisation of the ferric ion.[13] Titration of apotransferrin with neutral solutions of ferric chloride resulted in a sigmoid-shaped curve with no clear end point. Far more reliable results were obtained when the iron was presented to apotransferrin in the form of soluble ferric chelates.[75,76] The chelates used in these and subsequent studies included citrate, EDTA, ascorbate, and nitrilotriacetic acid (NTA). The rate at which iron is donated to apotransferrin is highly dependent upon the nature of the particular chelate. For example, it was shown that 100% saturation of apotransferrin with iron donated by ferric EDTA required at least 6 days and ferric citrate 20 hours, but when using ferric nitrilotriacetic acid (FENTA) the reaction was completed in less than 10 s.[13,75,76]

The reaction of apotransferrin with neutral solutions of FENTA has now been well characterised. In the presence of bicarbonate the time course of the reaction is biphasic. The first phase of the reaction is complete within a few tenths of a second and results in the formation of a Fe^{3+}–NTA–Tf complex. The second phase of the reaction (10 s) follows first-order kinetics and results in the formation of a new stable complex of Fe^{3+}–bicarbonate–Tf. By following the reaction of apotransferrin at 470 nm with increasing additions of FENTA, a clear end point is reached when one molecule of transferrin has bound two atoms of iron. Solutions of FENTA provide stable monomeric ferric chelates and have been used in many subsequent studies of iron binding by transferrin. Clearly, the results obtained from these experiments have to be treated with some degree of caution since NTA is not a normal physiological component of the body and cannot be the true biological iron chelator. It is simply a very convenient, stable, and rapid iron donor for *in vitro* studies.

Transferrin can bind a maximum of two atoms of iron, and therefore has within its structure two specific iron-binding sites. Within the bilobar architecture of the protein, these two sites have been located, one in each lobe. The generally accepted nomenclature for these two sites is to refer to the site within the N-lobe (residues 1 to 330) as the N-site, and the site within the C-lobe (residues 350 to 679) as the C-site. In many early reports in the literature, these two sites have been referred to as the B-site and A-site, respectively. Alternative labels that have been given to the two sites, and that still appear occasionally in the scientific literature, are given below:

N-site	C-site
Site-B	Site-A
Acid-labile site	Acid-stable site
Fe_N–transferrin	Fe_C–transferrin
Fe–transferrin	Transferrin–Fe

4. Apotransferrin and the Three Iron-Transferrin Complexes

The discovery that transferrin binds two atoms of iron at separate and specific sites posed the obvious question, "Why does the molecule have two metal-binding sites?" The simplest answer to this question, as suggested by Williams et al.,[32] is that the modern transferrin molecule (M.W. 80,000) is a protein that has doubled its size by an event of gene duplication from an ancestral monosited iron-binding protein (M.W. 40,000). The evolutionary significance of this occurrence has resulted in an iron-transport protein that is capable of delivering iron to the tissues via the blood plasma, whilst at the same time being of a sufficient size to prevent the protein, and more importantly its bound iron, from being filtered and subsequently lost from the body via the kidneys.

An alternative answer to the same question is that the existence of a two-sited iron carrier implies that there must be an important biological role for such a structure, one that could not be carried out by a monosited iron-transport protein. Over the last 30 years, a considerable amount of effort has been expended in attempting to distinguish between the two iron-binding sites, both at the physicochemical and the functional levels. The scientific literature abounds with reports of differences between the two iron-binding sites with respect to a whole range of characteristics, including binding constants, the effect of pH on iron binding and release, the effect of ATP and 2,3-diphosphoglycerate on iron release, the conformational stability of the sites in the presence of denaturing agents such as urea, and the nonrandom distribution of iron between the two sites. Resulting from these observations, there have been a number of suggestions as to the possible (and different) biological roles of the N- and C-sites. Without doubt the most famous hypothesis is the one suggested by Fletcher and Heuhns in the late 1960s.[77,78] This model proposed that the two sites were functionally distinct, such that one site preferentially directed its iron to immature red cells (reticulocytes) for the purpose of haemoglobin synthesis, whilst the other site directed its iron atom to liver cells for the purpose of storage. Attempts to validate or disprove the Fletcher-Heuhns hypothesis have led to an abundance of contradictory reports in the literature over the last 25 years.

The question of site equivalence vs. nonequivalence still remains unresolved, certainly at the functional level. In terms of *in vitro* studies, there is no doubt that the two iron-binding sites have many different properties and physical characteristics. Indeed, Chasteen[74] has argued that it would be very unusual if this were not the case. Even for a hypothetical transferrin with perfect homology of amino acid sequence between the two halves of the molecule, site inequivalence would exist, since for a duplicated molecule, joined head to tail, the structure would lack elements of symmetry relating one site to the other. Thus, in principle, the two halves of such a hypothetical protein could still contain functionally different iron-binding sites. Chasteen has further reasoned that since in the real transferrin molecule the two halves of the protein share only 40% sequence homology, this implies that at the remaining 60% of the positions, a different amino acid side chain is present in the two halves. Even assuming that the relatively few amino acid side chains that are the probable ligands involved in iron binding have remained the same at the two sites, the molecular environments in which the sites are situated in the two halves of the protein are likely to be significantly different. As a result, one might have already anticipated that differences between the two sites should be evident. This is now supported by a wealth of experimental evidence that has been summarised in a number of review articles.[28,70,73,74,80] Whether or not the various physicochemical differences between the two iron-binding sites of human transferrin are of any biological significance in the *in vivo* situation remains to be established. Whilst the balance of evidence available at the present time suggests that they are not, the question still remains unresolved. Consequently, this is still an area of active research.

The fact that transferrin has two separate iron-binding sites implies that under conditions of differing iron saturation, the protein could exist in four distinct molecular forms:

1. Apotransferrin — no iron bound .... **Tf**
2. Monoferric transferrin with one iron
    bound at the N-site .... **Fe–Tf**
3. Monoferric transferrin with one iron
    bound to the C-site .... **Tf–Fe**
4. Diferric transferrin with two atoms
    of iron bound............................... **Fe$_2$–Tf**

As a consequence, a molecule of transferrin would have four separate intrinsic site-binding constants (k) as shown by the following scheme:

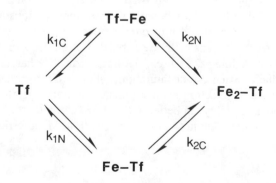

Here, k_{1C} is the constant for the binding of iron to the C-site when the N-site is empty; k_{1N} is the constant for the binding of iron to the N-site when the C-site is empty; k_{2C} is the constant for the binding of iron to the C-site when the N-site is already occupied by an atom of iron; and k_{2N} is the constant for the binding of iron to the N-site when the C-site is already occupied by an atom of iron.

In the first quantitative study of the binding of iron to a transferrin (ovotransferrin), Warner and Weber[81] in 1953 attempted to measure the thermodynamic binding constants K_1 (binding of one iron) and K_2 (binding of the second iron). From their results they concluded that the binding of the second iron was much more favourable than the binding of the first iron. In other words, iron binding was nonequivalent and cooperative. Using more refined techniques of equilibrium dialysis, these results were challenged 10 years later by Aasa et al.,[82] who discovered that iron binding to the two sites was equivalent, at least within a factor of 10. The implication of this finding, namely that the binding of iron to each of the two sites was similar, was that transferrin should exist in four possible molecular forms; apotransferrin, two different monoferric structures, and diferric transferrin. Results obtained by the equilibrium dialysis technique cannot by themselves provide more than the overall thermodynamic binding constants K_1 and K_2.[83] The relationship between these values and the four intrinsic site constants is as follows:

$$K_1 = k_{1a} + k_{1b}$$

$$K_2^{-1} = k_{2a}^{-1} + k_{2b}^{-1}$$

Much of the early work attempting to address the question of equivalence or nonequivalence of the two iron-binding sites of transferrin was hampered by an inability to measure the iron occupancy of the two sites separately. What was required was a method that could separate and quantify the four different molecular forms of transferrin generated under equilibrium conditions of differing iron saturation. Such a technique was reported for the first time in 1976 by Makey and Seal[84] and was to act as the catalyst for many of the subsequent comparative studies of the two iron-binding sites that will be discussed later in this chapter. The principle of the Makey and Seal method is based upon the fact that the binding of iron to transferrin protects the protein against unfolding (denaturation) by 6 M urea, and secondly, the binding of each atom of iron (with bicarbonate) releases three protons and increases the net negative charge of the molecule by one. When a mixture of the four molecular forms of transferrin are subjected to electrophoresis in polyacrylamide gels containing 6 M urea, apotransferrin (Tf) has the lowest anodal mobility due to extensive denaturation, whereas diferric transferrin (Fe$_2$–Tf) has the greatest protection against denaturation and therefore possesses the highest anodal mobility. In between these two extremes the monoferric transferrins will migrate, but not to the same position. Monoferric transferrin with

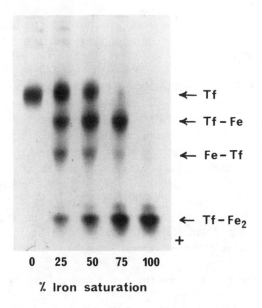

FIGURE 13. Polyacrylamide urea-gel electrophoresis of human transferrin at varying degrees of iron saturation, using the method of Makey and Seal.

iron at the C-site (Tf–Fe) migrates more slowly towards the anode than does the monoferric species with iron at the N-site (Fe–Tf). The cause of this differential mobility of the two monoferric transferrins is thought to reflect, at least in part, the relative ease with which the unprotected lobe (no iron bound) unfolds in the presence of urea.[85] The C-lobe of human transferrin with 11 disulphide bridges is more resistant to urea denaturation than the N-lobe, which has only 8 disulphide bridges.

The separation of the four molecular species of human transferrin by the urea-polyacrylamide gel of Makey and Seal can be seen clearly in Figure 13.

Although electrophoresis in the presence of 6 M urea is the method most commonly employed to separate the four forms of transferrin, anion-exchange chromatography[86] and isoelectric focussing[87] are alternative techniques capable of distinguishing between the monoferric transferrins Fe–Tf and Tf–Fe.

5. Iron-Binding Sites — Similarities and Differences

The first clear evidence of physicochemical differences between the two iron-binding sites of transferrin came in 1975 with the demonstration of the effects of pH on iron binding and release by Princiotto and Zapolski[88] and by Lestas.[89] Both groups described how, as the pH of a diferric solution of transferrin was lowered, iron was released in two steps. This implied that one of the two sites was acid labile (this was subsequently shown to be the N-site), whereas the other site (C-site) was relatively acid stable. Fully saturated diferric transferrin looses 50% of its bound iron when the pH is reduced to 5.7. The residual 50% remains firmly attached to the transferrin molecule, and it requires a further reduction of pH to below 5.0 before this iron begins to dissociate from the protein. Conversely, the effect of pH on the binding of iron by apotransferrin is selective. Princiotto and Zapolski[88] labelled transferrin at pH 5.0 with ^{56}Fe, then raised the pH to 7.4 and saturated the transferrin with ^{59}Fe. When the pH was subsequently lowered, the isotope bound at high pH (^{59}Fe) dissociated preferentially. The isotope bound at low pH (^{56}Fe) remained attached until the pH was reduced to below 5.5. The selective labelling of the two iron-binding sites of transferrin provided a very important tool for subsequent biological studies. In addition, the differential effect of pH on the two iron-binding sites finally laid to rest the previously accepted view that the two sites were equivalent and independent.

The inequivalence of the two iron-binding sites of human transferrin has now been demonstrated with respect to a range of different physicochemical parameters. A brief selection is given in Table 4 .

6. Distribution of Iron between the Two Binding Sites *In Vitro* and *In Vivo*

Differences between the two iron-binding sites of human transferrin have been revealed by a variey of thermodynamic, kinetic, and spectroscopic techniques (Table 4). For example, the intrinsic site constants alone suggest that the C-site (k_{1c} 6 × 10^{22} M^{-1}) should preferentially bind iron in comparison to the N-site (k_{1n} 1 × 10^{22} M^{-1}). Binding to the C-site is also favoured at low pH or when the iron is donated by $Fe^{3+}-NTA$. On the other hand, preferential binding to the N-site occurs at higher pH or when the iron donor is ferric chloride or citrate. In addition, binding to the N-site is strongly favoured in the presence of sodium chloride. All of these results have been obtained from *in vitro* studies, making it very difficult to predict how the balance of these contrasting properties is likely to affect the iron occupancy of the two sites in the *in vivo* situation, where the saturation of transferrin in normal plasma rarely exceeds 35%.

In the *in vivo* situation, are the two sites equivalent, noncooperative and therefore randomly occupied by iron, or are they nonequivalent, possibly cooperative with differential iron occupancy? This question has been an area of controversy for many years and is still not fully resolved. Once it became possible to separate and quantify the four molecular forms of transferrin (Tf, Fe–Tf, Tf–Fe, and Fe_2–Tf) by urea/polyacrylamide gel electrophoresis[84] or by isoelectric focussing,[87] the question of random vs. nonrandom occupancy of the two sites could be addressed.

In vitro studies, in which samples of pure transferrin at different iron saturations were separated and quantified, clearly demonstrated that pH significantly influenced the equilibrium distribution of iron between the two binding sites.[102] From these results it was possible to calculate the ratio of the four intrinsic site constants at different levels of iron saturation. There was found to be a very close agreement between the molar ratios of the four

TABLE 4
Physicochemical Properties that Distinguish between the Two Metal-Binding Sites of Human Transferrin

Property	N-Site		C-Site		Ref.
Intrinsic site constants for Fe^{3+} M^{-1}.	k_{1N}	k_{2N}	k_{1C}	k_{2C}	28, 90
pH 6.7	1.4×10^{18}	2.4×10^{18}	2.9×10^{19}	4.8×10^{18}	
pH 7.4	6.8×10^{19}	2.8×10^{19}	4.0×10^{20}	1.6×10^{20}	
Plasma pH and $[HCO_3^-]$	1.0×10^{22}	4.2×10^{22}	6.0×10^{22}	2.4×10^{22}	
Effect of pH on iron binding	Acid-labile site pH 6.0		Acid-stable site pH 5.0		88, 89
Transferrin loading by different iron donors					
Fe^{3+}–NTA pH 7–8.5			Preferred site		22
Fe^{3+}–NTA pH 10	Preferred site				91
Fe^{3+}–citrate pH 7–8.5 oxalate					
chloride	Preferred site				22
Fe^{2+}–NH_4SO_4 ascorbate					
Fe^{3+} N(2-hydroxy-ethyl)imino diacetic acid			Preferred site		92
Effect of chloride on iron loading	NaCl increases the affinity of iron for the N-site; the effect is augmented by increased pH				93, 94
Effect of chloride on the rate or iron release	Rate of iron release reduced		Rate of iron release increased		95, 96
Effect of increasing urea concentrations on stability	Urea labile denatured at 4 M		Urea stable denatured at 4.5 M		85
Binding of Cu^{2+}					
Below pH 6	No		No		97, 98
pH 6.5	No		Yes		
pH 7.2	Yes		Yes		
Above pH 9.5	No		No		
Binding of Cu^{2+} in the absence of bicarbonate	Yes		No		99

TABLE 4 (continued)
Physicochemical Properties that Distinguish between the Two
Metal-Binding Sites of Human Transferrin

Property	N-Site	C-Site	Ref.
Binding of vanadate ion VO^{2+}			
pH 6	No	Yes	100
Above pH 7	Yes	Yes	
Spectroscopically determined differences between the two sites			
EPR signals from diferric and dichromic transferrins	Site differences		70 (review)
Laser excitation spectra of Eu^{3+} transferrin			
Peak	579.26 nm	579.88 nm	101
Lifetime of excited state	210 μs	310 μs	

molecular species as calculated from the site constants, and the molar ratios as measured by the electrophoretic technique. For example, at 50% iron saturation and at pH 7.4, the proportions were found to be 20% Tf, 18% Fe–Tf, 42% Tf–Fe, and 20% Fe_2–Tf. Apart from showing that under the particular set of *in vitro* conditions used for this experiment, occupancy at the C-site was favoured in the ratio 2:1, the data also demonstrated an important principle, namely that at 50% saturation the proportions of apotransferrin and diferric transferrin are equal. Not only are they equal from the experimental evidence, but they must be so on theoretical grounds, regardless of whether or not the proportions of the two monoferric species are different. It can be demonstrated easily that the proportions of the apotransferrin and diferric transferrin at 50% iron saturation must be equal:

Let the molar fractions of the four species be X_{Tf}, X_{Fe-Tf}, X_{Tf-Fe}, and X_{Fe_2-Tf}. Therefore, the maximum number of atoms of iron that will be bound to each species will be

$$0 \text{ for } X_{Tf}$$
$$1 \text{ for } X_{Fe-Tf}$$
$$1 \text{ for } X_{Tf-Fe}$$
$$2 \text{ for } X_{Fe_2-Tf}$$

$$\% \text{ Saturation} = \frac{\text{the sum of the number of iron atoms bound to each of the 4 species}}{\text{the maximum number of atoms of iron that can be bound}} \times 100$$

$$= \frac{X_{Fe-Tf} + X_{Tf-Fe} + 2X_{Fe_2-Tf}}{2} \times 100$$

Let the percent saturation be equal to **50**:

$$50 = \frac{X_{Fe-Tf} + X_{Tf-Fe} + 2X_{Fe_2-Tf}}{2} \times 100 \qquad (1)$$

Since the sum of the molar ratios equals unity:

$$X_{Tf} + X_{Fe-Tf} + X_{Tf-Fe} + X_{Fe_2-Tf} = 1$$

$$X_{Fe-Tf} + X_{Tf-Fe} = 1 - X_{Tf} - X_{Fe_2-Tf} \qquad (2)$$

By substituting for $(X_{Fe-Tf} + X_{Tf-Fe})$ from Equation 2 in Equation 1, at 50% saturation:

$$50 = \frac{1 - X_{Tf} - X_{Fe_2-Tf} + 2X_{Fe_2-Tf}}{2} \times 100$$

$$1 = 1 - X_{Tf} - X_{Fe_2-Tf} + 2X_{Fe_2-Tf}$$

$$X_{Tf} = X_{Fe_2-TF}$$

At 50% iron saturation, the proportions of apotransferrin (X_{Tf}) and diferric transferrin (X_{Fe_2-Tf}) are equal.

The results obtained by Chasteen and Williams[102] were from *in vitro* studies. What is clearly far more relevant, from a physiological point of view, is the proportion of the four molecular species present in circulating human plasma. This should provide vital information as to whether or not the two binding sites, as judged by the ratio of the two monoferric transferrins, show equal (random) or unequal (nonrandom) iron occupancy, under the conditions of pH and ionic strength that prevail in the *in vivo* situation.

Huebers et al.[103] measured the proportion of the four transferrin species in the plasma from seven healthy subjects. They found that, irrespective of the plasma iron saturation, the proportions of the N- and C-monoferric trans-ferrins were equal. From these results it was argued that since the distribution of iron between the two sites appeared to be random, iron binding *in vivo* was not a selective process.

On the other hand, Williams and Moreton,[93] van Eijk and van Noort,[104] and Zak and Ainsen[105] have all reported a contrary finding. The three groups, who between them analysed a total of 63 plasma samples, demonstrated a preferential occupancy by iron for the weaker binding N-site. The average distribution of the four molecular species in normal human plasma[93] was found to be 39.2% Tf, 22.9% Fe–Tf, 11.2% Tf–Fe, and 26.7% Fe$_2$–Tf, indicating a significant preference for the N-site (N:C = 2:1). Furthermore, it has been found that N-site occupancy is increased in plasma that has been incubated at 37°C, whereas storage of plasma at −15°C or dialysis against buffer at pH 7.4 causes a significant change in the iron distribution, with preferential binding switched to the C-site. Zak and Ainsen[105] commented in their supporting study that since the conditions of sample collection, storage, and analysis might alter the distribution of iron between the two sites, this might explain the conflicting results reported by Huebers et al.[103] In a much earlier report of nonrandom iron distribution in human transferrin, the identification of the preferred site (N or C) was not confirmed.[106]

The balance of evidence from these *in vivo* studies suggests that under the conditions prevailing in human plasma, the distribution of iron between the two binding sites on the transferrin molecule is neither equivalent nor random. This may simply reflect the balance of the opposing characteristics of the two sites that have been found from the many *in vitro* studies (Table 4). It does not necessarily imply that the two sites are functionally different with respect to their iron delivery at the tissue level, or any other property that might support the Fletcher-Heuhns hypothesis.

7. Chemistry of the Iron-Binding Sites

As long ago as the early 1940s it was realised that the iron-binding transferrins were proteins which, unlike the haemoglobins or the cytochromes, did not contain haem iron. This implied that the iron-binding ligands were the side chain residues of amino acids at each of the two sites, with an additional contribution from the synergistic anion-bicarbonate. The identity and location of the iron-binding ligands has been the subject of a considerable research effort during the last 40 years and has been reviewed at each stage in its history.[28,70,72–74,108–112]

The iron-binding sites are situated in equivalent locations within the cleft between the two domains of each of the two lobes of the protein molecule. Each iron atom is deeply buried, 10 Å below the protein surface, and this accounts in part for the great stability of the iron-transferrin complex. The two iron atoms of diferric transferrin have been estimated to be between 28 and 43 Å apart, a distance sufficient to rule out the possibility that the iron centres could interact directly with one another.

The strong preference shown by the sites for highly positive cations implies that the sites themselves must be of an anionic nature. Analysis of the EPR spectra of iron-saturated transferrin reveals that the ferric ion is under the high-spin form with orthorhombic symmetry, suggesting that the iron has six attachment points to the protein. This hexacoordination has been confirmed by extended X-ray absorption fine-structure studies (EXAFS).[113] The search for the six ligands at the iron-binding sites, most of which have always been presumed to be negatively charged at physiological pH, has been carried out using a variety of techniques. These have included chemical-modification studies with group-specific reagents, UV and fluorescence difference spectroscopy, EPR, NMR, EXAFS, and, most recently, high-resolution X-ray diffraction. Many of the early studies, especially those involving chemical or spectrophotometric techniques, only provided evidence of the identity of most of the putative ligands, with very little information as to their locations within the protein. Further evidence of the positions of the ligands within the molecule has come from the comparative studies on the amino acid sequences of different transferrins. This approach has been based on the hypothesis that the amino acid residues involved in iron binding are very likely to be present in conserved positions within the polypeptide chains of different transferrin molecules.

In 1985, and as a result of the evidence available at that time, Montreuil et al.[114] proposed a general model for the iron-binding sites of transferrins. This postulated that iron was bound to two tyrosine residues and two histidine residues, with the fifth coordination site occupied by a molecule of water, and the sixth site by the synergistic bicarbonate ion attached to an arginine residue. At the time, this model seemed to best accommodate the experimental evidence that was available, and it replaced an earlier model suggested 18 years before by Windle et al.[115] involving three tyrosines, two histidines, and bicarbonate.[115]

High-resolution X-ray diffraction pictures of lactoferrin[56] and transferrin[57] became available for the first time 2 years after the publication of Montreuil's model. This breakthrough at last enabled researchers to look in detail at the chemistry and structure of the iron-binding sites. The results supported most of the proposals of Montreuil et al., with one notable exception. Iron coordination to two tyrosines and one histidine was confirmed, but there was no evidence for the direct involvement of a second histidine residue, despite the proximity of a second histidine to the iron atom. Instead, the X-ray data strongly indicated the involvement of the carboxylate group of an aspartic acid residue. This was all the more surprising since none of the chemical or spectroscopic studies of the previous 40 years had indicated a role for aspartic acid in iron binding. Finally, the X-ray pictures confirmed that there was a region of high electron density spanning the two remaining *cis*-octahedral positions of the bound iron atom. This could be attributed to a bicarbonate anion or a molecule of water, or more likely a molecule of each. X-ray studies at a resolution far higher than those currently available (3.2 Å) will be needed to confirm these options. However, the role of bicarbonate (or carbonate) bound to an arginine is not in dispute, and evidence for the involvement of a molecule of water is supported by earlier NMR[116] and EXAFS[117] studies.

A diagrammatic representation of the iron-binding sites of human transferrin, indicating the identity and location of the residues involved at both the N- and the C-sites, is shown in Figure 14. For comparison, the two earlier models are also shown. As to the sequence of events involved in the process of iron binding, evidence is only fragmentary. It is likely that the first step involves the binding of the synergistic anion (bicarbonate or carbonate). This event would serve to neutralise the positive electrostatic charges on the basic

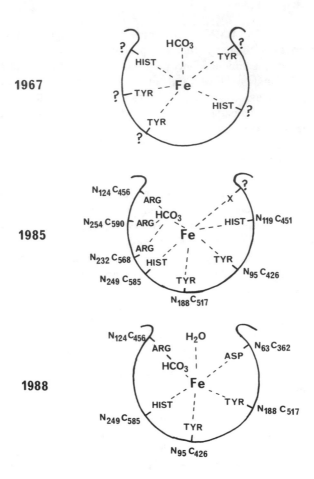

FIGURE 14. Diagrammatic representations of the proposed structures (1967, 1985, and 1988) for the iron-binding sites of human transferrin, showing the amino acid residues thought to be involved and their positions within the polypeptide chain.

side chains near the iron site, particularly the arginine residue (N-124 or C-456). This in turn would facilitate the approach of the positively charged ferric ion into the cleft between the two domains of each lobe. Once into the metal-binding pocket, the iron could then form stable coordination links with the relevant amino acid side chains acting as iron ligands. It has been suggested[112] that the iron first binds to the three ligands located in Domain II (two tyrosine, one histidine). Finally, to complete the process, the iron binds to the aspartic acid residue from Domain I as this domain closes over the iron site. Such a mechanism would help to explain the significant conformational change that transferrin undergoes during the process of iron binding.[106]

E. IRON RELEASE

In order for transferrin to act as an effective physiological carrier of iron, the molecule must not only be able to bind iron with high affinity, and thereby eliminate the toxic effects of free iron, but it must also be capable of releasing the bound iron at the tissues. It has already been described in a previous section of this chapter how *in vitro* studies have demonstrated that the protein has two high-affinity iron-binding sites with similar binding constants (1 to $6 \times 10^{22} M^{-1}$) for ferric ions presented to the apotransferrin molecule in the form of various soluble chelates. Once the iron-loaded transferrin circulating in the blood plasma reaches the target cell, it is convenient to consider its subsequent fate in three separate stages, and thereby pose three questions:

1.   What is the route of uptake of the iron-transferrin complex, once it has reached the plasma membrane of the target cell?
2.   How is the very strong coordination link between Fe^{3+} and the ligands at the iron-binding site broken in order to facilitate the release of iron?
3.   What is the intracellular fate of an atom of iron immediately following its release from the "iron cage" of transferrin, but before it becomes incorporated into its final molecular destination?

Question 1 will be considered in detail in Chapter 7 when the "transferrin-to-cell cycle" is discussed. This will incorporate an account not only of the plasma membrane transferrin receptor, but also the possible role of the asialoglycoprotein receptor in the uptake of transferrin by certain tissues. In the following sections discussion will be confined to questions 2 and 3. Very little is known at the present time about the mechanisms of iron release from transferrin *in vivo*. However, a considerable amount of information has been accumulated from *in vitro* studies in which iron-saturated transferrin has been exposed to a wide range of environments in order to ascertain which factors facilitate the release of the bound iron. It is still a matter of conjecture as to which, if any, of these factors might be operating within cells in the *in vivo* situation. In all, at least four separate mechanisms appear to be able to bring about the release of iron from the iron-transferrin complex;[73] acidification of the iron-binding ligands of the molecule; coordination of the bound iron by an alternative ligand (ligand exchange); reduction of the bound iron from Fe^{3+} to Fe^{2+}; and attack on, or replacement of, the synergistic anion-bicarbonate.

1. Acidification

The release of iron from human transferrin is most readily achieved *in vitro* by lowering the pH to between 5.0 and 5.5 in order to destabilise the metal-protein bond, with complexing agents present to sequester the released iron. In the case of human transferrin, if the pH is gradually lowered, the release of the iron is clearly seen to be biphasic,[88,89] with a rapid release of the iron atom bound to the N-site as the pH falls to 5.7, followed by a more gradual release of the iron bound to the C-site once the pH has been reduced to below 5.2. Not all animal transferrins behave in a similar fashion. In some cases (for example pig, cow, and goat), the difference in acid lability of the two sites is even more distinct, whereas in other examples (snake, turkey, and duck) the rates of iron release from the two sites, upon acidification of the molecule, have been found to be the same.[18]

The rate of iron release from diferric transferrin, brought about by acidification, is influenced by the ionic environment. High concentrations of sodium chloride facilitate iron release from the acid-stable C-site, whilst at the same time stabilising the iron-protein bond at the acid-labile N-site.[95] At very low ionic strength, iron release from both sites is severely impeded, implying that at zero ionic strength (clearly a situation that could not exist *in vivo*) no iron would be released from either site.[28]

The mechanism by which protons destabilise the iron-transferrin complex is not fully understood, yet it is quite clear that the rate of iron release is proportional to the hydrogen ion concentration, since the binding constants for iron are markedly reduced at low values of pH.[90] The increased tendency for transferrin to release its iron at low pH can be attributed to the increased positive charge of the protein, particularly the protonation of one or more of the amino acid side chains that act as ligands at the iron-binding site — aspartic acid, tyrosine, or histidine. The synergistic anion-bicarbonate is a further candidate for protonation. The release of iron from transferrin at low pH is accompanied by the release of the bicarbonate ion, but it has not yet been shown conclusively in which order these two events occur. In addition to a mechanism of iron release brought about by the direct effect of protons on the iron-binding ligands, an indirect (allosteric) effect has also been postulated. A model for iron release involving an alteration in the conformation of the protein has recently been proposed[118] in which transferrin changes from a "closed" configuration (with a stable iron-protein bond) to an "open" configuration (with a weak iron-protein bond). The equilibrium between these two conformational states might be affected by the presence of protons.

2. Ligand Exchange in the Presence of Alternative Iron Chelators

From *in vitro* studies it is evident that proton-induced release of iron from the iron-transferrin complex is considerably facilitated by the presence of iron chelators. These molecules trap and sequester the iron once it has been released from the binding sites. It is probable that their presence is not simply to enhance that rate of iron release, but is obligatory in order for the reaction to occur. In a detailed study on the effects of a wide range of small molecules on the rate of iron release from diferric transferrin, Morgan[119] concluded that the process involved an initial reaction between H^+ and the iron-transferrin complex, followed by the release of the iron under the action of the mediator or chelator. Several phosphatic compounds as well as known iron chelators were found to accelerate the process of iron release in the presence of protons. These included ATP, GTP, 2,3-DPG, inositol phosphate, pyrophosphate, citrate, EDTA, oxalate, and NTA. The greatest enhancement is brought about by inorganic pyrophosphate, closely followed by organic pyrophosphates such as ATP. At any given pH, iron release is increased to a maximum rate as the concentration of the mediator is raised. The data are consistent with the following general mechanism:

$$Fe^{3+}-Tf-CO_3^{2-} + H^+ + \text{chelator} \rightarrow Fe^{3+}-\text{chelator} + HCO_3^- + Tf$$

Chasteen,[74] in summarising the role of chelating agents, has suggested that the process probably occurs in a number of stages, some of which could involve the molecule of transferrin being converted from the stable "closed" conformational state to the reactive "open" configuration that has already been mentioned in the previous section.

The relevance of these studies to the cellular process of iron uptake and acquisition by cells is obvious. It is likely that small chelators play a role in the transport of iron within cells. Many of the mediators discovered by Morgan[119] are present in appreciable amounts in some cells. In some cases their concentrations have been found to influence iron uptake. For example, the rate of iron uptake by reticulocytes has been found to correlate with the ATP levels in these cells.[120] Also, the delivery of transferrin-bound iron to mitochondria is mediated by pyrophosphate.[121,122] It is within the mitochondria that the enzyme ferrochetalase catalyses the incorporation of Fe^{2+} into the porphyrin ring to form haem.

Most of the small molecules that have been shown to enhance the proton-catalysed release of iron from transferrin are perhaps better described as mediators rather than chelators. This is because their affinities for iron are considerably lower than the affinity shown by transferrin. There are, however, some powerful iron chelators that bind Fe^{3+} more strongly than transferrin. These include the bacterial siderophores such as desferrioxamine, which has been used for a number of years in the treatment of iron overload in humans. Desferrioxamine has a far stronger binding constant for iron than transferrin. In direct competition, desferrioxamine will preferentially bind free or weakly chelated iron. Yet it is known from *in vitro* studies that iron transfer from diferric transferrin to desferrioxamine occurs only very slowly. However, the rate is considerably enhanced in the presence of the same small-molecular-weight mediators that facilitate the release of iron from transferrin by protons. These include ATP, pyrophosphate, and citrate.[119] The barrier to iron removal from transferrin by desferrioxamine is a kinetic one, which can apparently be overcome by small-molecular-weight mediators.[123]

3. Reduction of Fe^{3+} to Fe^{2+}

Because of the comparative weakness with which transferrin binds Fe^{2+}, it is not surprising to find that a wide range of reducing agents increase the rate of iron release from transferrin by converting Fe^{3+} to Fe^{2+}. Many very effective agents include molecules that occur naturally within cells — cysteine, glutathione, NADH, and NADPH.[124] Whilst the rate of reductive iron removal is slow at physiological pH (7.4), it increases by two orders of magnitude if the pH is dropped to 6.1. In addition, the presence of small-molecular-weight mediators, such as pyrophosphate, along with a reducing agent, enhances the rate of iron removal in a synergistic way. Many *in vitro* studies of the redox chemistry of the iron bound to transferrin have shown that appreciable rates of metal release can be achieved under conditions that might prevail physiologically. It has recently been proposed that reticulocytes and hepatocytes have different mechanisms for iron uptake from transferrin.[125] It has been suggested that reticulocytes use the well-established membrane transferrin receptor-acidic endosome pathway, whilst hepatocytes use a redox-mediated plasma membrane process involving the reduction of transferrin-bound iron.[126] This will be discussed in Chapter 7.

4. Anion Attack or Exchange

Iron release from transferrin is associated with the release of the synergistic anion HCO_3^-. The protonation of the bound bicarbonate is thought to weaken the coordinate link between the iron and anion. Many alternative anions can replace bicarbonate in the $Tf-Fe^{3+}-$bicarbonate complex, and these have been extensively reviewed by Harris and Ainsen.[28] For example, oxalate can replace bicarbonate. When this occurs the iron remains attached to the transferrin at a lower pH than when bicarbonate is present.[127] The uptake of iron from the $Fe^{3+}-Tf-$oxalate complex is only 30% of that achieved using the normal $Fe^{3+}-Tf-$bicarbonate complex. On the other hand, no examples have yet been found of alternative synergistic anions that facilitate iron release and at the same time occur in physiological fluids. Therefore, anion exchange alone does not seem to be a mechanism for the release of iron from transferrin *in vivo*.

The conclusion that can be drawn from all the *in vitro* kinetic studies on iron release by transferrin is that no single mechanism alone — be it protonation, chelation, reduction, or anion attack — is likely to account for the release of iron from transferrin within cells. Some or all of these mechanisms, by acting in concert, need to be invoked in order to explain how transferrin is relieved of its iron during the very short time (less than 3 min) the molecule spends in most cells.[28]

REFERENCES

1. **Palmour, R. M. and Sutton, H. E.,** Vertebrate transferrins, molecular weights, chemical compositions, and iron-binding studies, *Biochemistry,* 10, 4026, 1971.
2. **Lee, M. Y., Heubers, H., Martin, A. W., and Finch, C. A.,** Iron metabolism in a spider, *Dugesiella hentzi , J. Comp. Physiol.,* 127, 349, 1978.

3. **Horn, E. C. and Kerr, M. S.**, The haemolymph proteins of the blue crab, *Callinectes sapidus, Comp. Biochem. Physiol.*, 29, 493, 1969.
4. **Ghidalia, W., Fine, J. M., and Marneux, M.**, On the presence of an iron-binding protein in the serum of the decapod crustacean *Macropipus puber, Comp. Biochem. Physiol.*, 41B, 349, 1972.
5. **Heubers, H. A., Heubers, E., Finch, C. A., and Martin, A. W.**, Characterisation of an invertebrate transferrin from the crab *Cancer magister* (Arthropoda), *J. Comp. Physiol.*, 148, 101, 1982.
6. **Topham, R., Cooper, B., Tesh, S., Godette, G., Bonaventura, C., and Bonaventura, J.**, Isolation, purification and characterisation of an iron-binding protein from the horseshoe crab *(Limulus polyphenus), Biochem. J.*, 252, 151, 1988.
7. **Landry, C. D. and Topham, R. W.**, Purification and characterisation of an iron-binding protein from the blue crab *(Callinectes sapidus), Comp. Biochem. Physiol.*, 97B, 831, 1990.
8. **Martin, A. W., Heubers, E., Heubers, H., Webb, J., and Finch, C. A.**, A monosited transferrin from a representative deuterostome: the Ascidian *Pyura stolonifera* (sub phylum Urochordata), *Blood*, 64, 1047, 1984.
9. **Applegate, V. C.**, Natural history of the sea lamprey, *U.S. Dep. Inter. Spec. Sci. Rep. Fish.*, 55, 1, 1950.
10. **Ainsen, P., Leibman, A., and Sia, C.**, Molecular weight and subunit structure of hagfish transferrin, *Biochemistry*, 11, 3461, 1972.
11. **Webster, R. O. and Pollara, B.**, Isolation and partial characterisation of transferrin in the sea lamprey, *Petromyzon marinus, Comp. Biochem. Physiol.*, 30, 509, 1969.
12. **Macey, D. J., Webb, J., and Potter, I. C.**, Iron levels and major binding proteins in the plasma of amniocytes and adults of the Southern hemisphere lamprey, *Geotria australis, Comp. Biochem. Physiol.*, 72A, 307, 1982.
13. **Bates, G. W. and Schlabach, M. R.**, The reaction of ferric salts with transferrin, *J. Biol. Chem.*, 248, 3228, 1973.
14. **Van der Heul, C., van Eijk, H. G., Wiltink, W. F., and Leijense, B.**, The binding of iron to transferrin and to other serum protein components at different degrees of saturation with iron, *Clin. Chim. Acta*, 38, 347, 1972.
15. **Meuller, J. O., Smithies, O., and Irwin, M. R.**, Transferrin variation in Columbidae, *Genetics*, 47, 1385, 1962.
16. **Giblett, E. R., Hickman, C. G., and Smithies, O.**, Serum transferrins, *Nature*, 183, 1589, 1959.
17. **Thymann, M.**, Identification of a new polymorphism as transferrin, *Hum. Genet.*, 43, 225, 1978.
18. **Welch, S. G.**, A comparison of the structure and properties of serum transferrin from 17 animal species, *Comp. Biochem. Physiol.*, 97B, 417, 1990.
19. **deJong, G., van Dijk, J. P., and van Eijk, H. G.**, The biology of transferrin, *Clin. Chim. Acta*, 190, 1, 1990.
20. **Parker, W. C. and Bearn, A. G.**, Alteration in the sialic acid content of human transferrin, *Science*, 133, 1014, 1960.
21. **Wang, A. and Sutton, H. E.**, Human transferrin C and D_1: chemical difference in a peptide, *Science*, 149, 435, 1965.
22. **Evans, R. W. and Williams, J.**, Studies of the iron binding of different iron donors to human serum transferrin and isolation of iron-binding fragments from the N- and C-terminal region of the protein, *Biochem. J.*, 173, 543, 1978.
23. **Cook, N. D., Simpson, R. J., Osterloh, K., and Peters, T. J.**, Rapid preparation of highly purified human transferrin, *Anal. Biochem.*, 149, 349, 1985.
24. **Welch, S. G. and Langmead, L.**, A comparison of the structure and properties of normal human transferrin and a genetic variant of human transferrin, *Int. J. Biochem.*, 22, 275, 1990.

25. **Oncley, J. L., Scatchard, G. G., and Brown, A.,** Physical-chemical characterisation of certain of the proteins of human plasma, *J. Phys. Chem.,* 51, 184, 1947.
26. **Roberts, R. C., Makey, D. G., and Seal, U. S.,** Human transferrin: molecular weight and sedimentation properties, *J. Biol. Chem.,* 241, 4907, 1966.
27. **Rosseneu-Motreff, M. Y., Soetewey, F., Lamote, R., and Peeters, H.,** Size and shape determination of apotransferrin and transferrin monomers, *Biopolymers,* 10, 1039, 1971.
28. **Harris, D. C. and Ainsen, P.,** Physical biochemistry of the transferrins, in *Iron Carriers and Iron Proteins,* T. Loehr, Ed., VCH Publishers, New York, 1989, chap. 3.
29. **Jeppson, J. O.,** Subunits of human transferrin, *Acta Chem. Scand.,* 21, 1686, 1967.
30. **Bezkorovainy, A. and Grohlich, G.,** The behaviour of native and reduced-alkylated human transferrin in urea and guanidine-HCl solutions, *Biochim. Biophys. Acta,* 147, 497, 1967.
31. **Mann, K. G., Fish, W. W., Cox, A. C., and Tanford, C.,** Single-chain nature of human serum transferrin, *Biochemistry,* 9, 1348, 1970.
32. **Williams, J., Grace, S. A., and Williams, J. M.,** Evolutionary significance of the renal excretion of transferrin half-molecule fragments, *Biochem. J.,* 201, 417, 1982.
33. **Parker, W. C. and Bearn, A. G.,** Human serum transferrin, *J. Exp. Med.,* 115, 83, 1962.
34. **Heimberger, N., Heide, K., Haupte, H., and Schultze, A. F.,** Amino acid composition of human TfC, *Clin. Chim. Acta,* 10, 293, 1964.
35. **Roop, W. E. and Putman, F. W.,** Purification and properties of human transferrin C and a slow moving genetic variant, *J. Biol. Chem.,* 242, 2507, 1967.
36. **Bezkorovainy, A., Rafelson, M. E., and Likhite, V.,** Isolation and partial characterisation of transferrin from normal human plasma, *Arch. Biochem. Biophys.,* 103, 371, 1963.
37. **Bezkorovainy, A., Grohlich, D., and Gerbeck, C. M.,** Some physical-chemical proterties of reduced-alkylated and sulphitolysed serum transferrin and hen's-egg albumin, *Biochem. J.,* 110, 765, 1968.
38. **Freenoy, N., Goussault, Y., and Bourrillon, R.,** Preparation de la transferrine du serum humain, *Clin. Chim. Acta,* 32, 243, 1971.
39. **Van Eijk, H. J., van Dijk, J. P., van Noort, W. L., Leijense, B., and Monfoort, C. H.,** Isolation and analysis of transferrin from different species, *Scand. J. Haematol.,* 9, 267, 1972.
40. **Sutton, M. R. and Brew, K.,** The sequence of residues 1 – 26 of human transferrin, *FEBS Lett.,* 40, 146, 1974.
41. **Montreuil, J. and Spik, G.,** Comparative studies of the carbohydrate and protein moieties of human serotransferrin and lactoferrin, in *Proteins of Iron Storage and Transport in Biochemistry and Medicine,* R. R. Crichton, Ed., North-Holland, Amsterdam, 1975, 27.
42. **Welch, S. G. and Skinner, A.,** A comparison of the structure and properties of human, rat and rabbit serum transferrin, *Comp. Biochem. Physiol.,* 93B, 417, 1989.
43. **Yang, F., Lum, J. B., McGill, J. R., Moore, C. M., Naylor, S. L., van Bragt, P. H., Baldwin, D., and Bowman, B.,** Human transferrin: cDNA characterisation and chromosomal localisation, *Proc. Natl. Acad. Sci. U.S.A.,* 81, 2752, 1984.
44. **Bezkorovainy, A. and Grohlich, D.,** Cyanogen bromide fragments of human serum transferrin, *Biochim. Biophys. Acta,* 310, 365, 1973.
45. **Sutton, M. R. and Brew, K.,** Purification and characterisation of the seven cyanogen bromide fragments of human serum transferrin, *Biochem. J.,* 139, 163, 1974.
46. **MacGillivray, R. T. A., Mendez, E., Sinha, S. K., Sutton, M. R., Lineback-Zins, J., and Brew, K.,** The complete amino acid sequence of human serum transferrin, *Proc. Natl. Acad. Sci. U.S.A.,* 79, 2504, 1982.
47. **Williams, J.,** The evolution of transferrin, *Trends Biochem. Sci.,* 7, 394, 1982.
48. **MacGillivray, R. T. A., Mendez, E., Shewale, J. G., Sinha, S. K., Lineback-Zins, J., and Brew, K.,** The primary structure of human serum transferrin, *J. Biol. Chem.,* 258, 3543, 1983.

49. **Schaeffer, E., Lucero, M. A., Jeltsch, J-M., Py, M-C., Levin, M. J., Chambon, P., Cohen, G. N., and Zakin, M.**, Complete structure of the human transferrin gene. Comparison with analogous chicken gene and human pseudogene, *Gene*, 56, 109, 1987.

50. **Metz-Boutigue, M., Jolles, J., Mazurier, J., Schoentgen, F., Legrand, D., Spik, G., Montreuil, J., and Jolles, P.**, Human lactoferrin: amino acid sequence and structural comparison with other transferrins, *Eur. J. Biochem.*, 145, 659, 1984.

51. **Rose, T. M., Plowman, G. D., Teplow, D. B., Dreyer, W. J., Hellstrom, K. E., and Brown, J. P.**, Primary structure of human melanoma-associated antigen p97 (melanotransferrin) deduced from the mRNA sequence, *Proc. Natl. Acad. Sci. U.S.A.*, 83, 1261, 1986.

52. **Baldwin, G. S. and Weinstock, J.**, Nucleotide sequence of porcine liver transferrin, *Nucleic Acids Res.*, 16, 8720, 1988.

53. **Williams, J., Ellerman, T. C., Kingston, I. B., Wilkins, A. C., and Kuhn, K. A.**, The primary structure of hen ovotransferrin, *Eur. J. Biochem.*, 122, 297, 1982.

54. **Moskaitis, J. E., Pastori, R. L., and Schoenberg, D. R.**, The nucleotide sequence of *Xenopus laevis* transferrin mRNA, *Nucleic Acids Res.*, 18, 6135, 1990.

55. **Mazurier, J., Aubert, J-P., Loucheux-Lefrevre, M-H., and Spik, G.**, Comparative circular dichroism studies of iron-free and iron-saturated human serotransferrin and lactoferrin, *FEBS Lett.*, 66, 238, 1976.

56. **Anderson, B. F., Baker, H. M., Dodson, E. J., Norris, G. E., Rumball, S., Waters, J. M., and Baker, E. N.**, Structure of human lactoferrin at 3.2 Å resolution, *Proc. Natl. Acad. Sci. U.S.A.*, 84, 1769, 1987.

57. **Bailey, S., Evans, R. W., Garratt, R. C., Gorinsky, B., Hasnain, C. H., Jhoti, H., Lindley, P. F., Mydin, A., Sarra, R., and Watson, J. L.**, Molecular structure of serum transferrin at 3.3 Å resolution, *Biochemistry*, 27, 5804, 1988.

58. **Magdoff-Fairchild, B. and Low, B. W.**, Preliminary X-ray crystallographic study of porcine transferrin, *Arch. Biochem. Biophys.*, 138, 703, 1970.

59. **Al-Hilal, D., Baker, E., Carlisle, C. H., Gorinsky, B., Horsburgh, R. C., Lindley, P. F., Moss, D. S., Schnieder, A., and Stimpson, R.**, Crystallisation and preliminary X-ray investigation of rabbit plasma transferrin, *J. Mol. Biol.*, 108, 255, 1976.

60. **Baker, E. N. and Rumball, S. U.**, Crystallographic data of human lactoferrin, *J. Mol. Biol.*, 111, 207, 1977.

61. **DeLucas, L. J., Suddath, F. L., Gains, R. A., and Bugg, C. E.**, Preliminary X-ray study of human transferrin, *J. Mol. Biol.*, 123, 285, 1978.

62. **Gorinsky, B., Horsburgh, C., Lindley, P. F., Moss, D. S., Parkar, M., and Watson, J. L.**, Evidence for the bilobal nature of diferric rabbit plasma transferrin, *Nature*, 281, 157, 1979.

63. **Pflugrath, J. W. and Quiocho, F. A.**, Sulphate sequestered in the sulphate-binding protein of *Salmonella typhimurium* is bound solely by hydrogen bonds, *Nature*, 314, 257, 1985.

64. **Roth, J.**, Subcellular organisation of glycosylation in mammalian cells, *Biochim. Biophys. Acta*, 906, 405, 1987.

65. **deJong, G., van Dijk, J. P., and van Eijk, H. G.**, The biology of transferrin, *Clin. Chim. Acta*, 190, 1, 1990.

66. **Schade, A. L., Reinhart, R. W., and Levy, H.**, Carbon dioxide and oxygen complex formation with iron and siderophilin, the iron binding component of human plasma, *Arch. Biochem. Biophys.*, 20, 170, 1949.

67. **Van Snick, J. L., Masson, P. L., and Hermans, J. F.**, The involvement of bicarbonate in the binding of iron by transferrin, *Biochim. Biophys. Acta*, 322, 231, 1973.

68. **Ainsen, P., Leibman, A., Pinkowitz, R. A., and Pollack, S.**, Exchangeability of bicarbonate specifically bound to transferrin, *Biochemistry*, 12, 3679, 1973.

69. **Schlabach, M. R. and Bates, G. W.**, The synergistic binding of anions and Fe^{3+} by transferrin, *J. Biol. Chem.*, 250, 2182, 1975.

70. **Harris, D. C. and Ainsen, P.**, Physical biochemistry of transferrin, in *Iron Carriers and Iron Proteins*, T. M. Loehr, Ed., VCH Publishers, New York, 1989, chap. 3.

71. **Harris, W. R.**, Thermodynamic binding constants of the zinc-human transferrin complex, *Biochemistry*, 22, 3920, 1983.
72. **Bezkorovainy, A.**, Chemistry and metabolism of transferrin, in *Biochemistry of Nonheme Iron*, Plenum Press, New York, 1980, chap. 4.
73. **Ainsen, P. and Listowsky, I.**, Iron transport and storage proteins, *Annu. Rev. Biochem.*, 49, 357, 1980.
74. **Chasteen, N. D.**, Transferrin: a perspective, *Adv. Inorg. Biochem.*, 5, 201, 1983.
75. **Bates, G. W., Billups, C., and Saltman, P.**, The kinetics and mechanism of iron (III) exchange between chelates and transferrin [1], *J. Biol. Chem.*, 242, 2810, 1967.
76. **Bates, G. W. and Wernicke, J.**, The kinetics and mechanism of iron (III) exchange between chelates and transferrin [4], *J. Biol. Chem.*, 246, 3679, 1971.
77. **Fletcher, J. and Heuhns, E. R.**, Significance of the binding of iron by transferrin, *Nature*, 215, 584, 1967.
78. **Fletcher, J. and Heuhns, E. R.**, Function of transferrin, *Nature*, 218, 1211, 1968.
79. **Legrand, D., Mazurier, J., Montreuil, J., and Spik, G.**, Structure and spatial configuration of the iron-binding sites of transferrin, *Biochimie*, 70, 1185, 1988.
80. **Brock, J. H.**, in *Metalloproteins*, P. Harrison, Ed., McMillan, London, 1985, 183.
81. **Warner, R. C. and Weber, I.**, The metal combining properties of conalbumin, *J. Am. Chem. Soc.*, 75, 5094, 1953.
82. **Aasa, R., Malmstrom, B. G., Saltman, P., and Vanngard, T.**, The specific binding of iron (III) and copper (II) to transferrin and conalbumin, *Biochim. Biophys. Acta*, 75, 203, 1963.
83. **Klotz, I. M. and Hunston, D. L.**, Protein interaction with small molecules, *J. Biol. Chem.*, 250, 3001, 1975.
84. **Makey, D. G. and Seal, U. S.**, The detection of four molecular forms of human transferrin during the iron binding process, *Biochim. Biophys. Acta*, 453, 250, 1976.
85. **Evans, R. W. and Williams, J.**, The electrophoresis of transferrins in urea/polyacrylamide gels, *Biochem. J.*, 189, 541, 1980.
86. **Strahler, J. R., Rosenblum, B. B., Hanash, S., and Butkunas, R.**, Separation of transferrin types in human plasma by ion-exchange high-performance liquid chromatography, *J. Chromatogr.*, 266, 281, 1983.
87. **Van Eijk, H. G., Van Noort, W. L., and Van der Heul, C.**, Analysis of the iron-binding sites of transferrin by isoelectric focussing, *J. Clin. Chem. Clin. Biochem.*, 16, 557, 1978.
88. **Princiotto, J. V. and Zapolski, E. J.**, Differences between the two iron-binding sites of transferrin, *Nature*, 255, 87, 1975.
89. **Lestas, A. N.**, The effect of pH on human transferrin: selective labelling of the 2 iron binding sites, *Br. J. Haematol.*, 32, 341, 1976.
90. **Ainsen, P., Leibman, A., and Zweier, J.**, Stochiometric site characteristics of iron bound to human transferrin, *J. Biol. Chem.*, 253, 1930, 1978.
91. **Van Eijk, H. J., Van Noort, W. L., Kroos, M. J., and Van der Heul, C.**, Iron binding to human transferrin, *J. Clin. Chem. Clin. Biochem.*, 18, 563, 1980.
92. **Zapolski, E. J. and Princiotto, J. V.**, Binding of iron from nitrilotriacetate analogues by human transferrin, *Biochemistry*, 19, 3599, 1978.
93. **Williams, J. and Moreton, K.**, The distribution of iron between the metal binding sites of transferrin, *Biochem. J.*, 185, 483, 1980.
94. **Williams, J., Chasteen, N. D., and Moreton, K.**, The effect of salt concentration on the iron binding properties of human transferrin, *Biochem. J.*, 201, 527, 1982.
95. **Baldwin, D. A. and DeSousa, D.**, The effects of salts on the kinetics of iron release from N-terminal and C-terminal monotransferrins, *Biochem. Biophys. Res. Commum.*, 99, 1101, 1981.
96. **Folajtar, D. A. and Chasteen, N. D.**, Measurement of the nonsynergistic anion binding to transferrin by EPR difference spectroscopy, *J. Am. Chem. Soc.*, 104, 5775, 1982.
97. **Zweier, J. L.**, An electron paramagnetic resonance study of single site copper complexes of transferrin, *J. Biol. Chem.*, 253, 7616, 1978.

98. **Zweier, J. L., Ainsen, P., Peisach, J., and Mims, W.,** Pulsed electron paramagnetic studies of the copper complexes of transferrin, *J. Biol. Chem.,* 254, 3512, 1979.

99. **Zweier, J. L. and Ainsen, P.,** Studies on transferrin with the use of Cu^{2+} as an electron paramagnetic resonance spectroscopic probe, *J. Biol. Chem.,* 252, 6090, 1977.

100. **Harris, D. C.,** Different metal binding properties of the two sites of human transferrin, *Biochemistry,* 16, 560, 1977.

101. **O'Hara, P. B. and Bersohn, R.,** Resolution of the two metal binding sites of human serum transferrin by low-temperture excitation of bound europium (III), *Biochemistry,* 21, 5269, 1982.

102. **Chasteen, N. D. and Williams, J.,** The effect of pH on the equilibrium distribution of iron between the metal binding sites of human transferrin, *Biochem. J.,* 193, 717, 1981.

103. **Huebers, H. A., Josephson, B., Huebers, E., Csiba, E., and Finch, C. A.,** Occupancy of the iron binding sites of human transferrin, *Proc. Natl. Acad. Sci. U.S.A.,* 81, 4326, 1984.

104. **Van Eijk, H. G. and Van Noort, W. L.,** The non-random distribution of transferrin iron in fresh human sera, *Clin. Chim. Acta,* 157, 299, 1986.

105. **Zak, O. and Ainsen, P.,** Non-random distribution of iron in circulating human transferrin, *Blood,* 68, 157, 1986.

106. **Hovanessian, A. G. and Awdeh, Z. L.,** Gel isoelectric focussing of human serum transferrin, *Eur. J. Biochem.,* 68, 333, 1976.

107. **Ainsen, P.,** in *Inorganic Biochemistry,* G. Eichorn, Ed., Elsevier, New York, 1973.

108. **Baker, E. W., Rumball, S. V., and Anderson, B. F.,** Transferrin: an insight into the structure and function from studies on lactoferrin, *Trends Biochem. Sci.,* 12, 350, 1987.

109. **Crichton, R. R. and Charloteaux-Wauters, M.,** Iron transport and storage, *Eur. J. Biochem.,* 164, 485, 1987.

110. **Morgan, E. M.,** in *Molecular Aspects of Medicine,* Pergamon Press, Oxford, 1, 1981.

111. **Huebers, H. A. and Finch, C. A.,** The physiology of transferrin and transferrin receptors, *Physiol. Rev.,* 67, 520, 1987.

112. **Legrand, D., Mazurier, J., Montreuil, J., and Spik, G.,** Structure and spatial conformation of the iron-binding sites of transferrins, *Biochimie,* 70, 1185, 1988.

113. **Garratt, R. C., Evans, R. W., Hasnain, S. S., and Lindley, P. F.,** An extended-X-ray-absorption-fine-structure investigation of diferric transferrins and their iron-binding fragments, *Biochem. J.,* 233, 479, 1986.

114. **Montreuil, J., Mazurier, J., Legrand, D., and Spik, G.,** Human lactoferrin structure and function, in *Proteins of Iron Storage and Transport,* G. Spik, J. Montreuil, R. R. Crichton, and J. Mazurier, Eds., Elsevier, Amsterdam, 25, 1985.

115. **Windle, J. J., Weirsema, A. K., Clark, J. R., and Feeney, R. E.,** Investigation of the iron and copper complexes of avian conalbumin and human transferrin by electron paramagnetic resonance, *Biochemistry,* 2, 1341, 1963.

116. **Koenig, S. H. and Schillinger, W. E.,** Nuclear magnetic relaxation dispersion in protein solutions II — transferrin, *J. Biol. Chem.,* 244, 6520.

117. **Hasnain, S. S., Evans, R. W., Garratt, R. C., and Lindley, P. F.,** An extended X-ray-absorption-fine-structure study of freeze dried and solution ovotransferrin, *Biochem. J.,* 247, 369, 1987.

118. **Cowart, R. E., Kojima, N., and Bates, G. W.,** Exchange of Fe^{3+} between acetohydroxamic acid and transferrin, *J. Biol. Chem.,* 257, 7650, 1982.

119. **Morgan, E. H.,** Studies on the mechanism of iron release by transferrin, *Biochem. Biophys. Acta,* 580, 312, 1979.

120. **Kailis, S. G. and Morgan, E. H.,** Iron uptake by immature erythroid cells, *Biochem. Biophys. Acta,* 464, 389, 1977.

121. **Konoka, K. and Romslo, I.,** Studies on the mechanism of pyrophosphate-mediated uptake of iron from transferrin by isolated rat-liver mitochondria, *Eur. J. Biochem.,* 117, 239, 1981.

122. **Nilsen, T. and Romslo, I.,** Transferrin as a donor of iron to mitochondria. The effect of pyrophosphate and the relationship to mitochondrial metabolism and haem synthesis, *Biochem. Biophys. Acta,* 802, 448, 1984.

123. **Pollack, S., Vanderhoff, G., and Leisky, F.,** Iron removal from transferrin: an experimental study, *Biochem. Biophys. Acta,* 497, 481, 1977.

124. **Kojima, N. and Bates, G. W.,** Reduction and release of iron from $Fe^{3+}-Tf-CO_3^{2-}$, *J. Biol. Chem.,* 254, 8847, 1979.

125. **Thorensten, K.,** Hepatocytes and reticulocytes have different mechanisms for the uptake of iron from transferrin, *J. Biol. Chem.,* 263, 16837, 1989.

126. **Thorensten, K. and Romslo, I.,** Uptake of iron from transferrin by isolated rat hepatocytes. A redox-mediated plasma membrane process, *J. Biol. Chem.,* 263, 8844, 1988.

127. **Najarain, R. C., Harris, D. C., and Ainsen, P.,** Oxalate and spin-labelled oxalate as probes of the anion binding sites of human transferrin, *J. Biol. Chem.,* 253, 38, 1978.

Chapter 5

TRANSFERRIN BINDING OF ELEMENTS OTHER THAN IRON

I. INTRODUCTION

The structure and properties of human transferrin have evolved in order that the molecule can carry out a range of specific functions within the internal environment of cells and tissue fluids. The characteristics and geometry of the two metal-binding sites will have arisen, during the process of molecular evolution, in order to accommodate the ferric ion (Fe^{3+}) within a suitably tailored environment. This "iron cage" has to be able to bind Fe^{3+} and subsequently protect the iron from the hazards of hydrolysis whilst the element is being transported between tissues. At the same time, the firm grip of the iron-binding ligands must also be capable of being broken in order that the element can eventually be released within cells to continue the journey to its ultimate molecular destination. The structure and properties of the molecule that allow transferrin to fulfill this vital biological role have been discussed in the previous chapter.

The binding of Fe^{3+} within the "iron cage" of transferrin can in many respects be likened to the binding of the substrate by an enzyme at its "active site". This latter event, which in most cases is a process exhibiting a high degree of specificity, relies upon a recognition between, on the one hand, amino acid side chain ligands at the active site of the enzyme protein, and on the other hand, a variety of structural features within the substrate molecule. In the case of the iron-transferrin interaction, what are the particular features of the ferric ion, and are they sufficiently unique so as to preclude the binding of any of the other elements to the metal-binding site? Fe^{3+} whilst attached to iron-transport proteins is in the "high-spin" state. All five of the valence electrons are unpaired, each one occupying a separate one of the five d-orbitals within the M-shell. This is the most stable electronic configuration, known as the ground state. Within the "iron cage" the stereochemistry of the ferric ion is octahedral, with a coordination number of 6. It has already been described in Chapter 4 how these six coordination sites are linked within the iron-transferrin complex to tyrosines (2), histidine (1), aspartate (1), bicarbonate (1), and water (1). In terms of size, the "iron cage" has to be large enough to allow for the entrance, binding, and subsequent exit of a positively charged Fe^{3+} ion with a radius of 0.65 Å.

With these characteristics in mind, a brief inspection of the size, charge, and electronic configuration of the other 102 elements in the periodic table would probably lead one to propose that transferrin ought to be capable of binding many other elements in addition to iron. During the last 30 years, this prediction has been substantiated by a wealth of experimental evidence. In total, 29 elements in addition to iron have been shown to bind specifically to one or both of the metal-binding sites of transferrin. These elements include representatives from four parts of the periodic table — group III metals, d-block transition elements, lanthanides, and actinides (Figure 1). The main criterion that has been used in order to distinguish "specific" binding from the "nonspecific" attachment of metal ions to transferrin is that specificity

	1a	2a	3b	4b	5b	6b	7b	8b			1b	2b	3a	4a	5a	6a	7a	8a
1	1 H																	2 He
2	3 Li	4 Be		TRANSITION		ELEMENTS							5 B	6 C	7 N	8 O	9 F	10 Ne
3	11 Na	12 Mg											13 Al	14 Si	15 P	16 S	17 Cl	18 Ar
4	19 K	20 Ca	21 Sc	22 Ti	23 V	24 Cr	25 Mn	26 Fe	27 Co	28 Ni	29 Cu	30 Zn	31 Ga	32 Ge	33 As	34 Se	35 Br	36 Kr
5	37 Rb	38 Sr	39 Y	40 Zr	41 Nb	42 Mo	43 Tc	44 Ru	45 Rh	46 Pd	47 Ag	48 Cd	49 In	50 Sn	51 Sb	52 Te	53 I	54 Xe
6	55 Cs	56 Ba	57 La	72 Hf	73 Ta	74 W	75 Re	76 Os	77 Ir	78 Pt	79 Au	80 Hg	81 Tl	82 Pb	83 Bi	84 Po	85 At	86 Rn
7	87 Fr	88 Ra	89 Ac															

Lanthanides	58 Ce	59 Pr	60 Nd	61 Pm	62 Sm	63 Eu	64 Gd	65 Tb	66 Dy	67 Ho	68 Er	69 Tm	70 Yb	71 Lu
Actinides	90 Th	91 Pa	92 U	93 Np	94 Pu	95 Am	96 Cm	97 Bk	98 Cf	99 Es	100 Fm	101 Md	102 No	103 Lr

FIGURE 1. The Periodic Table showing the elements (highlighted) that bind to one or both of the metal-binding sites of human transferrin.

is characterised by the firm binding of a maximum of two atoms of the element in question. There are a few examples from amongst the 29 elements, to be discussed later in this chapter, where only one atom of the element is capable of being bound to a molecule of transferrin. This is thought to reflect differences in both the size and binding affinities of the two metal-binding sites, wherein large ions, such as praeseodymium, are precluded from binding to one of the two sites. A second characteristic of "specific" binding is the requirement for a synergistic anion, usually bicarbonate.

Table 1 summarises some of the data that has been published regarding the binding of iron and 29 other elements to transferrin. The characteristics listed include the number of atoms bound, the charge and radius of the ion, and, where information is available, the thermodynamic binding constants K_1 and K_2. Under normal circumstances, serum transferrin is only about 35% saturated with iron. This leaves a substantial capacity for the binding of other metals, assuming that the binding of an alternative metal is sterically and thermodynamically possible. However, apart from iron, where the case is well proven, simply demonstrating iron binding does not imply that transferrin necessarily has a role to play in transport or metabolism of the element in question. Indeed, many of the examples on the list are certainly not elements essential for normal body metabolism, even in trace amounts.

The remainder of this chapter will be devoted to a brief description of the evidence for, and characteristics of, the binding of these 29 elements to

TABLE 1
The 31 Elements that Bind to Transferrin

Element	Atomic number (Z)	Maximum number bound	Ionic radius (Å)	Binding constants log K_1 and log K_2	Ref.
Group III Elements					
Aluminium	13 Al^{3+}	2	0.535	$K_1 = 12.9$, $K_2 = 12.3$	1, 3, 5, 72, 73, 74
Gallium	31 Ga^{3+}	2	0.620	$K_1 = 20.3$, $K_2 = 19.3$	3, 5, 8, 75, 76
Indium	49 In^{3+}	2	0.800		10, 11, 12, 13
Thallium	81 Tl^{3+}		0.885		14
d-Block Transition Elements					
Scandium	21 Sc^{3+}	2	0.745		17
Vanadium	23 V^{3+}		0.640		21, 22, 23, 77, 78
	VO^{2+}				
Chromium	24 Cr^{3+}	2	0.615		24, 25
Manganese	25 Mn^{3+}	2	0.645		25, 26, 29, 31
Iron	26 Fe^{3+}	2	0.645	$K_1 = 22.8$, $K_2 = 21.5$	
Cobalt	27 Co_3^{+}	2	0.610		25
Nickel	28 Ni^{2+}	2	0.690	$K_1 = 4.1$, $K_2 = 3.23$	29, 35, 36
Copper	29 Cu^{2+}	2	0.730		29, 41– 45, 79, 80
Zinc	30 Zn^{2+}	2	0.740	$K_1 = 8.0$, $K_2 = 6.6$	29, 46– 52, 82
Ruthenium	44 Ru^{4+}	?	0.620		83
Cadmium	48 Cd^{2+}	2	0.950	$K_1 = 5.95$, $K_2 = 4.86$	29, 54
Hafnium	72 Hf^{4+}	2	0.710		55
Platinum	78 Pt^{2+}	2	0.800		56, 57
Lanthanides					
Praeseodymium	59 Pr^{3+}	1	0.990		58
Neodymium	60 Nd^{3+}	2	0.985	$K_1 = 6.09$, $K_2 = 5.04$	58, 63
Samarium	62 Sa^{3+}	2	0.958	$K_1 = 7.13$, $K_2 = 5.39$	58, 63
Europium	63 Eu^{3+}	2	0.958		58, 64
Gadolinium	64 Gd^{3+}	1/2?	0.947	$K = 6.8$	59, 63
Terbium	65 Tb^{3+}	2	0.923		58, 60, 61, 65
Holmium	67 Ho^{3+}	2	0.901		53, 58
Erbium	68 Er^{3+}	2	0.890		53, 58

TABLE 1 (continued)
The 31 Elements that Bind to Transferrin

Element	Atomic number (Z)	Maximum number bound	Ionic radius (Å)	Binding constants log K_1 and log K_2	Ref.
			Actinides		
Thorium	90 Th^{4+}	2	0.940		53, 69
Protactinium	91 Pa^{4+}	?	1.025		70
Neptunium	93 Np^{4+}	?	1.010		71
Plutonium	94 Pu^{4+}	?	0.870		66, 68
Americium	95 Am^{3+}	?	0.975		63
Curium	96 Cm^{3+}	?	0.970		63

serum transferrin. It will become apparent that in only a few cases, such as zinc and manganese, and possibly chromium, nickel, and vanadium, is there evidence that transferrin might be involved in the physiological binding and transport of any nutritionally essential element, other than iron. Many of the other examples within the list have proved to be very useful and informative in studies on transferrin structure. For example, the lanthanides have provided many valuable fluorescent probes for electron paramagnetic resonance (EPR) analysis. Some of the other elements in the list, by virtue of their ability to bind to transferrin and form stable complexes, have been useful in many areas of diagnostic medicine. Radioactive isotopes of gallium and indium are used as radiological markers for a variety of tumours. Finally, there are the members of the actinide series (Z = 90 to 103), all of which are unstable and radioactive. There is evidence that transferrin is at least one of the vehicles by which these highly toxic substances, like, for example, plutonium, are distributed throughout the body after exposure to damaging radiation.

II. GROUP III ELEMENTS

A. ALUMINIUM (Al^{3+})
Aluminium is now recognised as being the toxic agent responsible for both the microcytic anaemia and the encephalopathy that sometimes affects patients undergoing maintenance haemodialysis for chronic renal failure. Many of these patients, as a result of dialysis against large volumes of fluids containing the normal trace amounts of aluminium, accumulate the element. Plasma levels of aluminium as high as 20 $\mu M/L$ have been recorded (normal value = 1 $\mu M/L$). In 1983, Trapp[1] confirmed earlier suggestions, namely that the bulk of the plasma aluminium in the dialysis patients and normal controls was protein bound, and only a small proportion was maintained in solution as a complex with plasma citrate. The binding protein was identified as transferrin. Trapp concluded that the aluminium ion (Al^{3+}) was bound to

at least one of the metal-binding sites of transferrin in a reaction that was dependent upon the presence of bicarbonate.

In a later and more extensive study, Martin et al.[2] confirmed that transferrin was the strongest aluminium binder in human plasma. Furthermore, it was clearly demonstrated that transferrin was capable of binding Al^{3+} at both of the metal-binding sites with the successive binding constants being measured as $\log K_1 = 12.9$ and $\log K_2 = 12.3$. These values were somewhat lower than previous estimates that had been based on calculations from the Fe–Tf constants.[3] The aluminium-binding constants are considerably lower than those for iron ($\log K_1 = 22.8$, $\log K_2 = 21.5$), suggesting that Al^{3+} is unable to coordinate with all the ligands at the metal-binding site. This conclusion is consistent with the smaller ionic radius of Al^{3+}. Nevertheless, since most of the transferrin molecules in plasma are not fully saturated with iron, the residual metal-binding capacity of the protein is considerable, amounting to about 50 $\mu M/L$. Therefore, without even invoking the need for plasma citrate as an aluminium chelator, transferrin alone has the capacity to carry not only all the aluminium present in normal plasma, but even the elevated amounts found in the plasma of haemodialysis patients.

Whilst aluminium has not yet been shown to have an essential role in normal body metabolism, the ability of transferrin to bind and deliver the element to cells and tissues, even those across the blood-brain barrier, has important implications in the aetiology of aluminium toxicity. An area of considerable interest at the present time is the possible role of aluminium in the pathogenesis of a variety of neurological disorders. These include not only the aluminium-induced encephalopathies such as those associated with haemodialysis or industrial exposure to aluminium, but also a range of neuropathies, including Parkinsonian dementia and Alzheimer's disease. The latter is a particularly insidious and ultimately fatal form of dementia affecting as many as 1% of the population. The possible association between plasma transferrin, the accumulation of aluminium within the brain, and Alzheimer's disease will be discussed in Chapter 10.

B. GALLIUM (Ga^{3+})

In nature, gallium is often found associated with aluminium in mineral deposits. In fact, the existence of the element was predicted by Mendeleef and called eka-aluminium before it was discovered in 1875 and renamed gallium. Like aluminium, gallium is extremely toxic and does not appear to have any role to play in normal body metabolism. The radioactive isotope Ga-67 is widely used as an imaging agent for a variety of soft-tissue tumours. Even though the radioisotope is usually administered as a citrate complex, once in the blood, gallium rapidly and avidly binds to transferrin.[4] The characteristics of the transferrin-gallium complex have been extensively studied by Harris and Pecoraro.[5] Two atoms of gallium, as Ga^{3+} ions, are bound to transferrin, one at each site. There is an obligatory requirement for bicarbonate. The binding constants have been measured ($\log K_1 = 20.3$, $\log K_2 = 19.3$) and found to be only slightly weaker than those for iron. The high affinity that transferrin has for gallium is at least partly due to the similarities in size of the two ions (Fe^{3+} = 0.64 Å, Ga^{3+} = 0.62 Å) and possibly explains why gallium is such a toxic element. It will readily bind to the free sites of plasma transferrin, which subsequently facilitates the movement of gallium across cell membranes using the same receptor-mediated mechanism as that for iron.[6] Tumour cells express increased numbers of these transferrin receptors in order to meet the demands for iron associated with rapid growth. This characteristic, in association with the known toxicity of gallium, has been exploited in the field of tumour therapy,[7] with the administration of gallium nitrate as a cancer therapeutic agent. The rationale behind this approach is that the gallium will be rapidly bound by plasma transferrin and delivered preferentially to the tumour cells, where gallium disrupts normal cellular iron incorporation and metabolism. An unfortunate and often frequent side effect of gallium therapy is gallium-induced anaemia. The transferrin-gallium disruption of normal haemoglobin production has been shown to be due to an inhibition of iron incorporation into the developing erythroid cell precursors.[8]

Because of the many chemical similarities between gallium and aluminium, gallium has frequently been used, particularly in the form of the isotope Ga-67, as an analogue of aluminium in order to study the uptake and distribution of aluminium within the body.[9]

C. INDIUM (In^{3+})

Indium (In-111) now has a widespread use in nuclear medicine as an imaging agent, particularly with the introduction of indium-labelled monoclonal antibodies. Previously, radioactive indium has been used as a method for the estimation of plasma volume.[11] The ability of transferrin to bind indium was first demonstrated by *in vitro* studies in 1969.[11] At plasma indium concentrations above 35 $\mu M/L$, transferrin becomes fully saturated and the indium then binds to other plasma globulins. The indium-transferrin and iron-transferrin complexes bind to reticulocyte membranes with an equal affinity, although the subsequent cellular uptake of indium is low (10%) in comparison with iron.[12] In a recent study it has been shown that transferrin binds a maximum of two atoms of indium,[13] and although the binding constants have yet to be reported, indirect evidence based upon metal-substitution experiments indicates that In^{3+} binds to transferrin with an affinity comparable to that of Fe^{3+}.

D. THALLIUM (Tl^{3+})

Thallium is one of the most toxic metals known to man, and although 90 years ago it was used for the treatment of night sweats in tuberculosis, its considerable toxicity was soon realised, such that today it has no place in modern therapeutics.

In vitro studies have shown that thallium (Tl^{3+}) binds strongly to both of the metal-binding sites of transferrin, with bicarbonate as the synergistic anion.[14] The radioactive isotope (Tl-205) has been used to prepare mono- and dithallium transferrin derivatives. [205]Tl NMR spectroscopy has proved to be a useful probe to monitor the occupancy of the metal-binding sites. NMR signals from the two sites are well separated and have indicated that thallium shows a greater affinity for the C-site than the N-site over a wide pH range.[14]

III. d-BLOCK TRANSITION ELEMENTS

A. SCANDIUM (Sc^{3+})

Scandium, as the lightest of the d-block elements, has not yet been shown to have any role to play in normal body metabolism. However, some degree of interest in the possible mechanisms by which scandium might be transported in the body was generated as a result of the discovery that scandium is produced *in vivo* from the decay of the ^{47}Ca that has been used in the study of human calcium metabolism. Radioactive scandium (^{46}Sc) has also been detected in the fallout following atomic explosions.[15] Following an earlier report that scandium (Sc^{3+}) binds to the globulin fraction of human plasma,[16] Ford-Hutchinson and Perkins[17] initiated a detailed *in vitro* and *in vivo* study. Within an hour following the injection of scandium into rabbits, 95% of the element was found to be bound to transferrin. Human transferrin was shown to bind two atoms of scandium, one at each of the two iron-binding sites. No evidence has yet been reported regarding the value of the binding constants, or whether the scandium-transferrin complex can be internalised by human cells.

B. VANADIUM (V^{3+} AND VO^{2+})

Whilst vanadium appears to be an essential element in some animal species (chicken, rat), its role in man has yet to be confirmed.[18] Far more is known about the toxicity of vanadium, and concern has been expressed regarding vanadium as an environmental pollutant.[19] The vanadium cation (V^{3+}) is unstable in aqueous solutions, becoming rapidly oxidised to oxovanadium (VO^{2+}). Chasteen et al.[20] showed that VO^{2+} binds specifically to both the metal sites of human transferrin. However, the anion requirements are slightly unusual. With oxalate as a synergistic anion, VO^{2+} binds to both sites even at pH 6.0, whereas at this pH, and in the presence of bicarbonate, the vanadyl ion is only bound to one site.[21] VO^{2+}–Tf complexes, by virtue of their EPR properties, have provided useful information concerning the conformation of the metal-binding sites. More recently it has become possible to prepare stable V^{3+}-transferrin complexes, and these also exhibit strict 2:1 metal/protein ratios, with an obligatory requirement for the bicarbonate anion.

Human plasma contains very little vanadium (0.1 nM/L), all of which is bound to transferrin. A two-way exchange of vanadium between transferrin and ferritin has recently been demonstrated.[23]

C. CHROMIUM (Cr^{3+})

Until 35 years ago, interest in chromium was confined to its toxic effects. However, the element is now considered to be essential for normal growth and development.[19] Although the precise role of chromium in human metabolism has yet to be elucidated, Cr^{3+} has been identified as an essential dietary factor for the maintenance of normal glucose tolerance. Blood plasma contains between 10 and 100 nM/L of chromium, of which more than 99% is associated with the protein transferrin.[24] The two metal-binding sites of transferrin each form a specific complex with one Cr^{3+} ion, and the requirement for bicarbonate appears to be absolute. The EPR spectrum of the chromium-transferrin complex clearly distinguishes between the two metal sites.[25] No other candidates have been proposed as transport vehicles for chromium in human blood.

D. MANGANESE (Mn^{3+})

Manganese was first shown to be required by plants and microorganisms more than 60 years ago. The essential requirement for this element by animals was demonstrated somewhat later. A number of human enzymes specifically require manganese, and these include enolase and pyruvate carboxylase, the latter containing four Mn^{2+} ions. Human blood contains between 100 and 200 nM/L of manganese, most of which is found within the red blood cells. The plasma manganese level is about 20 nM/L. Transferrin was shown to bind Mn^{3+} by Ainsen et al.[25] in 1969, with two atoms attached to the molecule, one at each of the specific metal-binding sites. During the last 30 years there has been considerable disagreement over which of the plasma proteins was principally responsible for the carriage of manganese in the blood. Not only have transferrin[26,27] and albumin[28,29] been proposed, but there was even an earlier suggestion that plasma contained a unique manganese-carrying protein, given the name transmanganin.[30] Within the last 2 years the situation has been clarified with the publication of a detailed study, both *in vitro* and *in vivo,* of manganese transport.[31] It now seems clear that transferrin is the major, and possibly only, plasma carrier protein for manganese, whether the element is introduced into the body orally or intravenously.

E. COBALT (Co^{3+})

The toxicity of cobalt-containing ores has been known for centuries, long before the element was discovered in 1735. Many of the salts of cobalt are highly coloured and have been used throughout history as pigments. Even in Roman times, the makers of vermillion took precautions against breathing its fatal dust.[19] Cardiac muscle is particularly sensitive to the accumulation of cobalt. The cardiomyopathy that follows industrial exposure to cobalt is associated with a very large increase in the level of this element in heart muscle cells.

Cobalt is a nutritionally essential element for sheep and cattle, since it is required for the synthesis of vitamin B_{12} by the microorganisms present in the rumen of these animals. Although humans will ingest small amounts of cobalt in their diet, over and above that which is already present in dietary B_{12}, there is no evidence to indicate that this extra cobalt is nutritionally essential. However, because of the similarities in size and electronic configuration of the cobalt and ferric ions, it is no surprise that transferrin is capable of binding and transporting cobalt. Ainsen et al.[25] have shown that human transferrin will bind two atoms of cobalt in the presence of bicarbonate. The binding constants were not reported. Whilst this characteristic of transferrin may not serve an important role in normal human metabolism, it probably explains how this toxic element is distributed to the tissues after accidental exposure to high levels of cobalt.

F. NICKEL (Ni^{2+})

Nickel is a relatively recent addition to the list of nutritionally essential elements. In a normal mixed diet, most of the average daily intake (0.2 to 0.5 mg) is provided from vegetable sources. The absorption of dietary nickel is poor (2 to 5%), a property that the element shares with iron. The precise biological roles of nickel have yet to be fully elucidated. Significant concentrations of nickel have been found in human nucleic acids.[32] In addition, a number of enzymes, particularly those associated with the reactions of ammonia and amide groups, are known to be metalloenzymes where nickel can substitute for other transition elements (zinc and manganese) at the active site.[33] Because dietary nickel is poorly absorbed, nickel toxicity from ingested food is very rare. However, industrial exposure to nickel and its compounds, particularly the volatile nickel carbonyl, is a far more serious matter. Nickel accumulation causes extensive tissue damage, particularly to the lungs. Skin hypersensitivity reactions are common, and there have been suggestions that nickel is a potential carcinogen.

The plasma nickel concentration is in the range 20 to 80 nM/L, but the mechanism by which nickel is transported in the blood has not been fully resolved. An early report[34] suggested that 40% of plasma nickel is bound to albumin, 15% to an unidentified small molecular chelator, and the remaining 45% to a unique nickel-transport globulin, given the name nickelplasmin. The molecular weight of nickelplasmin was estimated to be 70,000, a size not entirely dissimilar to that of transferrin. However, the ability of this molecule to bind elements other than nickel was not reported. Transferrin was first shown to bind nickel ions (Ni^{2+}) in 1969.[35] In a recent study by Harris,[36] human transferrin was shown to have the ability to bind a maximum of two atoms of nickel, with the characteristic requirement for bicarbonate. Binding constants were measured and found to be very low (log K_1 = 3.2, log K_2 = 2.5). A possible factor accounting for this low affinity is the divalent nature of the nickel cation. Nickel is unique amonst the metals that form complexes with transferrin in that the element exhibits preferential binding to the N-site.

In view of the low binding constants and the evidence that other plasma proteins bind nickel,[34] the contribution transferrin makes to the normal transport and distribution of nickel remains unresolved.

G. COPPER (Cu^{2+})

The vital and important roles played by copper in mammalian metabolism are well known and require no further comment. It is also well established that copper in plasma is found complexed to at least three transport vehicles — albumin, amino acids, and ceruloplasmin. Whilst albumin and plasma amino acids are thought to be the true copper-transport complexes, copper bound to ceruloplasmin is not exchangable *in vivo,* and this protein is best considered as a mobile store, regulating total body copper concentrations. In addition, ceruloplasmin exhibits a variety of catalytic properties, including a ferro-oxidase activity thought to be necessary for the oxidation of iron (Fe^{2+} to Fe^{3+}) before it is incorporated into transferrin. With this battery of well-characterised copper transporters available, there seems little need to invoke a role for plasma transferrin in the process of copper transport. Nevertheless, the binding of copper to transferrin has been the subject of considerable research activity over the last 40 years.

Less than 3 years after the discovery of transferrin by Schade and Caroline[37] in 1946, the ability of the protein to bind two atoms of copper in place of the iron was reported by Surgenor et al.[38] Bicarbonate is an obligatory requirement for the formation of Cu^{2+}-transferrin. Although the affinity of transferrin for copper is comparatively weak, these early spectrophotometric studies indicated that the number of ligands involved in the formation of the Cu^{2+} complex was less than the number required for Fe^{3+} binding.[39,40] Whereas iron binding is associated with the release of three protons, only two are released when each copper atom binds to the metal site. Much of the work that has followed has investigated various spectral properties of the Cu^{2+}-transferrin complex in an attempt to determine the mode of binding of the metal ions, the number and identity of the binding ligands, and the type of interaction, if any, between the two metal-binding sites. A variety of techniques have been used, including visible spectra and electron-spin resonance (ESR),[41] EPR,[42-44] and electron-nuclear double resonance.[45]

H. ZINC (Zn^{2+})

Zinc is a nutritionally essential element in mammalian metabolism. The body of an adult contains about 2 g of zinc and the element is distributed amongst all cells and tissues, functioning at the active sites of a wide variety of enzymes. Blood plasma zinc concentrations (15 to 25 $\mu M/L$) are very similar to those of iron. However, unlike iron, zinc is not susceptible to hydrolysis. Nevertheless, at neutral pH, and even in dilute solutions, zinc would be readily precipitated by the concentrations of bicarbonate in normal plasma. There is therefore a need for a mechanism to transport zinc in a soluble form.

Many studies in the early 1970s demonstrated that following the addition of [15]Zn to human plasma, zinc was bound to three proteins: albumin, α-2-macroglobulin, and transferrin. Evans and Winter[46–48] showed that dietary zinc, absorbed from the intestine, was transported to the liver in the portal blood, bound predominantly to transferrin. In the venous blood leaving the liver, most of the zinc was associated with either albumin or the α-2-macroglobulin fraction. The role of transferrin in zinc transport was challenged by Chesters and Will[49] on the basis that the zinc-transferrin binding constant that they had measured (log K = 5.9) was far too low to compete with albumin, whose zinc-binding constant was already known (log K = 7.0).[50] Furthermore, direct competitive studies between these two proteins for zinc seemed to support this conclusion.[51]

In 1983, Harris[52] reexamined the problem by attempting to estimate what the values of the zinc-transferrin binding constants would be at the concentration of bicarbonate in normal plasma. All previous estimates had been obtained at levels of bicarbonate far below those found in blood plasma. Harris concluded that transferrin was capable of binding two atoms of zinc (Zn^{2+}), one at each of the metal-binding sites, and that the binding of each zinc atom was associated with the release of two protons. The two binding sites exhibit slightly different affinities for zinc at pH 7.4 and 27 mM bicarbonate. The stronger of the two, the C-site, has a zinc-binding constant (log K) of 8.0, whereas at the weaker N-site the value is 6.6. From these results, Harris concluded that at the normal serum concentrations of albumin (19 μM/L) and transferrin (64 μM/L), 60% of the available plasma zinc would bind to albumin, whilst 40% would be transferrin bound.

Whilst it is clear that, unlike the situation with iron, transferrin is not the sole mechanism for zinc transport in the blood, there is now strong evidence to support the view that transferrin makes a significant contribution to the movement of zinc around the body.

I. CADMIUM (Cd^{2+})

Cadmium and zinc are similar in both atomic structure and chemical properties. The two elements frequently occur together in nature. However, whilst zinc is known to be an essential element, cadmium has no known function in human metabolism. Cadmium is extremely toxic,[19] and the very low levels that are normally found in plasma (0.5 nM/L) result from the intake of an element present in trace amounts in most foods. Apart from accidental industrial exposure, a further source of the element is from cigarette smoke, which contains significant levels of cadmium.

Cadmium binding to human transferrin was demonstrated by Pecoraro et al.[53] in 1981. The binding constants for cadmium were measured by equilibrium studies carried out by Harris and Madsen,[54] and found to be log K_1 = 5.95 and log K_2 = 4.86. These values are slightly lower than those for the similar divalent cation zinc, but this probably reflects the larger size of the cadmium ion. Transferrin binds two atoms of cadmium (Cd^{2+}), one at each of the metal sites, with the release of two protons for each Cd^{2+} bound. There is an obligatory requirement for bicarbonate. An important consequence of the cadmium-binding studies was the clear demonstration that an ion as large as cadmium (0.95 Å) is still able to enter and bind at the metal-binding sites of transferrin. Harris and Madsen concluded that since cadmium binding was not precluded by steric hindrance, the radioactive actinide thorium, of an equivalent size (0.94 Å), ought to be capable of being bound to serum transferrin. It was suggested that thorium might serve as a suitable analogue for the far more hazardous element plutonium.

J. HAFNIUM (Hf^{4+})

Hafnium is a toxic metal with no known biological function. The binding of hafnium to serum transferrin was studied by Then et al.,[55] since hafnium is thought to behave similarly to plutonium in its metabolism and its interaction with biochemical ligands of cells and tissues. As a substitute for plutonium in biological studies, the handling of ^{181}Hf as a β-emitter is far less restricted. Transferrin binds two atoms of hafnium (Hf^{4+}), one at each metal site, and the synergistic binding of bicarbonate is required in order to form a stable Hf–Tf complex.

K. PLATINUM (Pt^{2+})

Platinum is not an essential element in mammalian metabolism, and consequently plasma levels are extremely low (0.2 to 0.4 nM/L). The toxicity of platinum has been attributed to its ability to inhibit cell division. As a result, compounds of platinum have undergone a number of clinical trials in certain human malignancies — bladder cancer, ovarian cancer, and testicular cancer.[19] The binding of platinum to human transferrin was first reported by Stjernholm et al.[56] in 1978. The purpose of this investigation was to develop a more therapeutically effective means of delivering platinum to tumour cells by way of a platinum-transferrin complex. EPR examination of the complex indicated that the platinum ion was bound in the +2 oxidation state to both of the metal-binding sites of human transferrin. The *in vitro* binding of a variety of platinum compounds to human transferrin has been confirmed by Sykes et al.[57]

IV. LANTHANIDES

The first detailed study of the binding of the rare earth ions (lanthanides) to human transferrin was reported by Luk[58] in 1971. The lanthanides have no known biological function in mammalian metabolism. However, since most of the lanthanide ions are highly fluorescent, they have been used in many studies over the last 20 years as site-specific probes for the two metal sites of transferrin. Such studies have provided useful information concerning the following characteristics of the molecule of transferrin:

1.   Distance between the two metal-binding sites
2.   Interaction between the two sites
3.   Possible ligands involved in metal binding
4.   Influence of the size of different metal ions on the binding affinity (steric hindrance)
5.   Conformation and equivalence of the two sites

Some of the physical techniques that have been used in these studies include UV difference absorption spectroscopy,[55,58,59] fluorescence spectroscopy,[58,60] circular polarisation luminescence,[61] ESR,[62] nuclear magnetic relaxation dispersion,[62] and EPR difference spectroscopy.[59]

A. PRAESEODYMIUM (Pr^{3+})

Pr^{3+} is the largest of the lanthanide ions that have so far been shown to bind to transferrin. Luk[58] was able to demonstrate weak binding of one atom of praeseodymium, and inferred that the two metal sites of transferrin were neither identical nor equivalent, since one of the sites was unable to accommodate and bind the Pr^{3+} ion.

B. NEODYMIUM (Nd^{3+}) AND SAMARIUM (Sm^{3+})

Conditional binding constants for the complexation of both Nd^{3+} and Sm^{3+} by human serum transferrin have been reported by Harris.[63] Each element binds to both of the metal sites, but the C-site complex is thermodynamically more stable. The values of the site constants (Table 1) have been measured at very low concentrations of bicarbonate (0.2 mM), since at higher concentrations transferrin binding is severely inhibited due to the formation of lanthanide-carbonato complexes.

C. EUROPIUM (Eu^{3+})

Derivatives of human transferrin have been prepared in which Eu^{3+} replaces iron at either one or both of the metal-binding sites.[58,64] At low temperatures (77 K), two separate and sharp absorption lines have been detected by means of laser-induced fluorescence of the bound europium. The lifetimes of the excited states of the Eu^{3+} ions bound at the N- and C-sites are significantly different, and this has been taken to indicate charge differences of the liganding groups at the two sites.[64]

D. GADOLINIUM (Gd^{3+})

The ability of human transferrin to bind gadolinium (Gd^{3+}) was first demonstrated by O'Hara and Koenig.[62] Observed changes upon metal binding in both the UV absorption of ligated tyrosine residues and the solvent proton magnetic relaxation rates have been interpreted as indicating the binding of two gadolinium ions, one at each metal site. However, these studies were complicated by nonspecific gadolinium binding at pH 7.0, and by the complexation of the Gd^{3+} with the synergistic anion bicarbonate. In addition, the study also provided evidence for the involvement of a molecule of water at the metal-binding site. Zak and Ainsen[59] have independently examined the binding of gadolinium by transferrin, using an alternative analytical technique — EPR difference spectroscopy. They confirmed that gadolinium binds to the C-site of transferrin, albeit with an affinity that precludes the possibility that transferrin could bind Gd^{3+} in plasma. However, they were unable to demonstrate conclusively the binding of Gd^{3+} to the N-site.

E. TERBIUM (Tb^{3+})

Terbium binding to human transferrin was demonstrated by Luk[58] in 1971. The molecule binds two atoms of terbium, one at each of the metal-binding sites. It was noted that the fluoresence of the Tb^{3+} ions was enhanced by a factor of 10^5 upon binding to transferrin. This characteristic has been exploited in subsequent studies to measure the distance between the metal-binding sites and the identity of the binding ligands.[58,61,65,66] By measuring the energy transfer between an excited terbium ion bound at one site and a ferric ion bound at the other, the intersite distance has been estimated at 36 Å.[60]

F. HOLMIUM (Ho^{3+}) AND ERBIUM (Er^{3+})

The binding of two atoms of holmium and erbium to each of the metal sites of human transferrin was reported by Luk,[58] and has subsequently been confirmed by Pecoraro et al.[53] Of all the lanthanide ions, holmium and erbium, being the smallest of the group, bind most readily to transferrin.

V. ACTINIDES

A. THORIUM (Th^4), PROTACTINIUM (Pa^{4+}), NEPTUNIUM (Np^{4+}), PLUTONIUM (Pu^{4+}), AMERICIUM (Am^{3+}), AND CURIUM (Cm^{3+})

Every known isotope of the actinide series of elements ($Z = 90$ to 103) is radioactive, and the half-lives are such that only thorium-232, uranium-235, uranium-238, and possibly plutonium-244 could have survived since the formation of the solar system. All other members of the actinide group are short-lived radioactive isotopes that either arise during the natural process of radioactive decay of uranium and plutonium or are produced artificially (transuranium elements).

The ability of transferrin to bind plutonium was confirmed by Boocock and Popplewell in 1965.[66] The same authors[67] subsequently demonstrated that transferrin also bound americium, a product of β-decay from plutonium-241. It has subsequently been confirmed that plutonium (Pu^{4+}) follows similar metabolic pathways to the ferric ion in mammalian systems, eventually being deposited on bone surfaces or incorporated into the iron-storage protein ferritin. It has been confirmed that transferrin is the principal plutonium-binding protein in the blood plasma and the cell cytoplasm.[68] Because of the radiation hazards of the transuranium elements, particularly those associated with nuclear power and nuclear weapons, it has become increasingly important to study the distribution of the actinides in biological systems. Harris et al.[69] have demonstrated that thorium also binds to transferrin, and because this particular actinide is less hazardous than plutonium, it has been recommended as a suitable model for plutonium-metabolism studies.

Between thorium and plutonium in the actinide series are the elements protactinium and neptunium. Transferrin has been identified as the principal carrier of both of these elements.[70,71]

Finally, because of the extremely hazardous properties of curium, Cm^{3+} binding to serum transferrin has never been demonstrated experimentally. However, Harris[63] has attempted to estimate the likely binding constant for curium by extrapolating from the data obtained from the trivalent lanthanides neodymium and samarium. A value of log K_1 = 6.5 was suggested for both curium (Cm^{3+}) and americium (Am^{3+}).

REFERENCES

1. **Trapp, G. A.,** Plasma aluminium is bound to transferrin, *Life Sci.,* 33, 311, 1983.
2. **Martin, R. B., Savory, J., Brown, S., Berthoff, R. L., and Wills, M. R.,** Transferrin binding of Al^{3+} and Fe^{3+}, *Clin. Chem.,* 33, 405, 1987.
3. **Cochran, M., Neoh, S., and Stephens, E.,** Aluminium interaction with ^{67}Ga uptake by human plasma and transferrin, *Clin. Chim. Acta,* 132, 199, 1983.
4. **Clausen, J., Edeling, C. J., and Fogh, J.,** ^{67}Ga binding to human serum proteins and tumour components, *Cancer Res.,* 34, 1931, 1974.
5. **Harris, W. R. and Pecoraro, V. L.,** Thermodynamic binding constants for gallium-transferrin, *Biochemistry,* 22, 292, 1983.
6. **Larson, S. M., Rasey, J. S., Allen, D. R., Nelson, W. J., Grunbaum, Z., Harp, G., and Williams, D. L.,** Common pathway for tumour cell uptake of gallium-67 and iron-59 via a transferrin receptor, *J. Natl. Cancer Inst.,* 64, 41, 1980.
7. **Warrell, R. P., Coonley, C. J., Strauss, D. J., and Young, C. W.,** Treatment of patients with advanced malignant lymphomas using gallium nitrate administered as a seven-day continuous infusion, *Cancer,* 51, 1982, 1983.
8. **Chitambar, C. R. and Zivkovic, Z.,** Inhibition of haemoglobin production by transferrin-gallium, *Blood,* 69, 144, 1987.
9. **Farrar, G., Morton, A. P., and Blair, J. A.,** The intestinal absorption and tissue distribution of aluminium, gallium and scandium: a comparative study, *Biochem. Soc. Trans.,* 15, 1164, 1987.
10. **Wochner, R. D., Adatepe, M., van Amburg, A., and Potchen, E. J.,** A new method for estimation of plasma volume with the use of the distribution space of 113-In-transferrin, *J. Lab. Clin. Med.,* 75, 711, 1970.
11. **Hasnain, F., McIntyre, P., Poulose, K., Stern, H. S., and Wagner, H. N.,** Binding of trace amounts of indium-113 m to plasma transferrin, *Clin. Chim. Acta,* 24, 69, 1969.
12. **Beamish, M. R. and Brown, E. B.,** A comparison of the behaviour of 111-indium and 59-Fe-labelled transferrin on incubation with human and rat reticulocytes, *Blood,* 43, 703, 1974.
13. **Evans, R. W. and Ogwang, W.,** Interaction of Indium with transferrin, *Biochem. Soc. Trans.,* p. 833, 1988.

14. **Bertini, I., Luchinat, C., and Mesori, L.,** [205]Tl as an NMR probe for the investigation of transferrin, *J. Am. Chem. Soc.,* 105, 1347, 1983.
15. **Krieger, H. L. and Groche, D.,** The occurrence of scandium-46 in radioactive fallout, *Science,* 131, 40, 1960.
16. **Rosoff, B., Stand, F., and Spencer, H.,** Rare earth binding to serum proteins and nucleic acids, *Fed. Proc., Fed. Am. Soc. Exp. Biol.,* 21, 421, 1962.
17. **Ford-Hutchinson, A. W. and Perkins, D. J.,** The binding of scandium ions to transferrin *in vivo* and *in vitro, Eur. J. Biochem.,* 21, 55, 1971.
18. **Schwarz, L. and Milne, D. B.,** Growth effects of vanadium in the rat, *Science,* 174, 426, 1971.
19. **Berman, E.,** in *Toxic Metals and Their Analysis,* Heyden, London, 1980.
20. **Chasteen, N. D., White, L. K., and Campbell, R. F.,** Metal site conformational states of vanadyl human serotransferrin complexes, *Biochemistry,* 16, 363, 1977.
21. **Campbell, R. F. and Chasteen, N. D.,** An anion binding study of vanadyl (IV) human serotransferrin, *J. Biol. Chem.,* 252, 5996, 1977.
22. **Bertini, I., Canti, G., and Luchinat, C.,** Preparation and characterisation of the vanadium (III) derivative of transferrin, *Inorg. Chim. Acta,* 67, L21, 1982.
23. **Sabbioni, E., Rade, J., and Bertolero, F.,** Relationship between iron and vanadium metabolism: the exchange of vanadium between transferrin and ferritin, *J. Inorg. Biochem.,* 12, 307, 1980.
24. **Hopkins, L. L. and Schwarz, K.,** Chromium (III) binding to serum proteins, specifically siderophilin, *Biochim. Biophys. Acta,* 90, 484, 1964.
25. **Ainsen, P., Aasa, R., and Redfield, A. G.,** The chromium, manganese, and cobalt complexes of transferrin, *J. Biol. Chem.,* 244, 4628, 1969.
26. **Keeper, R. L., Barak, A. J., and Boyett, J. D.,** Binding of manganese and transferrin in rat serum, *Biochim. Biophys. Acta,* 221, 390, 1970.
27. **Scheuhammer, A. M. and Cherian, M. G.,** Binding of manganese in human and rat plasma, *Biochim. Biophys. Acta,* 840, 163, 1985.
28. **Nandedkar, A. K. N., Nurse, C. E., and Friedberg, F.,** Mn[' '] binding by plasma protein, *Int. J. Pept. Protein Res.,* 5, 279, 1973.
29. **Lau, S-J. and Sarkar, B.,** Comparative studies of manganese (II)-, nickel (II)-, zinc (II)-, copper (II)-, cadmium (II)-, and iron (III)-binding components in human cord and adult sera, *Can. J. Biochem. Cell. Biol.,* 62, 449, 1984.
30. **Cotzais, G. C. and Bertinchamps, A. J.,** Transmanganin, the specific manganese carrying protein in human plasma, *J. Clin. Invest.,* 39, 979, 1960.
31. **Davidsson, L., Lonnerdal, B., Sandstrom, B., Kunz, C., and Keen, C. L.,** Identification of transferrin as the major plasma carrier protein for manganese introduced orally or intravenously or after in vitro addition in the rat, *J. Nutr.,* 119, 1461, 1989.
32. **Wacker, W. E. C. and Vallee, B. L.,** Nucelic acids and metals, *J. Biol. Chem.,* 234, 3259, 1959.
33. **Dixon, N. E., Gazzola, C., Blakeley, R. C., and Zerner, B.,** Metal ions in enzymes using ammonia and amides, *Science,* 191, 1144, 1976.
34. **Nomota, S., McNeely, M. D., and Sunderman, F. W.,** Isolation of a nickel-α-2-macroglobulin from rabbit serum, *Biochemistry,* 10, 1647, 1971.
35. **Tsangaris, J. M., Chang, J. W., and Martin, R. B.,** Cupric and nickel ion interaction with protein as studies by circular dichroism, *Arch. Biochem. Biophys.,* 130, 53, 1969.
36. **Harris, W. R.,** Estimation of the ferrous-transferrin binding constants based on thermodynamic studies of nickel (II)-transferrin, *J. Inorg. Chem.,* 27, 41, 1986.
37. **Schade, A. L. and Caroline, L.,** An iron-binding component in human plasma, *Science,* 104, 340, 1946.
38. **Surgenor, D. M., Koechlin, B. A., and Strong, L. E.,** The replacement of siderophilin iron by copper, *J. Clin. Invest.,* 28, 73, 1949.
39. **Schade, A. L., Reinhart, R. W., and Levy, H.,** Carbon dioxide and oxygen complex formation with iron and siderophilin, *Arch. Biochem. Biophys.,* 20, 170, 1949.

40. **Warner, R. C. and Weber, I.,** The metal combining properties of conalbumin, *J. Am. Chem. Soc.*, 75, 5094, 1953.
41. **Aasa, R., Malmstrom, B. G., Saltman, P., and Vanngard, T.,** The specific binding of iron (III) and copper (II) to transferrin and conalbumin, *Biochim. Biophys. Acta*, 75, 203, 1963.
42. **Windle, J. J., Weirsema, A. K., Clark, J. R., and Feeney, R. E.,** Investigation of the iron and copper complexes of avian conalbumins and human transferrins by electron paramagnetic resonance, *Biochemistry*, 2, 1341, 1973.
43. **Zweier, J. L.,** An electron paramagnetic resonance study of single site copper complexes of transferrin, *J. Biol. Chem.*, 253, 7616, 1978.
44. **Froncisz, W. and Ainsen, P.,** The EPR spectra of copper transferrin complexes at 2-4 GHZ, *Biochim. Biophys. Acta*, 700, 55, 1982.
45. **Roberts, J. E., Brown, T. G., Hoffman, B. M., and Ainsen, P.,** Electron-nuclear double resonance of copper complexes of human transferrin, *Biochim. Biophys. Acta*, 747, 49, 1983.
46. **Evans, G. W. and Winter, T. W.,** Zinc transport by transferrin in rat portal blood, *Biochem. Biophys. Res. Commun.*, 66, 1218, 1975.
47. **Evans, G. W. and Winter, T. W.,** Zinc transport by transferrin in rat portal blood plasma, *Biochem. Biophys. Res. Commun.*, 71, 339, 1976.
48. **Evans, G. W.,** Transferrin function in zinc absorption and transport, *Proc. Soc. Exp. Biol. Med.*, 151, 775, 1976.
49. **Chesters, J. K. and Will, M.,** The affinity of human transferrin for zinc, *Br. J. Nutr.*, 46, 111, 1981.
50. **Giroux, E. L. and Henkin, R. I.,** Competition for zinc amongst serum albumin and amino acids, *Biochim. Biophys. Acta*, 273, 64, 1972.
51. **Charlwood, P. A.,** The relative affinity of transferrin and albumin for zinc, *Biochim. Biophys. Acta*, 581, 260, 1979.
52. **Harris, W. R.,** Thermodynamic binding constants of the zinc-human serum transferrin complex, *Biochemistry*, 22, 3920, 1983.
53. **Pecoraro, V. L., Harris, W. R., Carrano, C. J., and Raymond, K. N.,** Siderophilin metal coordination. Difference Ultraviolet Spectroscopy of di-, tri-, and tetravalent metal ions with ethylenebis [(0-hydroxyphenyl)glycine], *Biochemistry*, 20, 7033, 1981.
54. **Harris, W. R. and Madsen, L. J.,** Equilibrium studies of the binding of cadmium (II) to human serum transferrin, *Biochemistry*, 27, 284, 1988.
55. **Then, G. M., Appel, H., Duffield, J., Taylor, D. M., and Thies, W-G.,** In vivo and in vitro studies of hafnium-binding to rat serum transferrin, *J. Inorg. Biochem.*, 27, 255, 1986.
56. **Stjernholm, R., Warner, F. W., Robinson, J. W., Ezekiel, E., and Katayama, N.,** Binding of platinum to human transferrin, *Bioinorg. Chem.*, 9, 277, 1978.
57. **Sykes, T. R.,** In vitro binding of platinum compounds to human transferrin, *Res. Commun. Chem. Pathol. Pharmacol.*, 50, 387, 1985.
58. **Luk, C. K.,** Study of the nature of the metal binding sites and estimate of the distance between the metal binding sites in transferrin using trivalent lanthanide ions as fluorescent probes, *Biochemistry*, 10, 15, 1971.
59. **Zak, O. and Ainsen, P.,** Spectroscopic and thermodynamic studies on the binding of gadolinium (III) to human serum transferrin, *Biochemistry*, 27, 1075, 1988.
60. **O'Hara, P., Yeh, S. M., Meares, C. F., and Bersohn, R.,** Distance between metal-binding sites in transferrin: energy transfer from bound terbium (III) to iron (III) of manganese (III), *Biochemistry*, 20, 4704, 1981.
61. **Gafni, A. and Steinberg, I. Z.,** Optical activity of terbium ions bound to transferrin and conalbumin studied by circular polarization of luminescence, *Biochemistry*, 13, 800, 1974.

62. **O'Hara, P. B. and Koenig, S. H.**, Electron spin resonance and magnetic relaxation studies of gadolinium (III) complexes with human transferrin, *Biochemistry*, 25, 1445, 1986.

63. **Harris, W. R.**, Binding constants for neodymium (III) and samarium (III) with human serum transferrin, *Inorg. Chem.*, 25, 2041, 1986.

64. **O'Hara, P. B. and Bersohn, R.**, Resolution of the two metal binding sites of human serum transferrin by low-temperature excitation of bound europium (III), *Biochemistry*, 21, 5269, 1982.

65. **Teuwissen, B., Masson, P. L., Osinski, P., and Heremans, J. F.**, Metal-combining properties of human lactoferrin. The possible involvement of tyrosyl residues in the binding sites, *Eur. J. Biochem.*, 31, 239, 1972.

66. **Boocock, G. and Popplewell, D. S.**, Distribution of plutonium in serum proteins following intravenous injection in rats, *Nature*, 208, 282, 1965.

67. **Boocock, G. and Popplewell, D. S.**, In vitro distribution of americium in human blood serum proteins, *Nature*, 210, 1283, 1966.

68. **Lehman, M., Culig, H., and Taylor, D. M.**, Identification of transferrin as the principal plutonium binding protein in blood serum and liver cytosol of rats, *Int. J. Radiat. Biol.*, 44, 65, 1983.

69. **Harris, W. R., Carrano, C. J., Pecoraro, V. L., and Raymond, K. N.**, Siderophilin metal coordination. Complexation of thorium by transferrin: structure-function implications, *J. Am. Chem. Soc.*, 103, 2231, 1981.

70. **Taylor, D. M.**, Identification of transferrin as the main binding site for protactinium in rat blood serum, *Int. J. Radiat. Appl. Instrum. (B)*, 14, 27, 1987.

71. **Wirth, R.**, Identification of transferrin as the principal neptunium-binding protein in the blood serum of rats, *Int. J. Nuc. Med. Biol.*, 12, 327, 1985.

72. **Cochran, M.**, The competitive equilibrium between aluminium and iron for the binding sites of transferrin, *FEBS Lett.*, 176, 129, 1984.

73. **Donovan, J. W. and Ross, K. D.**, Nonequivalence of the metal binding sites of conalbumin. Calorimetric and spectrophotometric studies of aluminium binding, *J. Biol. Chem.*, 250, 6022, 1975.

74. **Cochran, M.**, Direct spectrophotometric determination of the two site binding of aluminium to transferrin, *Life Sci.*, 40, 2337, 1987.

75. **Hara, T.**, On the binding of gallium to transferrin, *Int. J. Nucl. Med. Biol.*, 1, 152, 1974.

76. **Tomimatsu, Y.**, Spectrophotometric evidence for perturbation of tryptophan in Al(III) and Gal(III) binding to human serum transferrin, *FEBS Lett.*, 71, 299, 1976.

77. **Chasteen, N. D., White, L. K., and Campbell, R. F.**, Metal site conformational states of vanadyl (IV) human serotransferrin complexes, *Biochemistry*, 16, 363, 1977.

78. **Bertini, I.**, Spectral characterisation of vanadium-transferrin systems, *J. Inorg. Biochem.*, 25, 57, 1985.

79. **Zweier, J., Ainsen, P., Peisach, J., and Mims, W. B.**, Pulsed electron paramagnetic studies of the copper complexes of transferrin, *J. Biol. Chem.*, 254, 3512, 1979.

80. **Aasa, R. and Ainsen, P.**, An electron paramagnetic resonance study of the iron and copper complexes of transferrin, *J. Biol. Chem.*, 243, 2399, 1968.

81. **Phillips, J. L.**, Specific binding of zinc transferin to human lymphocytes, *Biochem. Biophys. Res. Commun.*, 72, 634, 1976.

82. **Chesters, J. K.**, Zinc transport proteins in plasma, *Br. J. Nutr.*, 46, 111, 1981.

83. **Som, P.**, 97-Ruthenium-transferrin uptake in tumour and abcess, *Eur. J. Nucl. Med.*, 8, 491, 1983.

Chapter 6

THE TRANSFERRIN GENE — STRUCTURE, REGULATION, AND TISSUE EXPRESSION

I. CHROMOSOME ASSIGNMENT, GENE STRUCTURE, AND EVOLUTION

A. LINKAGE GROUP AND CHROMOSOMAL LOCATION

It has been the long-established aim of biologists to map the human chromosomes, and thereby to identify the positions and sequence of the individual genes that comprise the entire human genome. The methods that have been used to achieve this goal have changed dramatically over the last 40 years. Initially, the approach was to employ the classical genetic methods of the day, namely to follow the inheritance of characteristics controlled by two separate gene loci through a number of generations in a family. The closer together the two genes are on the same chromosome, the more likely that the two genes will travel together (linked) from one generation to the next. The further apart the two genes, the greater the probability that they will become separated from one another during the process of "crossover" that occurs at meiosis. In order to measure the recombination frequency between two selected gene loci, and thereby ascertain whether they are closely linked on the same chromosome, both of the loci must exhibit genetic (allelic) variation. This is necessary in order that individual allelic genes can be identified. By use of this procedure during the period from 1953 to 1970, the human genome map began to be unravelled, although at a very slow rate. In most of the cases where linkage between gene loci was established, it has not been possible to assign the gene locus to a particular chromosome.

A significant advance, and one that accelerated the process of gene mapping, was the development of the technique of somatic cell hybridisation. When cells from two different species (A and B) are fused, the hybrid cell frequently retains a complete set of the chromosomes from one of the species (A), whilst rejecting all but one of the chromosomes from the other species (B). When the hybrid cells are grown in culture, many of the gene products coded for by the single chromosome from species B are synthesised along with a full complement of species A proteins. If two or more B-specific gene products can be identified, then it can be assumed with reasonable certainty that the loci involved must be located on the same chromosome. Furthermore, if the identity of the single chromosome from species B could be ascertained, then the B species linkage group could be assigned to a particular chromosome. Somatic cell hybridisation experiments made a significant contribution to the task of mapping the human genome. By the middle of the 1970s the human chromosome map had about 70 gene loci located.

On a conservative estimate, the human genome, with its 3×10^9 nucleotides, probably codes for a repertoire of about 30,000 different proteins. This implies a minimum of 30,000 structural gene loci. Clearly, in order to map the remaining 99.75% of the structural gene loci, a major technological advance was required. In the last 10 years new techniques have become available to the molecular biologist, particularly in the area of genetic engineering, which have made the prospect of mapping the entire human genome a distinct possibility. Gene-specific probes, cloned from genomic DNA or synthesised from mRNA, can be used to directly "stain" individual chromosomes in an attempt to answer the question, Is the gene locus for protein X present on this particular chromosome? Furthermore, the techniques of DNA nucleotide sequencing have become available, routine, and susceptible to automation. This now makes it possible, setting aside the financial implications, to sequence the entire human genome.

Genetic (allelic) variation of human transferrin was first reported in 1957.[1] Linkage between the gene locus for transferrin and the gene locus for the plasma enzyme cholinesterase E_1 was established 9 years later using the method of recombinant-frequency analysis.[2] This was one of the first linkage relationships to be established in man. A further 16 years elapsed before a third member was added to this linkage group, namely the gene locus for the copper-containing protein ceruloplasmin.[3] Neither the order of these three gene loci (transferrin, ceruloplasmin, cholinesterase E_1) nor their chromosomal locations could be determined on the evidence available at that time.

However, in the meantime the techniques of gene cloning had been developed and were being applied to the problem of human transferrin. Yang et al.[4] were able to construct a 17-mer oligonucleotide probe based on the known amino acid sequence of human transferrin. The region selected was from amino acids 309 to 314, since this sequence contained two methionine residues, an amino acid that is coded for by a single unique triplet codon. The labelled oligonucleotide was used to probe a cDNA library constructed from human liver mRNA. From this library, a 2.3-kb human transferrin cDNA was isolated and sequenced. The characteristics of human transferrin cDNA will be described in the next section.

Radiolabelled transferrin cDNA has been utilised for chromosomal mapping by *in situ* hybridisation on human mitotic chromosome spreads and somatic cell hybrids.[4] The human transferrin gene is located on the long arm of chromosome 3 in the region 3q21-25. Genes coding for two other members of the transferrin family are also located on the long arm of chromosome 3. The human lactoferrin gene has been mapped at 3q21-23[5] and the gene for the melanoma antigen (p97) at 3q28-29.[6] The extensive amino acid sequence homology between these three iron-binding proteins has already been discussed, and the proximity of their genes on chromosome 3 is further evidence supporting the hypothesis that they have evolved from a common ancestral gene by a process of gene duplication. Within the same gene cluster on chromosome 3, the gene locus for the cell membrane transferrin receptor has been mapped at 3q22-26.[7,8] Although the transferrin molecule and the transferrin receptor protein can be considered, in some respects, to be functionally related in that part of one molecule must be able to recognise part of the other (ligand-receptor binding), there is no suggestion that the two gene loci are evolutionarily related or that the synthesis of their respective gene products are in any way coordinated.

The transferrin gene is also closely linked to two other genes encoding proteins that bind metals, ceruloplasmin that binds copper, and α_2-human

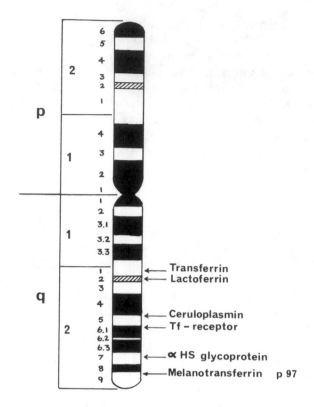

FIGURE 1.   The regional assignment of transferrin-related genes on human chromosome 3.

serum glycoprotein (AHSG) that binds calcium and barium. Neither protein is homologous to transferrin. The ceruloplasmin gene has been mapped to 3q25[9] and the AHSG gene to 3q27-29.[10] The locations of the six gene loci are shown diagrammatically in Figure 1.

B. TRANSFERRIN cDNA STRUCTURE

In February 1984, Uzan et al.[11] reported the first successful isolation and sequencing of a human transferrin cDNA. The molecule was approximately 1000 bp in length, and from its sequence it was deduced that the cDNA corresponded to that part of the transferrin mRNA that coded for approximately 40% of the transferrin protein — residue 403 to the C-terminal amino acid at position 679. There was an additional 3′ noncoding region of 166 nucleotides.

Yang et al.,[4] 3 months later, published the complete nucleotide sequence of a 2324-bp cDNA, encoding the entire transferrin protein. The primary structure of plasma transferrin consists of 679 amino acid residues, and this is encoded, within a single reading frame, by a sequence of 2037 nucleotides starting with a GTC triplet for the N-terminal valine, and ending with a CCT

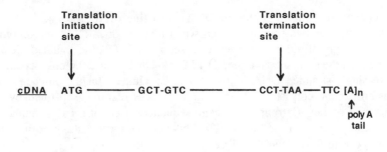

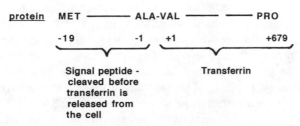

FIGURE 2. Human transferrin cDNA structure (simplified).

triplet for the C-terminal proline (Figure 2). At the 3′ end of the coding sequence of the cDNA, CCT is immediately followed by the full-stop codon TAA. The cDNA molecule then continues with a further 54 nucleotides, terminating with a poly-A tail. At the 5′ end of the cDNA, a methionine-initiation codon (ATG) is located 19 triplets upstream of the N-terminal valine codon (GTC). Initiation of protein synthesis at the ATG codon results in the production of a transferrin molecule with an extra 19-amino acid sequence at the N-terminal end of the protein. Before secretion of the transferrin into the bloodstream occurs, this signal peptide is excised by proteolytic digestion.[12] The shortening of the initial translation product (698 amino acids) is obligatory, since inhibition of this event prevents the secretion of the mature transferrin protein (679 amino acids) by the liver cells. It has been suggested that the 19-residue signal sequence is necessary for the proper translocation of the mRNA-ribosome-transferrin complex from the cytoplasm to the endoplasmic reticulum in preparation for the addition of the oligosaccharide chains.[13] A similar 3′-flanking region, coding for a 19-residue signal peptide, has been detected in the cDNAs for chicken ovotransferrin[14] and frog transferrin.[15]

C. TRANSFERRIN GENE STRUCTURE

A protein composed of 679 amino acids plus an additional 19-residue leader sequence requires an mRNA molecule containing a minimum of 2094 nucleotides. This implies that the transferrin gene, excluding any regulatory elements, must contain a similar number of bases. The first transferrin gene to be cloned from a genomic DNA library was that for chicken ovotransferrin. Cochet et al.[16] cloned the gene and discovered that the entire coding sequence was contained within a stretch of DNA consisting of 10,300 bp. This discrepancy in size was soon explained when hybrids of mRNA and genomic DNA were visualised by electron microscopy. The picture obtained clearly showed that the structure consisted of 17 RNA-DNA hybrid regions, separated by 16 single-stranded DNA loops. It was concluded that the chicken ovotransferrin gene consists of 17 coding sequences (exons), separated by 16 noncoding regions (introns). The exon sequences account for less than 25% of the entire gene. At the time (1979), this was the most striking example of a split gene to have been described.

The first reports of a partial structure of the human transferrin gene appeared in 1985. Park et al.[17] utilised two different cDNA probes to detect, and subsequently isolate and sequence, two overlapping genomic DNA clones. The genomic DNA region extended over a 24,000-bp sequence. Despite the large size of the polynucleotide, it was found to be responsible for encoding only 70% of the amino acid sequence of human transferrin. When the sequence was compared with the established sequence of transferrin mRNA, it was concluded that this particular fragment of the transferrin gene contained 12 exons and 13 introns. By analogy with the chicken transferrin gene, the 12 exons corresponded to exon 3 through to exon 14. Whilst the lengths of these 12 analogous exons are very similar in both genes, the intron sequences within the human gene are considerably longer. A larger fragment of the transferrin gene was subsequently isolated,[18] and this was shown to extend from exon 3 through to the final exon 17. In 1983, Adrian et al.[19] published the evidence that completed the final parts of the jigsaw, namely the nucleotide sequence of a 14,000-bp genomic DNA fragment that contained the first eight exons of the human transferrin gene. In addition, this particular length of DNA contained a 3600-bp sequence upstream (5') from the initiation site.

By 1986, the complete sequence of the human transferrin gene could be deduced by piecing together published sequences from three overlapping genomic fragments.[17-19] The sequence of the entire gene was confirmed independently in 1987 by Schaeffer et al.[20] with the characterisation of four overlapping fragments that encompassed the complete coding region of the human transferrin gene. The gene consists of 33,500 bp, organised into 17 exons separated by 16 noncoding intron sequences. Their sizes and positions are shown in Figure 3 and Table 1. Exon 1 contains the coding sequence for the first 15 amino acids of the signal peptide. The remaining four residues of the signal peptide are coded by the first four triplets of exon 2. The last exon (number 17) codes for the terminal 19 amino acids of transferrin as well as an untranslated region at the end of the mRNA, finishing with the poly-A tail.

The picture of the human transferrin gene is not only complete with respect to both the exon and intron sequences, but in addition, a considerable length of the 5'-flanking region, upstream of the initiation site, has now been sequenced.[21] It is likely that the 5'-flanking region contains not only the common promoter sites, such as TATA and GC boxes, but also contains nucleotide sequences that respond to a range of cellular factors that regulate transferrin

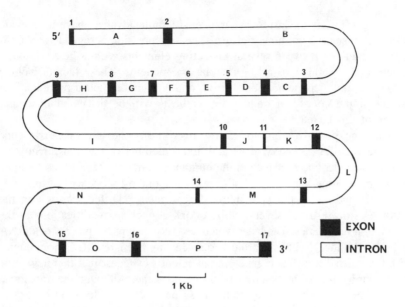

FIGURE 3. The human transferrin gene (drawn to scale), showing the positions and sizes of the exons and introns.

TABLE 1
The Structure of the Human Transferrin Gene

Exon	Number of bases	Region of amino acid sequence	Intron	Number of bases
1	93	−19 to −5	A	2100
2	173	−4 to 53	B	5000
3	106	54 to 90	C	750
4	177	91 to 149	D	685
5	133	150 to 193	E	810
6	56	194 to 212	F	675
7	179	213 to 271	G	765
8	178	272 to 331	H	1070
9	155	332 to 382	I	4900
10	94	383 to 414	J	900
11	33	415 to 425	K	1300
12	156	426 to 477	L	1400
13	136	478 to 522	M	2400
14	65	523 to 544	N	5300
15	185	545 to 605	O	1600
16	190	606 to 660	P	2600
17	206	661 to 679		

gene expression. In the last few years, considerable advances have been made in our understanding of how transferrin gene expression is regulated by multiple interactions between several *cis*-acting elements within the 5'-flanking region, and several *trans*-acting cellular components. These factors include steroid and polypeptide hormones, iron, and a range of nuclear proteins. The subject of the control of transferrin synthesis will be discussed in a later section of this chapter.

One unexpected finding to emerge from the studies on transferrin gene structure was the discovery of an additional member of the transferrin gene family. A nucleotide sequence in the human genome has been found to show considerable homology (72%) with the corresponding sequences of exons 7, 8, 9, 10, and 12 of the human transferrin gene.[20] Differences within the reading frame result in several stop codons as well as modifications at the exon-intron boundaries. The latter would severely disrupt the process of mRNA splicing. Although only a partial sequence has been reported, homologies with the normal transferrin gene are sufficient to suggest that this new gene is a "nonprocessed" human transferrin pseudogene. Although the transferrin pseudogene has been mapped to chromosome 3, its exact location in respect to the other members of the transferrin family whose gene loci are on the same chromosome (Figure 1) has not yet been identified.[22]

D. EVOLUTION OF THE TRANSFERRIN GENE

In earlier chapters reference has been made to the extensive amino acid sequence homology, not only between the two lobes of the transferrin protein (N and C), but also between the various members of the siderophilin family — plasma transferrin, lactoferrin, and melanoma-associated antigen p97. Even in the absence of any data on the structure of the respective genes, it has been postulated that the modern-day transferrin protein has arisen by a process of gene duplication from an ancestral gene coding for a protein containing approximately 350 amino acids, and with a molecular weight (40,000) of about half of its present-day counterpart. Now that the nucleotide sequence of the transferrin gene and the intron/exon structure is known, it is possible to suggest how a process of gene duplication might have given rise to the human transferrin gene.

From the gene structure, it is clear that certain pairs of exons exhibit considerable homology both in terms of their size and nucleotide sequence. Of the 17 exons, the following pairs share structural and functional homology: 2/9, 3/10, 5/13, 6/14, 7/15, and 8/16. Exon 1 codes for the first 15 amino acids of the 19-residue signal peptide, and would therefore not be expected to have a counterpart in the C-lobe of transferrin. Exon 17 codes for part of the nontranslated region of the mRNA, ending in the poly-A tail. Again, this particular exon would not be expected to be present in the N-lobe part of the gene. A simple model suggesting a possible origin for the present-day transferrin gene is depicted in Figure 4. Under this scheme it is proposed that an ancestral gene, coding for a 40,000-M.W. protein, contained nine exon sequences (1 to 9), with the first exon encoding the signal peptide and the last

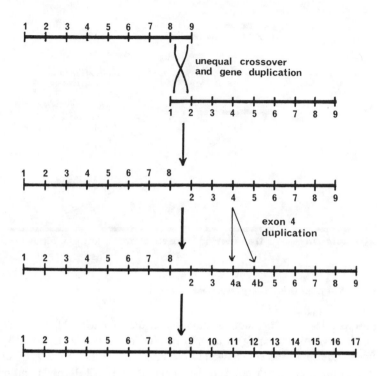

FIGURE 4. A possible mechanism by which the present day transferrin gene (17 exons) evolved from a smaller ancestral precursor (9 exons) by a process of unequal crossover and gene duplication.

exon coding for the 3′-untranslated region of the transferrin mRNA. A gene-duplication event, resulting from unequal crossover between intron [1-2] and intron [8-9], generated a 16-exon gene. At a later stage in evolution it appears that exon 4 in the second half of the gene has become split into two smaller exons (4a and 4b in Figure 4) by a new intervening intron sequence of nucleotides. The final structure has resulted in an unequal distribution of exons between the two halves of the duplicated gene. The N-lobe region of the protein, including the signal peptide, is encoded by exons 1 to 8 inclusive. The C-lobe is encoded by exons 2, 3, 4a, 4b, 5, 6, 7, 8, and 9. These nine exons are now renumbered 9 to 17 (Figure 4).

The product of the duplicated gene locus is considered to be the ancestor from which all the members of the siderophilin family, including the recently discovered transferrin pseudogene, have subsequently evolved. Each individual gene locus will have arisen by a process of complete gene duplication and separation, followed by a series of independent mutations. Bowman et al.[10] have suggested a scheme for the evolution of these genes (Figure 5). Despite the differences that have arisen in both the intron and exon sequences of these genes, their encoded protein products have retained functional homology. In addition, the four gene loci have remained closely linked on the long arm of chromosome 3.

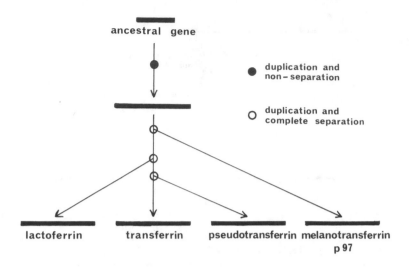

FIGURE 5.   A suggested route by which the genes of the transferrin family could have evolved.

Before leaving this short discussion on the evolution of the transferrin gene, it is worth returning to a topic briefly mentioned in Chapter 3. This concerns the small-molecular-weight proteins that are the products of a group of tranforming genes for chicken B-cell lymphomas (ChBlym-1) and human B-cell Burkitt lymphomas (HuBlym-1). The nucleotide sequences of these transforming genes, which in their activated states induce the development of cell and tissue neoplasia, have been determined. The ChBlym-1 and HuBlym-1 genes have been found to exhibit extensive homology with the nucleotide sequence of exon 2 from the human transferrin gene.[23,24] The proteins encoded by both transforming genes are small — 65 and 58 amino acids, respectively. The amino acid sequences of the two proteins are similar to the amino acid sequence at the N-terminal end of human transferrin. It is this homology that has led to ChBlym-1 and HuBlym-1 being classified as siderophilins, despite the fact that neither protein binds iron. Exon 2 encodes residues 1 to 53 in the N-lobe of transferrin. Its analogue in the C-lobe is exon 9, encoding residues 332 to 382. From the X-ray crystallographic analysis of transferrin, Bailey et al.[25] have mapped the areas of the transferrin molecule, encoded by these exons, to surface regions of the protein remote from the iron-binding sites. Bailey et al. have furthermore suggested that these exons might have originated in the transforming genes and have subsequently become incorporated into the transferrin gene by a process of exon shuffling. The polypeptide sequence could have retained a function that is independent of iron binding. The homology of the lymphoma-derived transforming proteins with part of the transferrin molecule has generated considerable interest and speculation. Transforming proteins possibly act by overstimulating cell proliferation. Transferrin has been known for many years to be an essential factor for cell growth and division. Whether the transferrin molecule fulfills this role by a mechanism other than supplying iron to cells is a subject of considerable debate. The growth factor role of transferrin will be considered in a later section of this chapter.

II. TRANSFERRIN SYNTHESIS AND TISSUE DISTRIBUTION, AND THE CONTROL OF EXPRESSION OF THE LIVER TRANSFERRIN GENE

The body of an adult 70-kg man contains about 17 g of transferrin. At any one time, only a very small proportion of this total will be present inside cells — either at the final stages of synthesis prior to secretion, or whilst passing through cells at some stage of the intracellular iron cycle (Chapter 7). The majority of the body transferrin content is equally divided between the intravascular (plasma) and extravascular fluid compartments. Since the volume of the intravascular compartment (3.5 L) is substantially smaller than the extravascular compartment (12.5 L), the concentration of transferrin is far higher in plasma (2.5 g/L) than in any of the other body fluids in which it has been detected — interstitial fluid, cerebrospinal fluid, pleural fluid, tears, seminal plasma, milk, amniotic fluid, and bile.

Of the 8 g of transferrin present in the plasma pool, approximately 10% is catabolised in a period of 24 hours.[26] Only a small proportion of this breakdown takes place in the liver. Most transferrin catabolism occurs during the intracellular iron cycle whilst the molecule is delivering iron to the intracellular sites of iron storage or utilisation. Each molecule of transferrin spends between 7 and 15 minutes inside the target cell before being released back into the circulation at the cell membrane[13] in order to acquire and transport further atoms of iron. A transferrin molecule traverses many such cycles during its lifetime in the circulation (12 to 15 days). Whilst inside cells, most molecules of transferrin are kept separate from the proteolytic enzymes of the lysosomes by mechanisms which are only partially understood. Nevertheless, some molecules will not escape partial proteolytic digestion, and once damaged they are likely to be rapidly catabolised. In contrast to most other plasma proteins, desialylation has little effect on the rate of transferrin catabolism.[27] While desialylation of transferrin does occur *in vivo,* the protein can be resialylated in the hepatocyte and returned to the circulation.[28]

In order to balance the daily loss of about 1 g of transferrin from the plasma pool, an equal amount of transferrin is synthesised and secreted into the circulation each day.[29] The organ responsible for the synthesis of most of the plasma transferrin is the liver. This production occurs primarily within the hepatocyte cells, which have been shown to contain high concentrations of transferrin mRNA[30] as well as a significant pool of newly synthesised transferrin.[31] This intracellular pool of transferrin within hepatocytes is rapidly depleted when transferrin synthesis is stimulated.[32] Whilst the liver is unquestionably the principal organ of plasma transferrin synthesis, small contributions to the plasma pool will come from the many extrahepatic tissues that have been shown to be capable of synthesising transferrin. These sites include brain, lymphocytes, Sertoli cells in the testes, mammary gland, spleen, lung, heart, kidney, and muscle. Whilst the synthesis of transferrin at these nonhepatic sites makes very little contribution to the plasma pool, there is evidence that for some cells and tissues the ability to synthesise transferrin, independent of the liver, is of great importance. This is particularly true where physical barriers effectively separate the tissues from the transferrin in the plasma (blood-brain barrier, blood-testis barrier). Extrahepatic transferrin synthesis, its control, and physiological importance will be discussed in the last section of this chapter.

A. HEPATOCYTE TRANSFERRIN SYNTHESIS AND SECRETION

The pathway of transferrin synthesis within the hepatocyte cell starts in the nucleus with the transcription of the transferrin gene by RNA polymerase, and finishes at the plasma membrane with the secretion of the mature glycoprotein composed of 679 amino acids bearing two N-linked oligosaccharide chains attached at asparagine residues 413 and 611.

The initial transcript from the transferrin gene is a 33.5-kb RNA molecule containing both exon and intron sequences. Within the nucleus the 16 intron sequences are removed and the resultant mRNA (2.3 kb), with a 5' cap and a 3' sequence ending with a poly-A tail, is exported across the nuclear membrane into the cytoplasm. Translation of the mRNA at the ribosome begins at an initiation codon 19 triplets upstream of the codon for the N-terminal valine of the mature transferrin polypeptide. The primary translation product is therefore a polypeptide chain 19 amino acids longer than the molecule that finally appears in the plasma. This short N-terminal signal peptide is retained throughout the subsequent passage of the protein through the rough endoplasmic reticulum (RER) and the Golgi system, and it appears to be essential in order to direct the protein on this journey.[13] Before secretion of the glycoprotein at the hepatocyte membrane, the signal peptide is removed by proteolytic enzmes.[12,14]

The purpose of the journey through the RER and Golgi system is in order for the polypeptide to acquire the two oligosaccharide chains. N-Glycosylation begins in the RER, whilst the polypeptide is still attached to the ribosome, and follows a pathway that is common for all glycoproteins with N-linked oligosaccharide chains.[33] The process, shown schematically in Figure 6, starts with the synthesis of a lipid intermediate, dolichol-phosphoriboxyl-oligosaccharide, with the stepwise addition of activated (UDP) sugar residues. The lipid-linked precursor is then transferred to the polypeptide chain, in a reaction catalysed by a membrane-bound oligosaccharyl transferase. This reaction is extremely specific, and the transfer of the glycan chain only occurs at asparagine residues within a sequence Asn–X–Ser/Thr (Cys), where X is any amino acid except proline or aspartic acid. In the case of human transferrin, only two possible glycosylation sites are available (413 and 611), and both are utilised. Whilst still within the RER, the oligosaccharide chains are trimmed, with the loss of three glucose and one mannose residue.

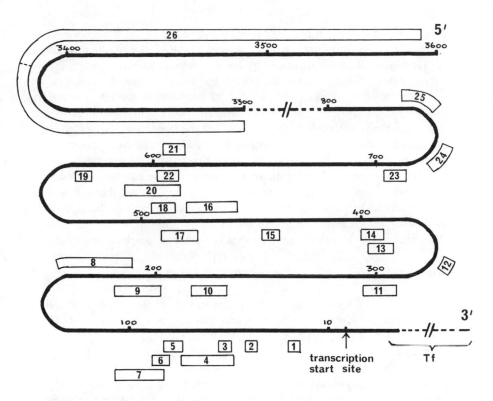

FIGURE 6. A diagrammatic representation of the 5'-flanking region of the human transferrin gene showing the location of the various regulatory elements referred to in the text. Sites: **1**, TATA box;[19] **2**, SP1 recognition site;[19] **3**, Metal-response element;[19] **4**, PR1 region;[40] **5**, Metal-response element;[21] **6**, Metal-response element;[19] **7**, PR2 region (CCAAT binding protein);[40] **8**, CR1 region (Tf–NF–1 factor);[40] **9**, Progesterone-receptor element;[21] **10**, **11**, Metal-response element;[21] **12**, DNA enhancer (*cis*-acting);[21] **13**, Metal-response element;[19] **14**, DNA enhancer (*cis*-acting);[21] **15**, Metal-response element;[21] **16**, DR1 region;[40] **17**, Cyclic AMP regulatory domain;[21] **18**, Homology with interleukin-2 and γ-interferon promoter;[19] **20**, DR2 region;[40] **21**, DNA enhancer (*cis*-acting);[21] **22**, SP1 recognition site;[21] **23**, **24**, **25**, Glucocorticoid receptor;[19] **26**, Upstream enhancer region, two functional domains.[83]

The next phase of the glycan chain synthesis occurs as the glycoprotein passes through the three sequential compartments of the Golgi system (*cis, medial*, and *trans* compartments). It is during this stage of the pathway that glycan heterogeneity is produced, affecting all parts of the branched molecule, with the exception of a core structure consisting of three mannose and two *N*-acetyl glucosamine residues. The modifications that the noncore parts of the glycan structure are subjected to result from the action of a battery of enzymes within the Golgi system. Some of these enzymes remove different sugar residues, whilst others add sugars to the oligosaccharide chains. It is at this phase that the common pathway for N-linked glycosylation that started in the RER diverges. At least four separate and structurally distinct classes of N-linked oligosaccharides, built on a common core, have been recognised:

a high mannose type, a complex type, a hybrid type, and a poly-*N*-acetyl-lacosamine type. It appears that the particular type of glycan chain acquired by the glycoprotein is influenced by the polypeptide moiety itself.[12] Transferrin contains two glycans of the complex class. However, even within the complex class, the degree of branching and the nature of the terminal sugars can vary extensively. In the case of transferrin, each of the two glycans can have either two, three, or four branches, but the biantennary structure is by far the most common. Whilst most of the newly synthesised glycans have branches terminating in a sialic acid residue, occasionally molecules are secreted where a branch lacks sialic acid, or more rarely a galactose or *N*-acetyl glucosamine residue.[12] The result of this variability is that there is no one single chemical structure that can accurately describe each of the molecules of transferrin that are secreted into the plasma at the hepatocyte membrane. The most predominant molecular species is a polypeptide chain of 679 amino acids bearing two biantennary, complex-type glycan chains, with each of the four branches (two per glycan) terminating in a negatively charged sialic acid residue.

The structural variability of the transferrin found in the plasma pool is further enhanced by additional posttranslational modifications that occur throughout the life-span (10 to 15 days) of the molecule. During this time, each molecule will be taken up by cells and recycled back to the plasma pool many times as transferrin fulfills its role as an iron transporter. Loss of sugar residues from the glycan chains, particularly the terminal sialic acids, coupled with amino acid side chain modifications (amidation, deamidation, oxidation), will further add to the microheterogeneity of the plasma transferrin. Although research has indicated that a considerable degree of control is exerted on the mechanisms of polypeptide and glycan synthesis, much of the microheterogeneity exhibited by plasma transferrin is likely to be the result of random processes over which the body has little control. The functional significance of the many molecular forms of plasma transferrin is still a matter of much speculation. There is some evidence that the proportions of the various glycan chain structures vary considerably in different pathological states. This subject will be discussed in Chapter 10.

The pathway of transferrin synthesis in the hepatocyte is typical of that for any glycoprotein destined for export into the plasma: polypeptide synthesis followed by oligosaccharide chain assembly, attachment and modification in the RER and Golgi system, signal peptide removal, and, finally, secretion at the plasma membrane. However, it should be remembered that the same cell (hepatocyte) is also able to synthesise the transferrin receptor protein. Evidence has recently been produced from experiments on human hepatoma cells[34] that transferrin and the transferrin receptor can interact during the process of biosynthesis. It is only those molecules of newly synthesised transferrin that have acquired iron that are capable of binding to the transferrin-receptor dimer. This interaction is thought to occur in the Golgi system at a late stage in the transferrin synthesis pathway. Neither the route taken by the transferrin-transferrin receptor complex from the Golgi system, nor the functional significance of these observations, has yet been elucidated. The case of transferrin as an example of the interaction between a receptor and its protein ligand during the course of biosynthesis is the first of its kind to be reported. It has been suggested that it may serve as a model for other situations where receptors and their corresponding ligands are synthesised within the same cell.[34]

B. CONTROL OF HEPATOCYTE TRANSFERRIN SYNTHESIS

The transferrin gene is present in the nucleus of all cells, and yet it is only within a limited range of cell types that the gene is expressed at significant levels. This tissue specificity is most dramatically demonstrated by means of measuring the concentration of transferrin mRNA in the cytoplasm of different tissues. Idzerda et al.[35] have reported the transferrin mRNA content of rat tissues as follows: liver, 6500 molecules per cell; testis, 114 per cell; brain, 83 per cell; spleen, 11 per cell; and kidney, 5 per cell. Clearly, intracellular factors must be operating within the hepatocyte in order to stimulate the tissue-specific expression of the gene.

Over and above this high background level of hepatocyte-specific transferrin gene expression, liver transferrin synthesis, and thereby the concentration of the protein in the plasma, is significantly affected by a range of extracellular signals. The best documented examples of these include body iron status and a range of hormones, particularly the steroids. The regulation of transferrin synthesis within the hepatocyte occurs at the level of transcription, and factors that stimulate synthesis, such as the steroid hormones, do so by enhancing the expression of the gene as evidenced by increased levels of transferrin mRNA. This is in contrast to the mechanism thought to be involved in the regulation of the synthesis of the transferrin receptor. In this case, control is effected at the level of translation by modulating the stability of the receptor mRNA molecules.

The effect of body iron status on the level of plasma transferrin was first observed over 40 years ago. Iron deficiency results in increased levels of plasma transferrin, and the measurement of this increase (total iron-binding capacity) is commonly used as an aid to the clinical diagnosis of the condition. The stimulatory effect of reduced iron levels on transferrin gene expression is confined to the liver gene, since transferrin mRNA levels in the brain, testis, spleen, and kidney are not enhanced when body iron stores are depleted. Pregnancy also results in an elevation of plasma transferrin levels. Whilst this was originally thought to be due solely to the iron deficiency incurred during gestation, there is now good evidence that changes in hormone levels during pregnancy directly stimulate transferrin synthesis. Lee et al.[36] have compared the effect of oestrogen and progesterone on the expression of the transferrin gene in chicken liver and oviduct. Whilst both steroid hormones induced a marked stimulation of ovotransferrin synthesis in the oviduct cells, only oestrogen was found to exert an effect on the liver gene.

In addition to oestrogen, a variety of other hormones, including cortisol and thyroxine, have been shown to increase the expression of the liver transferrin gene.[36] In contrast, the hormone glucagon decreases the rate of transferrin mRNA synthesis within the liver, and the secondary messenger cyclic AMP has been shown to cause a transient transcriptional inhibition.[37]

In order to define more precisely the mechanisms of action at the DNA level of the many factors that have been shown to affect transferrin gene expression, a detailed structure of the gene and its putative regulatory sites was needed. In the last few years, with the successful cloning and sequencing of the human transferrin gene, this has now become possible.

C. THE 5' PROMOTER REGION OF THE HUMAN TRANSFERRIN GENE, ITS SEQUENCE, AND POSSIBLE REGULATORY SITES

A substantial portion of human DNA immediately upstream (5') from the transcription-initiation site of the human transferrin gene has recently been cloned. The nucleotide sequence of the 620-bp 5'-flanking region has been reported by Lucero et al.,[21] and an even longer sequence, extending 1081 bp from the initiation site, has been published by Adrian et al.[19] It is very likely that situated within this stretch of DNA are the major regulatory regions of the transferrin gene. This would include promoters, positive and negative enhancers, regions conferring tissue-specific expression, and regulatory regions responsive to hormones and iron levels. The identification of possible regulatory regions has been the subject of extensive research over the last few years. The results from much of this work have recently been reviewed[11,13] and are summarised diagrammatically in Figure 6. In order to relate DNA structure (nucleotide sequence) with possible regulatory functions, a variety of different methodological approaches have been employed.

1. Nucleotide Sequence Homologies within the Promoter

Now that a considerable stretch of the nucleotide sequence 5' to the transferrin gene-initiation site has been elucidated, it has been possible to search the sequence for areas of homology with other known regulatory elements. Computer-aided searches of the 5'-flanking region of the human transferrin gene have revealed many short nucleotide sequences that closely match highly conserved regulatory elements associated with other mammalian genes. Lucero et al.[21] have identified a number of putative regulatory regions within a 620-bp sequence upstream from the initiation site. These included a TATA box close to the initiation site; two transcription factor (Sp1)-binding sequences; four copies of a putative metal (iron)-binding sequence sharing extensive sequence homology with similar regulatory elements in the promoter regions of the metallothionen gene;[38] a progesterone-receptor element; a glucocorticoid regulatory sequence; a cyclic AMP-binding domain; and several *cis*-acting DNA enhancers. In a similar study reported by Adrian et al.,[19] a longer sequence (1081 bp) was scanned for easily recognisable regulatory elements. Additional sites identified included three further glucocorticoid-binding sequences in the distal part of the promoter region, four copies (within intron-1) of the acute phase reaction signal CTGGGA,[39] and a 14-base sequence sharing extensive homology with regulatory regions of the interleukin-2 and γ-interferon genes. Whilst the identification of sequence homology does not provide direct evidence of the mechanism of transferrin gene regulation, it does at least indicate potential regulatory sites that can be further explored by alternative techniques.

2. DNase Footprint Analysis

A quite different approach to the identification of putative regulatory sites has been the technique of DNase-1 footprint analysis. This method works on the principle that regions of the gene at which regulatory proteins have been bound will be protected from digestion by the nuclease enzyme DNase-1. Brunel et al.,[40] using standard recombinant DNA procedures, have constructed plasmid vectors in which a 626-bp 5'-flanking region of the human transferrin gene has been ligated to the chloramphenicol acetyl transferase (CAT) gene from *Escherichia coli*. In this situation, the CAT gene acts as a reporter gene, responsive to the transferrin promoter. The constructed plasmids were used to transfect human hepatoma cells. Hepatocyte nuclear proteins were then isolated and tested for their ability to bind to the transferrin promoter and protect nucleotide sequences from DNase digestion. Five binding sites were identified (PR1, PR2, CR1, DR1, DR2), two of which (PR1 and DR1) were found to be essential for the liver-specific expression of the transferrin gene. From this and subsequent experiments, it has been possible to identify a number of *cis*-regulatory elements in the 5'-flanking region of the transferrin gene that by binding specific *trans*-acting factors (nuclear proteins) control the background level of expression of the transferrin gene in different tissues. The 3' deletion analysis of the transferrin promoter region, followed by transfection of the deleted vectors into hepatoma cells, suggested that the nucleotide sequence from -45 to -119 plays an essential role in the expression of the transferrin gene in liver cells.

3. *In Vitro* Transcription Following Site-Directed Mutagenesis

Using an *in vitro* transcriptional system, Mendelzon et al.[41] have recently reported results from a study of the liver-specific transcriptional activity of the normal 620-bp 5'-flanking region of the transferrin promoter, and the same promoter region after nucleotide modification by site-directed mutagenesis. Results from this *in vitro* study contrast slightly with those obtained by Brunel et al.[40] from *in vivo* experiments. The most significant difference was the observation that a TATA box and a nucleotide sequence capable of binding the liver nuclear protein Tf-LR1 are the only promoter elements needed in order to direct hepatocyte specific transcription of the transferrin gene *in vitro*. For *in vivo* transcription, additional promoter elements are required. Tf-LR1 resembles previously described liver nuclear proteins, variously labelled HNF-1, DBP, and LF-A1. The promoter-binding site for Tf-LR1 is in the proximal region of the 5'-flanking sequence and probably corresponds to the site PR1, described by Brunel et al.[40] (Figure 6).

4. Gene Expression in Transgenic Mice

A recent addition to the range of techniques used to study transferrin gene regulation has been the successful expression of human transferrin chimeric genes in transgenic mice.[42] Chimeric genes containing, respectively, 152, 622, and 1152 bp of the human transferrin gene 5'-flanking region have been ligated to the reporter gene CAT and introduced into the germ cells of mice. Different tissues from these transgenic mice were then tested for evidence of expression of the CAT gene under the control of the three different lengths of transferrin gene promoter. Transgenes containing the shortest of the promoter sequences (152 bp) were found to be poorly expressed in all tissues, indicating that the first 152 nucleotides of the promoter do not contain sufficient information to direct liver-specific expression. In contrast, transgenes containing the longer promoter sequences (622 or 1152 bp) were expressed at very high levels in both the liver and the brain, 1000-fold greater than in other mouse tissues. This observation suggests that information contained within the nucleotide sequence $[-152$ to $-622]$ of the transferrin gene-promoter region directs liver and brain transferrin gene expression. Adrian et al.[42] also investigated the effect of iron on the expression of liver CAT activity in these transgenic mice carrying different lengths of the transferrin-promoter region. Animals with the chimeric genes containing the longer promoter sequences (622 and 1152 nucleotides) exhibited significant decreases in the level of liver CAT activity following the administration of iron. This response mimics the decrease in plasma transferrin concentration seen in humans during iron overload, and supports the evidence from the sequence homology studies, namely that regions within the 5'-flanking sequence of the liver transferrin gene (heavy metal-response elements) can bind iron and thereby exert transcriptional inhibition on the adjacent transferrin gene. The mechanism of action of the metal-response regions within the transferrin promoter is clearly different from the homologous elements within the metallothionen promoter. In the case of transferrin, the binding of iron to these regulatory regions inhibits gene transcription, whereas in the case of metallothionen, the binding of zinc and cadmium to the metal-response elements stimulates mRNA transcription.[43]

The transgenic mouse model, as well as being used to study the expression of a chimeric gene (CAT reporter + transferrin promoter), has also been used to study the regulation of a complete transferrin gene. McKnight et al.[44] have injected the chicken transferrin gene, including substantial 5'- and 3'-flanking sequences, into the male pronucleus of fertilised mouse eggs. Many of the offspring were found to contain multiple copies of the chicken gene within their own genomes. Significant expression of the chicken transferrin gene was demonstrated, particularly within the mouse liver cells. In further experiments it has been shown that the chicken gene, when active in the transgenic mice, has retained not only those regulatory elements that control tissue-specific expression, but also the elements that are responsive to oestrogen administration.[45]

It now seems apparent that the expression of the liver transferrin gene is controlled by the interaction of a number of regulatory *cis*-acting elements within the 5'-flanking promoter region of the transferrin gene. This may be a reflection of the status of the gene — a highly conserved section of DNA, carefully tuned to respond to a wide range of physiological signals, including tissue type, iron levels, and several hormones. Regulatory elements in the proximal parts of the promoter region, responding to tissue-specific nuclear proteins, control the basal or background level of tissue expression. This would explain how a single copy of the transferrin gene in a liver cell nucleus comes to be expressed at rates in the order of 100 times greater than the same gene in the nucleus of other cells, such, for example, as the kidney.

In the more distal regions of the gene promoter, positive and negative regulatory elements, responding to signals such as iron and hormone levels, can further modulate the basal levels of gene expression.

So far the discussion on transferrin gene synthesis and its control has centred on one particular tissue — the liver. In the remaining sections of this chapter, the question of transferrin synthesis in nonhepatic tissues will be addressed.

III. TRANSFERRIN SYNTHESIS IN NONHEPATIC TISSUES, ITS PHYSIOLOGICAL ROLE, AND CONTROL OF EXPRESSION

A. MAMMARY GLAND

Mammalian milk contains two members of the siderophilin family — lactoferrin and transferrin. As has already been discussed in earlier chapters, these two molecules are the products of separate gene loci, they exhibit substantial differences in amino acid sequence and glycan structure, yet share the common characteristic of binding two atoms of iron. From the evidence on the structure of the transferrin and lactoferrin polypeptides and their respective genes, it seems clear that the two gene loci have evolved from a common ancestor. The relative proportions of the two siderophilins present in the milk of different species varies considerably.[46] Some examples are shown in Table 2. Human milk has a very high lactoferrin content (3 to 4 mg/mL), but contains only small amounts of transferrin (20 to 30 μg/mL). This situation is reversed in the case of both rats and rabbits, where the predominant iron-binding protein of the milk is transferrin and the lactoferrin content is negligible. It has usually been assumed that the structure of the transferrin in milk is identical in structure to that present in the plasma. However, an exception has recently been described in the case of the transferrin in mouse milk. The mouse is a species that exemplifies the intermediate category in Table 2, with approximately equal proportions of lactoferrin and

TABLE 2
The Transferrin and Lactoferrin Content
of Milk from a Variety of Mammals

	μg/mL		
	20–200	**200–2000**	**>2000**
Transferrin	Human	Mouse	Rabbit
	Cow	Guinea pig	Rat
	Pig		
	Goat		
	Horse		
	Dog		
Lactoferrin	Rabbit	Mouse	Human
	Rat	Guinea pig	
	Dog	Horse	
	Goat		
	Pig		
	Cow		

Note: Data taken from Reference 46.

transferrin in milk. The mouse milk transferrin, whilst having the same protein structure as the molecule in mouse plasma, differs from the latter with regard to the structure of the glycan chains.[47] There are no fucose residues on the glycan chains of mouse serum transferrin, whereas the milk transferrin, in common with the milk lactoferrin, contains fucose.

The tissue origin of the transferrin found in milk, particularly in those species like the rat where milk transferrin concentration is high, has been the subject of controversy. Early experimental evidence[48] implied that the mammary gland simply acted as a molecular sieve for the plasma proteins, and that during lactation transferrin synthesised in the liver was able to pass via the plasma into the milk. More recent experiments have refuted this suggestion. Jordan and Morgan[49] have conclusively demonstrated that mammary gland tissue slices from pregnant and from lactating rats are capable of the independent synthesis of transferrin. Furthermore, the process was quantified, and it was shown that during lactation the rate of transferrin synthesis by rat mammary gland epithelial cells was 1.5 to 3 times greater than that of the liver. Similar results have been reported for the synthesis of milk transferrin in mice, where it has additionally been found that transferrin synthesis by the mammary gland is regulated independently from that of other major milk proteins.[10] The control of expression of the mammary gland transferrin gene in rats is quite distinct from that of the liver gene locus. Grigor et al.[50] have measured the levels of transferrin mRNA in the liver and mammary glands of rats at different stages of lactation, and correlated this with the concentrations of transferrin in the plasma and milk. The studies were carried out on three groups of animals, maintained on different dietary regimes — high iron, normal iron, and iron free. It was found that whilst iron deficiency resulted in a significant increase in the levels of transferrin mRNA in the liver, leading to increased levels of transferrin in the plasma, there was no change in either the level of transferrin mRNA in the mammary gland or transferrin in the milk. These results are consistent with the milk transferrin concentrations and mammary transferrin-gene expression being independent of iron status. Although the transferrin gene in the mammary gland appears to lack the iron-response elements that are functional in its liver counterpart, the expression of the gene is nevertheless still regulated, probably by the levels of circulating hormones. During the period of lactation in the rat the levels of mammary gland transferrin mRNA and milk transferrin follow a biphasic pattern. Immediately prior to delivery the levels are high, but rapidly fall over the first 10 days post partum. The levels rise again at the later stages of lactation, when the rate of expression of the mammary gland gene is found to exceed that of the liver. Clearly, in those species where transferrin is a major milk protein, the capacity of the mammary gland to synthesise and secrete the molecule is of a similar order to that found in the liver. With this observation in mind, there seems little need to invoke the plasma as a source of milk transferrin.

Whilst the concentration of transferrin in human milk is relatively low in comparison to that of lactoferrin, the levels are nevertheless significantly higher in the milk secreted during the first few days following delivery.[46] The regulation of the human transferrin gene within the mammary gland awaits further study.

B. SERTOLI CELLS OF THE TESTIS

Transferrin synthesis within the testis was first reported by Thorbecke et al.[51] in 1973, and it was subsequently shown that the cells principally responsible for the synthesis of transferrin in the testis were the Sertoli cells.[52] Sertoli cells secrete most of the fluid component of the seminiferous tubules, thereby providing essential nutrients for the spermatids, spermatozoa, and dividing spermatocytes. The architecture of the testis is such that the tight junctions between adjacent Sertoli cells are thought to constitute a functional blood-testis barrier.[53] Rapidly dividing cells, such as spermatocytes, have a high demand for nutrients, including iron. If direct access to plasma transferrin-bound iron is denied by virtue of an effective blood-testis barrier, then local synthesis of transferrin by the Sertoli cells becomes of paramount importance. It has been suggested by Huggenvik et al.[54] that Sertoli cells synthesise and secrete transferrin into the seminiferous tubules in order to complete the bridge between plasma iron and the developing germinal cells.

Transferrin and the androgen-binding protein represent together a significant proportion of the total protein secreted by Sertoli cells, and they are known to be under independent hormonal control.[55] Most of the studies of transferrin synthesis and its control have been carried out *in vitro* using cultured Sertoli cells. Under these conditions transferrin gene expression is increased by a number of factors, including testosterone, insulin, follicle-stimulating hormone, epidermal growth factor, and vitamin A.[55,56] It has, however, been observed that the rate of transferrin synthesis by Sertoli cells in the artificial *in vitro* situation is significantly higher than *in vivo*.[57] Nevertheless, there is evidence from *in vivo* studies to suggest that the levels of transferrin mRNA in Sertoli cells are sufficient to account for a significant synthesis of transferrin under normal physiological conditions.[58] The importance of transferrin in seminal fluid, and its contribution to normal sperm development, has aroused considerable interest in recent years. There have been many reports demonstrating a correlation between the level of seminal plasma transferrin and both the number and fertilising capacity of human sperm cells.[59-61]

C. LYMPHOCYTES

In 1970, Soltys and Brody[62] discovered that human white cells were capable of synthesising transferrin, and that this capacity was confined to the T cell compartment of the lymphocyte fraction. Lum et al.,[63] 15 years later, and using radiolabelled transferrin cDNA probes, showed that the distribution of transferrin mRNA transcripts was restricted to one particular subset within the peripheral lymphocyte population — activated helper-inducer T4[+] cells. Neither transferrin nor transferrin mRNA are detectable in resting T4[+] cells, T8[+] cells, or B lymphocytes.

An essential feature of the immune response is the rapid clonal expansion of T4[+] lymphocytes. When T cells are activated, a cascade of events occur, leading ultimately to DNA synthesis and cell proliferation. Whilst many of the individual steps in the process have yet to be fully elucidated, some of the molecular changes that occur within the lymphocytes are known, and these include the expression of a plasma membrane receptor for interleukin-2 (T cell growth factor),[64] interleukin-2 synthesis,[65] and transferrin-receptor synthesis.[66] To this list can now be added the activation of the transferrin gene. Transferrin synthesis by T4[+] lymphocytes appears to be part of a normal autocrine reaction in which the growth factors and their respective membrane receptors serve as premitotic signals in part of the chain of events that lead to lymphocyte DNA synthesis and cell division. Lum et al.[63] have studied the timing of the expression of the four genes following lymphocyte activation, and from the experimental results have concluded that the sequence of gene activation is as follows: interleukin-2 → transferrin → interleukin-2 receptor → transferrin receptor. There is independent evidence that an interaction between interleukin-2 and its receptor is required before the transferrin gene can be fully expressed.[66] In addition, the transferrin synthesised by lymphocytes must also interact with its own receptor in order to provide successive stimulatory signals for lymphocyte proliferation.[67] This latter observation supports an earlier suggestion that transferrin may fulfill a role as a growth factor for both normal and malignant dividing cells, via a mechanism that is quite separate from its well-known iron-donating function.[68] The recent demonstration that areas of nucleotide sequence homology exist within the promoter regions of the genes for transferrin, the transferrin receptor, and interleukin-2[10] support this hypothesis.

Whilst the role of transferrin as a specific mitogenic signal is to some people still a matter of controversy, its essential role in delivering iron to proliferating lymphocytes is not in doubt, and has been well documented.[69,70] During the early stages of an immune response, following, for example, a bacterial infection, increased T cell proliferation, with an attendent demand for iron, is essential. It is likely, however, that the local concentration of iron will be severely depleted, both by the action of bacterial siderophores and the lactoferrin secreted by the host macrophages. The capacity of T cells to synthesise their own transferrin may therefore provide an essential source of available iron to support localised proliferation of lymphocytes.

Some years ago a report appeared suggesting that the molecule of transferrin synthesised by the T cells is structurally different from that of the normal 80,000-M.W. transferrin glycoprotein secreted by the liver into the blood plasma.[63] The lymphocyte version of transferrin appears to be a truncated version of the liver molecule, with a molecular weight of only 62,000. This reduction in size cannot simply be accounted for by an absence of glycan chains, and it was suggested that a shortened polypeptide chain was produced in the T cells as a result of an altered transcription from the lymphocyte transferrin gene.

D. NERVOUS TISSUE — CENTRAL AND PERIPHERAL

Transferrin mRNA synthesis in the human brain was first demonstrated in 1984 by Levin et al.[71] following earlier reports of the presence of the transferrin message in the brain of chickens.[36] The expression of the gene in the central nervous system (CNS) is confined to specific locations. In adults, the majority of the transferrin mRNA is confined to two sites, the oligodendrocytes[72] and the choroid plexus.[73,74] The cells of the choroid plexus, in particular, are capable of synthesising large amounts of transferrin, at least as much as liver cells on a per gram of tissue basis.[75] Additional sites of transferrin synthesis within the CNS include the thalamus, the medulla, and the developing neurones. Since it is the cells of the choroid plexus that are principally responsible for the synthesis and secretion of cerebrospinal fluid (CSF), it seems logical to conclude that the high concentration of transferrin found in the CSF has originated from the choroid plexus cells, and not from the circulating plasma. However, such a simple interpretation is made more difficult with the recent discovery by Tu et al.[76] that the cerebral distribution of transferrin mRNA exhibits a striking species specificity. Whilst demonstrating the presence of transferrin mRNA within the choroid plexus of mice, dogs, and rabbits, Tu et al., in contrast to other groups, were unable to detect the molecule in the choroid plexus of sheep, pigs, and humans.

With such conflicting experimental results, it is not surprising that the function of transferrin within the central and peripheral nervous systems is still the subject of considerable debate. The possibility that transferrin might have a special role to play within nervous tissue has recently been reviewed by Espinosa de los Monteros et al.[77] The presence of iron in the central and peripheral nervous systems is well established. However, the cellular distribution of the iron does not correlate well with either the distribution of transferrin[78] or the transferrin receptors.[79] Such observations have led to the obvious question: Do the cells of the nervous system obtain their iron from the transferrin present in the blood plasma by a selective transfer of the iron-laden plasma transferrin across the epithelial cells of the choroid plexus that comprise the blood-brain barrier, or, alternatively, is it just the iron that crosses the blood-brain barrier to be subsequently bound to the CSF transferrin that has been synthesised locally within the brain?

The presence and concentration of transferrin mRNA within the many different cell types that are found in the CNS vary considerably, and depend upon the particular stage of development of the animal, from embryo to adult. Early in embryogenesis, transferrin synthesis is particularly high within those cells undergoing active proliferation or differentiation; for example, neurons. Soon after birth the picture changes and the highest levels of transferrin gene expression are found associated with the oligodendrocytes, a specialised type of glial cell that is responsible for the formation of the myelin sheath around the developing neurones. Finally, in the adult the majority of transferrin synthesis occurs in the cells of the choroid plexus, associated with the blood-CSF barrier. It is the presence and possible role of the transferrin in the choroid plexus that has received much attention. Before the closure of the blood-brain barrier, an event thought to occur soon after birth, cells of the CNS have free access to the iron bound to plasma transferrin. Even once the barrier has been closed, there is evidence that transferrin produced outside the brain can still cross the capillary endothelial cells that constitute the blood-brain barrier, by means of specific receptor-mediated transport.[80] If this mechanism is both operative and efficient, why should the cells of the CNS continue to synthesise locally produced transferrin? At least three separate roles have been postulated. The experimental evidence and supporting arguments have been extensively discussed in a recent review.[77] In summary, the possible roles of the transferrin produced locally within the CNS are as follows:

1. To provide iron to cells deep within the CNS, where the blood-brain barrier prevents an adequate supply via the plasma transferrin. This is very similar to the argument that has been put forward to account for the synthesis of transferrin by the Sertoli cells of the testis.

2. To act as a specific autocrine signal for the process of neuronal differentiation and synapse formation, and also as an essential differentiation factor for oligodendrocytes. These events are postmitotic, and thought to be independent of the iron-donating properties of transferrin.

3. To fulfill the role of a premitotic trophic factor, stimulating cell division, both directly by supplying iron and indirectly by regulating the expression of other cellular genes. A trophic role for transferrin in the process

of lymphocyte activation has already been discussed in a previous section. A similar function for nerve-derived transferrin as a muscle trophic factor has received considerable attention over the last 15 years.

In 1979, Markelonis and Oh[81] isolated a substance from chicken sciatic nerve that was shown to promote the growth of muscle cells in culture. The substance was given the name sciatin.[81] It has now been shown conclusively that sciatin and transferrin are the same molecule. There is little doubt that transferrin is essential in order to maintain normal growth and development of muscle cells, both *in vitro* and *in vivo*. What has, however, been the subject of much controversy is whether the source of the transferrin is the blood plasma, or whether it is synthesised by neurones (sciatin) with their cell bodies in the spinal cord and subsequently secreted, following axonal transport, at the motor end plate. Ozawa[82] has recently reviewed much of the experimental evidence concerning the possible source of the transferrin supplied to skeletal muscle, and has calculated that nervous tissue alone would only be capable of supplying a very small fraction of the total amount of transferrin required by skeletal muscle, the majority being obtained from the tissue fluid surrounding muscle cells, by way of the plasma transferrin.

REFERENCES

1. **Smithies, O.**, Variations in human serum β-globulins, *Nature*, 180, 1482, 1957.
2. **Robson, E. B., Sutherland, I., and Harris, H.**, Evidence for linkage between the transferrin locus (Tf) and the serum cholinesterase locus (E₁) in man, *Ann. Hum. Genet.*, 29, 325, 1966.
3. **Weitkamp, L. R.**, Evidence for the linkage between the loci for transferrin and ceruloplasmin in man, *Ann. Hum. Genet.*, 47, 293, 1983.
4. **Yang, F., Lum, J. B., McGill, J. R., Moore, C. M., Naylor, S. L., VanBragt, P. H., Baldwin, W. D., and Bowman, B. H.**, Human transferrin: cDNA characterisation and chromosomal localisation, *Proc. Natl. Acad. Sci. U.S.A.*, 81, 2752, 1984.
5. **McCombs, J. L.**, Chromosomal localisation of human lactoferrin gene by *in situ* hybridisation, *Cytogenet. Cell Genet.*, 47, 16, 1988.
6. **Plowman, G. D., Brown, J. P., Enns, C. A., Schroder, J., Nikinmaa, B., Sussman, H. H., Hellstrom, K. E., and Hellstrom, I.**, Assigment of the gene for melanoma-associated antigen p97 to chromosome 3, *Nature*, 303, 70, 1983.
7. **Miller, Y. E., Jones, C., Scoggins, C., Morse, H., and Seligman, P.**, Chromosome 3q (22-ter) encodes the human transferrin receptor, *Am. J. Hum. Genet.*, 35, 573, 1983.
8. **Rabin, M., McClelland, A., Kuhn, L., and Ruddle, F. H.**, Regional localization of the human transferrin receptor gene to 3q26.2-qter, *Am. J. Hum. Genet.*, 37, 1112, 1985.
9. **Yang, F., Naylor, S. L., Lum, J. B., Cutshaw, S., McCombs, J. L., Naberhans, K. H., McGill, J. R., Adrian, G. S., Moore, G., Brandt, D. R., and Bowman, B. H.**, Characterisation, mapping and expression of the human ceruloplasmin gene, *Proc. Natl. Acad. Sci. U.S.A.*, 83, 3257, 1986.
10. **Bowman, B. H., Yang, F., and Adrian, G. S.**, Transferrin: evolution and genetic regulation of expression, *Adv. Genet.*, 25, 1, 1988.

11. **Uzan, G., Frain, M., Park, I., Besmond, C., Maessen, G., Trepat, J. S., Zakin, M. M., and Kahn, A.,** Molecular cloning and sequence analysis of cDNA for human transferrin, *Biochem. Biophys. Res. Commun.,* 119, 273, 1984.

12. **Schrieber, C., Dryburgh, H., Millership, A., Matsuds, Y., Inglis, A., Phillips, J., Edwards, K., and Maggs, J.,** The synthesis and secretion of rat transferrin, *J. Biol. Chem.,* 254, 12013, 1979.

13. **deJong, G., van Dijk, J. P., and van Eijk, H. G.,** The biology of transferrin, *Clin. Chim. Acta,* 190, 1, 1990.

14. **Thibodeau, S. N., Lee, D. C., and Palmiter, R. D.,** Identical precursors for serum transferrin and egg conalbumin, *J. Biol. Chem.,* 252, 3771, 1978.

15. **Moskaitis, J. E., Pastori, R. L., and Schoenberg, D. R.,** The nucleotide sequence of Xenopus laevis transferrin mRNA, *Nucleic Acids Res.,* 18, 6135, 1990.

16. **Cochet, M., Gannon, F., Hen, R., Maroteaux, L., Perrin, F., and Chambon, P.,** Organisation and sequence of the 17-piece chicken conalbumin gene, *Nature,* p. 282, 1979.

17. **Park, I., Schaeffer, E., Sidoli, A., Barelle, F. E., Cohen, G. N., and Zakin, M. M.,** Organisation of the human transferrin gene: direct evidence that it originated by gene duplication, *Proc. Natl. Acad. Sci. U.S.A.,* 82, 3149, 1985.

18. **Schaeffer, E., Huchenq, A., Park, I., Lucero, M. A., Cohen, G. N., Zakin, M. M., and Constans, J.,** Gene organisation and DNA polymorphism of the human transferrin gene, in *Protides of the Biological Fluids,* H. Peeters, Ed., Pergamon Press, Oxford, 1985, 131.

19. **Adrian, G. S., Korinek, B. W., Bowman, B. H., and Yang, F.,** The human transferrin gene: 5' region contains conserved sequences which match the control elements regulated by heavy metals, glucocorticoids and acute phase reaction, *Gene,* 49, 167, 1986.

20. **Schaeffer, E., Lucero, M. A., Jeltsch, J-M., Py, M-C., Levin, M. J., Chambon, P., Cohen, G. N., and Zakin, M. M.,** Complete structure of the human transferrin gene. Comparison with analogous chicken gene and human pseudogene, *Gene,* 56, 109, 1987.

21. **Lucero, M. A., Schaeffer, E., Cohen, G. N., and Zakin, M. M.,** The 5' region of the human transferrin gene: structure and potential regulatory sites, *Nucleic Acids Res.,* 14, 8692, 1986.

22. **Cohen-Haguenauer, O., Cong, V., Schaeffer, E., Zakin, M. M., Tand, M. F., Seroro, S., Stubnicer, A. C., Cohen, G. N., and Frezal, J.,** Chromosomal assignment of a human transferrin pseudogene to chromosome 3, Abst. 7th Int. Cong. Hum. Genet., Berlin, 1986, p. 618.

23. **Goubin, G., Goldman, D. S., Luce, J., Neiman, P. E., and Cooper, G. M.,** Molecular cloning and nucleotide sequence of a transforming gene detected by transfection of chicken B-cell lymphoma DNA, *Nature,* 302, 114, 1983.

24. **Diamond, A., Devine, J. M., and Cooper, G. M.,** Nucleotide sequence of a human Blym transforming gene activator in a Burkitt's lymphoma, *Science,* 225, 516, 1984.

25. **Bailey, S., Evans, R. W., Garratt, R. C., Gorinsky, B., Hasnaln, S., Horsburgh, C., Jhoti, H., Lindley, P. F., Mydin, A., Sarra, R., and Watson, J.,** Molecular structure of serum transferrin at 3.3 Å resolution, *Biochemistry,* 27, 5804, 1988.

26. **Morgan, E. H.,** Synthesis and secretion of transferrin, in *Plasma Protein Secretion by the Liver,* H. Glauman, T. Peters, and C. Redman, Eds., Vol. 4, Academic Press, New York, 1983, 96.

27. **Morell, A. G., Gregoriadis, G., and Scheinberg, I. H.,** The role of sialic acid in determining the survival of glycoproteins in the circulation, *J. Biol. Chem.,* 246, 1461, 1971.

28. **Regeoczi, E., Chimdemi, P. A., and Debanne, M. T.,** Partial resialylation of human asialotransferrin type 1 and 2 in the rat, *Can. J. Biochem. Cell Biol.,* 62, 853, 1984.

29. **Kernoff, L. M. and Baker, G.,** Direct measurement of transferrin synthesis rates in man using the ^{14}C carbonate method, *Anal. Biochem.,* 106, 529, 1980.

30. **McKnight, G. S., Lee, D. C., and Palmiter, R. D.,** Transferrin gene expression, *J. Biol. Chem.,* 255, 148, 1980.
31. **Vassy, J., Rissel, M., Kraemer, M., Fourier, J., and Guillouzo, A.,** Ultrastructural indirect immunolocalisation of transferrin in cultured rat hepatocytes permeablized with saponin, *J. Histochem. Cytochem.,* 32, 538, 1984.
32. **Heubers, H. A. and Finch, C. A.,** The physiology of transferrin and transferrin receptors, *Physiol. Rev.,* 67, 520, 1987.
33. **Sharon, N. and Lis, N.,** in *The Proteins,* H. Neurath, and R. L. Hill, Eds., Academic Press, New York, 1982, 1.
34. **Neefjes, J. J., Hengeveld, T., Tol, O., and Ploegh, H. L.,** Intracellular interaction of transferrin and its receptor during biosynthesis, *J. Cell. Biol.,* 111, 1383, 1990.
35. **Idzerda, R. L., Heubers, H., Finch, C. A., and McKnight, G. S.,** Rat transferrin gene expression: tissue-specific regulation by iron deficiency, *Proc. Natl. Acad. Sci. U.S.A.,* 83, 3723, 1986.
36. **Lee, D. C., McKnight, G. S., and Palmiter, R. D.,** The action of oestrogen and progesterone on the expression of the transferrin gene, *J. Biol. Chem.,* 253, 3493, 1978.
37. **Tuil, D., Vaulont, S., Levin, M. J., Munnich, A., Moguilewsky, A., Bourton, M. M., Brissot, P., Dreyfus, J. C., and Kahn, A.,** Transient transcriptional inhibition of the transferrin gene by cyclic AMP, *FEBS Lett.,* 189, 310, 1985.
38. **Stuart, G. W., Searle, P. F., and Palmiter, R. D.,** Identification of multiple regulatory elements in mouse metallothionen-1 promoter by assaying synthetic sequences, *Nature,* 317, 824, 1985.
39. **Fowlkes, D. M., Mullis, N. T., Comeau, L. M., and Crabtree, G. R.,** Potential basis for the coordinately expressed fibrinogen genes: homology in the 5' flanking regions, *Proc. Natl. Acad. Sci. U.S.A.,* 81, 2313, 1984.
40. **Brunel, F., Ochoa, A., Schaeffer, E., Boissier, F., Gillou, Y., Cereghini, S., Cohen, G. N., and Zakin, M. M.,** Interactions of DNA-binding proteins with the 5' flanking region of human transferrin gene, *J. Biol. Chem.,* 263, 10180, 1988.
41. **Mendelzon, D., Boisser, F., and Zakin, M. M.,** The binding site for the liver-specific transcription factor Tf-LF1 and the TATA box of the human transferrin gene promoter are the only elements necessary to direct liver-specific transcription *in vitro, Nucleic Acids Res.,* 18, 5717, 1990.
42. **Adrian, G. S., Bowman, B. H., Herbert, D. C., Weaker, F. J., Adrian, E. K., Robinson, L. K., Walter, C. A., Eddy, C. A., Riehl, R., Pauerstein, C. J., and Yang, F.,** Human transferrin; expression and iron modulation of chimeric gene in transgenic mice, *J. Biol. Chem.,* 265, 13344, 1990.
43. **Yagle, M. K. and Palmiter, R. D.,** Coordinate regulation of mouse metallothionen 1 and 2 genes by heavy metals and glucocorticoids, *Mol. Cell. Biol.,* 5, 291, 1985.
44. **McKnight, G. S., Hammer, R. E., Kuenzel, E. A., and Brinster, R. L.,** Expression of the chicken transferrin gene in transgenic mice, *Cell,* 34, 335, 1983.
45. **Hammer, R. E., Idzerda, R. L., Brinster, R., and McKnight, G. S.,** Estrogen regulation of the avian transferrin gene in transgenic mice, *Mol. Cell. Biol.,* 6, 1010, 1986.
46. **Masson, P. L. and Heremans, J. F.,** Lactoferrin in milk from different species, *Comp. Biochem. Physiol.,* 39B, 119, 1971.
47. **Leclerq, Y., Sawatzki, G., Weiruszerski, J. M., Montreuil, J., and Spik, G.,** Primary structure of the glycan chains from mouse serum and milk transferrins, *Biochem. J.,* 247, 571, 1987.
48. **Ezekiel, E.,** The iron-binding proteins in milk and the secretion of iron by the mammary gland in the rat, *Biochim. Biophys. Acta,* 107, 511, 1965.
49. **Jordan, S. M. and Morgan, E. H.,** Plasma protein synthesis by tissue slices from pregnant and lactating rats, *Biochim. Biophys. Acta,* 174, 373, 1969.
50. **Grigor, M. R., McDonald, F. J., Latta, N., Richardson, C. L., and Tate, W. P.,** Transferrin gene expression in the rat mammary gland. Independence of maternal iron status, *Biochem. J.,* 267, 815, 1990.

51. **Thorbecke, G. J., Liem, H. H., Knight, S., Cox, K., and Muller-Eberhard, U.,** Sites of formation of the serum proteins transferrin and hemopexin, *J. Clin. Invest.,* 52, 725, 1973.

52. **Skinner, M. and Griswold, M. D.,** Sertoli cells synthesise and secrete transferrin-like protein, *J. Biol. Chem.,* 255, 9523, 1980.

53. **Fawcett, D. W.,** Ultrastructure and function of the Sertoli cell, in *Handbook of Physiology: Male Reproductive System,* D. W. Hamilton and R. D. Grup, Eds., Vol. 5, American Physiological Society, Washington, D.C., 1975, 21.

54. **Huggenvik, J., Sylvester, S. R., and Griswold, M. D.,** Control of transferrin mRNA in Sertoli cells, *Ann. N.Y. Acad. Sci.,* 438, 1, 1985.

55. **Perez-Infante, V., Bardin, C. W., Gunsalus, G. L., Musto, N. A., Rich, K. A., and Mather, J. P.,** Differentiation of testicular transferrin and androgen-binding protein secretion in primary cultures of Sertoli cells, *Endocrinology,* 118, 383, 1986.

56. **Huggenvik, J. I., Idzerda, R. L., Haywood, L., Lee, D. C., McKnight, G. S., and Griswold, M. D.,** Transferrin messenger RNA: molecular cloning and hormonal regulation in rat Sertoli cells, *Endocrinology,* 120, 332, 1987.

57. **Lee, N. T., Chae, C. B., and Kierszenbaum, A. L.,** Contrasting levels of transferrin gene activity in cultured rat Sertoli cells and intact seminiferous tubules, *Proc. Natl. Acad. Sci. U.S.A.,* 83, 8177, 1986.

58. **Lum, J. B.,** Visualisation of mRNA transcription of specific genes in human cells and tissues using in situ hybridisation techniques, *Biotechniques,* 4, 32, 1986.

59. **Sveldo, C.,** Correlation of semen transferrin concentration and sperm fertilizing capacity, *Am. J. Obstet. Gynecol.,* 150, 528, 1984.

60. **Barthelemy, C.,** Seminal fluid transferrin as an index of gonadal function in infertile men, *J. Reprod. Fertil.,* 82, 113, 1988.

61. **Yoshida, K.,** Seminal plasma transferrin concentration in idiopathic oligozoospermia, *Urology,* 33, 395, 1989.

62. **Soltys, H. D. and Brody, J. I.,** Synthesis of transferrin by human peripheral blood lymphocytes, *J. Lab. Clin. Med.,* 75, 250, 1970.

63. **Lum, J. B., Infante, A. J., Makker, D. M., Yang, F., and Bowman, B. H.,** Transferrin synthesis by inducer T lymphocytes, *J. Clin. Invest.,* 77, 841, 1986.

64. **Robb, R. J., Munck, A., and Smith, K. A.,** T cell growth factor receptors: Quantitation, specificity and biological relevance, *J. Exp. Med.,* 154, 1455, 1981.

65. **Ruscetti, F. W., Morgan, D. A., and Gallo, R. C.,** Functional and morphological characterisation of human T cells continuously grown *in vitro, J. Immunol.,* 119, 131, 1977.

66. **Neckers, L. M. and Cossman, J.,** Transferrin receptor induction in mitogen-stimulated human T lymphocytes is required for DNA synthesis and cell division and is regulated by interleukin-2, *Proc. Natl. Acad. Sci. U.S.A.,* 80, 3494, 1983.

67. **Lum, J. B.,** Role of transferrin in cellular proliferation, Ph.D. thesis, University of Texas Graduate School of Biomedical Science, San Antonio, 1987.

68. **Seligman, P. A.,** Structure and function of the transferrin receptor, *Prog. Hematol.,* 13, 131, 1983.

69. **Brock, J. H.,** The effect of iron and transferrin on the response of serum-free cultures of mouse lymphocytes to concanavalin A and lipopolysaccharide, *Immunology,* 43, 387, 1981.

70. **Mainon-Fowler, T. and Brock, J. H.,** Effect of iron deficiency on the response of mouse lymphocytes to concanavalin A: the importance of transferrin-bound iron, *Immunology,* 54, 325, 1985.

71. **Levin, M. J., Tuil, D., Uzan, G., Dreyfus, J. C., and Kahn, A.,** Expression of the transferrin gene during development of non-hepatic tissues: high level of transferrin mRNA in fetal muscle and adult brain, *Biochem. Biophys. Res. Commun.,* 122, 212, 1984.

72. **Block, B., Popovici, T., Levin, M. J., Tuil, D., and Kahn, A.,** Transferrin gene expression visualised in oligodendrocytes of the rat brain using *in situ* hybridisation and immunochemistry, *Proc. Natl. Acad. Sci. U.S.A.,* 82, 6706, 1985.

73. **Block, B., Popovici, T., Chahman, S., Levin, M., Tuil, D., and Kahn, A.,** Transferrin gene expression in choroid plexus of the adult rat brain, *Brain Res. Bull.,* 18, 573, 1987.
74. **Aldred, A. R., Dickson, P. W., Marley, P. D., and Schrieber, G.,** Distribution of transferrin synthesis in brain and other tissues of the rat, *J. Biol. Chem.,* 262, 5293, 1987.
75. **Dickson, P. W., Aldred, A. R., Marley, P. D., Tu, G. F., Howlett, G. J., and Schreiber, G.,** High prealbumin and transferrin mRNA levels in the choroid plexus of the rat brain, *Biochem. Biophys. Res. Commun.,* 890, 895, 1985.
76. **Tu, G-F., Achen, M. G., Aldred, A. R., Southwell, B. R., and Schreiber, G.,** The distribution of cerebral expression of the transferrin gene is species specific, *J. Biol. Chem.,* 266, 6201, 1991.
77. **Espinosa de los Monteros, A., Pena, L. A., and de Vellis, J.,** Does transferrin have a special role to play in the nervous system?, *J. Neurosci. Res.,* 12, 125, 1989.
78. **Dwork, A. G., Schon, E. A., and Herbert, J.,** Non identical distribution of transferrin and ferric iron in human brain, *Neuroscience,* 27, 333, 1988.
79. **Hill, J. M., Ruff, M. R., Weber, C. B., and Pert, C. B.,** Transferrin receptors in rat brain: neuropeptide-like pattern and relationship to iron distribution, *Proc. Natl. Acad. Sci. U.S.A.,* 82, 4553, 1985.
80. **Jeffries, W. A., Brandon, M. R., Hunt, S. U., Williams, A. F., Gatter, K. C., and Mason, D. Y.,** Transferrin receptors on endothelium of brain capillaries, *Nature,* 312, 162, 1984.
81. **Markelonis, G. J. and Oh, T. H.,** A sciatic nerve protein has trophic effect on development and maintenance of skeletal muscle cells in culture, *Proc. Natl. Acad. Sci. U.S.A.,* 76, 2470, 1979.
82. **Ozawa, E.,** Transferrin as a muscle trophic factor, *Rev. Physiol. Biochem. Pharmacol.,* 113, 89, 1989.
83. **Boissier, F., Auge-Gouillou, C., Schaeffer, E., and Zakin, M. M.,** The enhancer of the human transferrin gene is organised in two structural and functional domains, *J. Biol. Chem.,* 266, 9822, 1991.

Chapter 7

THE TRANSFERRIN RECEPTOR AND THE CELLULAR UPTAKE OF IRON

I. INTRODUCTION

The role of transferrin as a vehicle for the transport of iron begins with the synthesis and secretion of the glycoprotein molecule by tissues such as the liver, continues with the acquisition of a maximum of two atoms of ferric iron, and terminates with the delivery of this essential element to a variety of body tissues. The stucture of transferrin, its physical and chemical properties, and the genetic and cellular control of its synthesis and secretion have been the subject of the earlier chapters of this book. The purpose of this chapter is to review current knowledge concerning the mechanisms of iron delivery, first to the cell membrane of iron-requiring tissues, and second to the intracellular sites where the element is either incorporated directly into iron-dependent systems (for example, enzymes and haem proteins), or becomes stored within the protein shell of ferritin. Much of the account will concern a specific cell membrane receptor that recognises and binds the iron-loaded transferrin molecule. If this interaction were to result in the direct uptake of inorganic iron across the cell membrane, with the concomitant release of apotransferrin from the receptor complex back into the blood plasma, then the role of transferrin would essentially be complete at this stage. However, as will be described in later sections of this chapter, this is far too simplistic a model to account for all the experimental evidence. In erythroid cells, following the initial interaction of the iron-loaded transferrin with the membrane receptor, the receptor-ligand complex is destined to become internalised by the cell and enters one or more intracellular pathways. These routes eventually lead to the release of the bound iron, the recycling of the receptor-apotransferrin complex back to the cell membrane, the splitting of the complex, and finally the return of the receptor into the membrane and the release of the apotransferrin into the intracellular fluids. Hence both the receptor and the transferrin molecules are reusable. From the evolutionary aspect, the delivery of iron via a circulating protein and a membrane receptor would appear to have ancient origins. The primitive invertebrate, *Pyura stolonifera,* thought to have originated about 200 million years ago, contains an analogue of mammalian transferrin. The protein has a molecular weight of 40,000, binds one atom of iron, and is coded for by a gene which is considered to be the precursor of the modern (duplicated) transferrin gene. Nevertheless, the iron-binding protein of *Pyura* is still recognised by transferrin receptors on mammalian reticulocytes such that its iron can be used for haemoglobin synthesis.[1] This implies that whilst the molecule of transferrin may have undergone substantial changes in structure during the process of evolution, the mechanisms of receptor recognition and internal cellular iron transport have remained essentially unaltered.

It is nearly 30 years since it was originally proposed by Jandl and Katz[2] that transferrin interacts with cells by binding to specific receptors on the cell membrane. During the last 3 decades a considerable amount of research has been devoted to the subject of the structure and biological role of the transferrin receptor of cell membranes, and how it participates in the cell iron cycle. Only a brief synopsis of the more important findings will be considered in this chapter, since the subject has been extensively reviewed on many occasions, particularly during the last 10 years.[3-10] As the details of the interaction between transferrin and its receptor have emerged, it has become increasingly clear that no one single mechanism can account for the uptake of iron by all the different tissues in a complex organism such as man. The description of an iron cycle involving transferrin, the transferrin receptor, and an acidic intracellular compartment or vesicle (endosome), may be adequate for cells such as the erythrocyte precursors of the bone marrow. However, there is recent evidence to suggest that in tissues such as the liver, iron uptake can occur by means of a variety of different pathways, some of which involve the interaction of transferrin with its specific receptor, whilst others use alternative receptor mechanisms, or possibly do not even use transferrin at all.

II. THE TRANSFERRIN RECEPTOR

A. DISCOVERY AND INITIAL IDENTIFICATION

Before discussing the experimental evidence for the existence of a specific transferrin receptor in cell membranes, it is worth considering some predictable characteristics of plasma iron and plasma transferrin by way of a few simple calculations based on the following well-established facts:

1. Plasma volume of an adult man   − 3000 mL
2. Plasma Tf concentration   = 2.5 mg/mL
3. Normal iron saturation of plasma Tf   = 30%
4. Half-life of plasma iron[11]   = 2 hours
5. Half-life of plasma Tf[11]   = 7–10 days
6. Amount of iron exchanged between   = 35 mg
   cellular compartments in 24 hours[12]

Since 1 mole of Tf binds a maximum of two atoms of iron, 80,000 g of transferrin binds a maximum of 112 g of iron.

The 7.5 g of Tf in plasma can bind a maximum of 10.5 mg of iron. At 30% saturation, this 7.5 g of Tf would carry 3.2 mg of iron.

Since the amount of iron taken up by different cellular compartments in the body during the course of 1 day is 35 mg, it would require a total of 82 g of Tf to deliver this iron.

If each molecule of Tf were to be destroyed by the cell once the iron had been delivered, then in a period of 24 hours the amount of new transferrin that would need to be synthesised in order to replace this loss (82 g) would represent approximately 11 times the total amount present in the plasma (7.5 g). In such an event, the calculated half-life of plasma Tf would be extremely short, probably between 1 and 2 hours.

CONCLUSION

Since the experimental evidence indicates that the actual half-life of plasma transferrin is between 7 and 10 days, each molecule of transferrin must be recycled, in an intact state, on many subsequent occasions during the course of delivery of iron to cells.

The first convincing evidence that iron-loaded transferrin was able to bind to cell membranes was published in 1963 by Jandl and Katz.[2] Reticulocytes (cells with a high iron requirement to support haemoglobin synthesis) were incubated at a low temperature with transferrin in which the iron and the protein had been separately labelled with radioactive tags. It was observed that whilst the majority of the iron was soon found in the cytoplasm of the cells, the bulk of the protein (apotransferrin) remained associated with the membrane fraction of the reticulocytes. From this observation it was inferred that the transferrin had become bound to a membrane receptor, and that the receptor was most likely a protein component of the membrane, since treatment of reticulocytes with trypsin abolished their ability to take up iron from transferrin. A simple iron-to-cell cycle was postulated. This envisaged an initial binding of iron-loaded transferrin to a membrane receptor, followed by release of the iron into the cell cytoplasm. The cycle would be completed by the dissociation of apotransferrin from the receptor and its return to the plasma in order to acquire more iron.

During the last 30 years our understanding of the iron-cell cycle has evolved considerably. The initial step of the simple scheme described by Jandl and Katz — transferrin binding to a membrane receptor — has remained valid. Likewise, the very last stage of the cycle — the return of the intact apotransferrin back to the plasma — is not disputed. It is the events that occur in the middle of the cycle that have had to be modified on the basis of new experimental evidence. It is now apparent that, certainly in the case of reticulocytes, once transferrin-receptor binding has taken place on the cell membrane, the entire complex (Tf–Fe–receptor) becomes internalised within the cell by a process of endocytosis. Only after this event has occurred is the iron released. In striking contrast with many other endocytosed ligands, transferrin is not degraded during its passage through the cell. Instead, it remains attached to its receptor until the receptor returns to the plasma membrane. It is only then that the molecule of apotransferrin dissociates from the receptor and is released back into the extracellular fluid.

Whilst transferrin binding remains the principal reference method for the identification of transferrin receptors on cell membranes, a more rapid, sensitive, and commonly used screening technique has been developed using monoclonal antibodies. The discovery of these antibodies was entirely fortuitous, arising out of work on mouse hybridomas. It was only later realised that it was the antigenic sites of the plasma membrane transferrin receptor of these cells that had triggered the antibody formation.[13,14] Many monoclonal antibodies have now been isolated and whilst it seems likely that they all recognise the same or structurally very similar membrane receptor, individual epitope recognition varies, with the result that some antibodies block the subsequent binding of transferrin, whereas others do not.[15] One of the most commonly used anti-Tf-receptor antibodies (OKT9) is frequently used as a reference against which other monoclonals are compared. As the range of available antibodies has expanded, so increasing doubt has been cast on the original concept of receptor homogeneity within tissues of the same species.[16] In a recent review, de Jong et al.[17] present evidence that structural and possibly functional heterogeneity of the transferrin receptor may be as extensive as the heterogeneity exhibited by the molecule of transferrin itself.

B. TISSUE DISTRIBUTION OF TRANSFERRIN RECEPTORS

The identification of cell membrane transferrin receptors in a wide variety of tissues has been carried out either by measuring the binding of labelled transferrin at low temperatures, or by the use of monoclonal antibodies. In most cases there has been found to be a good agreement between the qualitative and quantitative results obtained by either method.[18] In the rare situations where this has not been found to be the case, lack of detector specificity or variation in receptor reactivity has usually been the cause.[19,20] The tissues that have been found to express the largest numbers of transferrin receptors have been the erythrocyte precursors of the bone marrow, the placenta, and the liver. In addition, receptors have been identified, albeit at a wide range of concentrations, on the plasma membranes of many other tissues and cells,[8] including spermatocytes, Sertoli cells and seminiferous tubules of the testis, islet cells from the pancreas, the anterior pituitary, activated lymphocytes, endothelial cells in the brain, tumour cells (particularly rapidly dividing neoplasms), adipocytes, and a wide variety of cells grown in culture. In most of these examples there is a good agreement between the iron requirements of the cell and the density of membrane transferrin receptors.

In this regard, the presence of a large number of transferrin receptors in the liver would certainly be predicted, since this organ is second only to the erythroid bone marrow in its capacity to exchange iron with plasma transferrin. The literature abounds with reports indicating the presence of transferrin receptors from studies on liver cell suspensions, cultured hepatocytes, and whole-organ perfusions.[21] Of the three major cell types found in the liver (hepatocytes, Kupffer cells, and sinusoidal endothelial cells), the hepatocyte parenchymal cell is by far the most abundant. For this reason alone it has usually been assumed that these cells would be equipped with a plentiful supply of transferrin receptors on their plasma membranes. However, there have been a significant number of reports in the literature suggesting that hepatocyte cells may not actually have any transferrin receptors,[22,23] or, if they do, they are present in comparatively low numbers.[24] On the other hand, the endothelial and Kupffer cells of the liver appear to be richly supplied with transferrin receptors.[24] From these observations it has been suggested that the endothelial and Kupffer cells make a major contribution to the transferrin-bound uptake of iron by the liver. As to the hepatocytes, there is increasing evidence suggesting that these cells are able to acquire iron by at least five separate mechanisms:

1. Transferrin receptor-mediated endocytosis (the classic iron cycle)
2. Transferrin uptake via the asialoglycoprotein membrane receptor
3. Transferrin receptor-associated NADH reductase activity, with the reduction of transferrin-bound Fe^{3+} and the transport of the released Fe^{2+} across the hepatocyte membrane
4. A transferrin-independent system that is passive, saturable, and shared by other transition metal ions
5. Receptor-mediated uptake of ferritin, supplied to the hepatocytes by the Kupffer cells, following the degradation of effete red cells

The significance and relative contributions of these various suggested mechanisms for iron uptake by hepatocyte cells is still a matter of considerable controversy. The reasons why it has become necessary to invoke more than one route for the uptake of hepatocyte iron will be briefly discussed in the final section of this chapter.

C. TRANSFERRIN RECEPTOR NUMBERS AND THEIR LOCALISATION WITHIN CELLS

From ultrastructural studies on a variety of cell types, using as a probe both labelled transferrin and monoclonal antibodies, it has been possible to measure not only the number of transferrin receptors present, but also their relative distribution between the plasma membrane and cytoplasm. Nondividing cells are, in most cases, in a state of relatively stable iron balance, and this is reflected by the fact that the number of transferrin receptors remains fairly constant. On the other hand, cells undergoing replication, with the extra iron requirements associated with this process, show significant increases in the number of transferrin receptors. Examples of the latter situation include transformed lymphocytes[25] and tumour cells, particularly those with neoplastic characteristics.[26] A similar situation is found in whole tissues undergoing regeneration. The number of receptors on the residual liver cells following partial hepatectomy more than doubles within the first 24 hours after the operation.[27]

Since the number of transferrin receptors is directly correlated with the prevailing iron demands of the particular cell, estimates of absolute numbers are often found to be extremely variable. For example, rabbit reticulocytes have variously been reported to contain 100,000,[4] 130,000,[28] and 300,000[4] receptors per cell. In the case of rat liver endothelial cells, the variation is even more striking, ranging from 5000[29] to 2,000,000 per cell,[30] and in one paper a figure as high as 14,000,000 has been reported.[22]

Leaving aside the problems associated with measuring absolute receptor numbers, it is clear that at any one time only a proportion of the transferrin receptors are present on the cell membrane. The remainder are located within the cell substance, inaccessible to the macromolecular probes. In a study of adult rat hepatocytes, Rudolph et al.[31] estimated that of the total number of transferrin receptors per cell (130,000), only about one third (47,000) were associated at any one time with the plasma membrane. A similar distribution has been reported in human carcinoma cells.[32,33] The distribution pattern of the receptors on the cell membrane has been mapped at high resolution using monoclonal antibody-gold complexes. Some of the receptors are diffusely distributed across the entire surface of the cell, whilst others are found concentrated in the regions of the clathrin-coated pits.[34] The clustering of receptors within the clathrin-coated pits is indicative of the start of an endocytotic sequence, leading eventually to receptor uptake into the cell cytoplasm. In the case of the transferrin receptor, there is considerable evidence suggesting that cellular uptake occurs, albeit at a reduced rate, even in the absence of ligand (transferrin) binding.[33] There is a continuous shuttling of receptors between the surface and the interior of the cell, but the process is enhanced upon the binding of transferrin to the receptor.[32]

Once the process of endocytosis has occurred, transferrin receptors have been found in the cell cytoplasm associated with a variety of intracellular organelles[34] — endocytotic vesicles (endosomes), tubular elements of the Golgi system, and microtubular membrane elements thought to be part of the exocytotic mechanism of the cell. Transferrin receptors are rarely found within those intracellular vesicles that are destined to be degraded by the lysosomes, an observation that adds support to the proposal that transferrin receptors normally recycle back to the cell membrane to be used again. The time spent by the receptor within the cell cytoplasm, during which it is always complexed to a molecule of transferrin, has been estimated to be between 3 and 15 min.[17,35] This cycle may be repeated as many as 300 times before the receptor becomes finally degraded and needs to be replaced.[36]

Changes in receptor number have been most extensively studied in cells of the developing erythroid line from the bone marrow. These cells require iron not only for proliferation, but also exhibit very high demands for iron in order to synthesise haemoglobin. In a detailed study of rat erythroid cells, Iacopetta et al.[37] showed that there was a close correlation between transferrin receptor number and iron uptake. Early precursor stem cells in the bone marrow have very few receptors, since at that stage they are not yet programmed to produce haemoglobin. Significant numbers of receptors have appeared by the early normoblast stage (300,000 per cell) and increase to a maximum in the intermediate normablasts (800,000 per cell). From then on the receptor numbers decline, levelling off at about 100,000 per cell in the reticulocytes. By this stage in erythroid cell development, haemoglobin synthesis is almost complete. Once the reticulocytes have been released into the circulation to be transformed into mature erythrocytes, receptor number declines very rapidly, soon reaching undetectable levels. Since mammalian erythrocytes possess neither DNA nor any residual mRNA, further synthesis of the transferrin receptor is not possible.

D. ISOLATION AND STRUCTURAL ANALYSIS OF THE TRANSFERRIN RECEPTOR

Transferrin receptors have been detected on the plasma membranes of most proliferating, differentiating, or haemoglobin-synthesising cells. The receptor was first isolated and partially characterised from rabbit reticulocytes in 1978.[38,39] Within a year, the human transferrin receptor had been isolated from placental brush-border membranes.[40,41] Purification methods have now become rapid and efficient, particularly with the use of affinity chromatography techniques. Since at any one time, transferrin receptors can be in one of two possible states, occupied or vacant, both forms of the receptor can be trapped if two separate affinity columns are utilised. A detergent-solubilised membrane lysate is first passed through an affinity column containing an antibody to transferrin, thereby binding transferrin-occupied receptors. The column eluate is then passed through a second affinity column containing covalently bound diferric transferrin. This column binds the vacant or unoccupied transferrin receptors. The receptor is then eluted from both columns by chelating the iron with desferrioxamine (DFO).[42]

The human transferrin receptor is a disulphide-linked transmembrane dimer composed of two identical glycoprotein subunits. The molecular weight of the receptor dimer is 180,000. A schematic representation of the receptor, including its orientation within the plasma membrane, is shown in Figure 1. The detailed structure of the receptor has been the subject of a number of review articles,[8,35] and only a brief description will be given in this section.

The complete primary structure has been deduced from the cDNA sequence.[43] Each monomer consists of a polypeptide chain (M.W. 84,910) containing 670 amino acid residues. The N-terminal domain of the protein, comprising the first 61 amino acids, is located within the cytoplasm of the cell. The next 28 residues (62 to 89) span the lipid bilayer of the cell membrane, and this short peptide sequence consists almost entirely of uncharged, hydrophobic amino acid side chains. Finally, the long C-terminal domain, extending from residues 90 to 760 and containing the transferrin-binding site, is located on the extracellular side of the plasma membrane. Each dimeric receptor is thought to be capable of binding two molecules of transferrin. The two identical monomers, which together comprise a single receptor molecule, are joined by a covalent disulphide bond which is located in the extracellular domain, close to the membrane. Treatment of the purified receptor with reducing agents leads to the cleavage of this disulphide bridge, and the release of two 90,000-M.W. monomers. The difference in molecular weight between the isolated monomer (90,000) and its constituent polypeptide chain (84,910) is accounted for mainly by the presence of two *N*-asparagine-linked oligosaccharide chains and one O-linked oligosaccharide chain.[86] Two of these chains are of the high mannose variety, a characteristic of glycan chains at the early stages of biosynthesis. The third chain (O-linked), however, is a mature galactose-containing glycan. All three chains are attached to amino acid residues in the C-terminal extracellular domain of the receptor. The

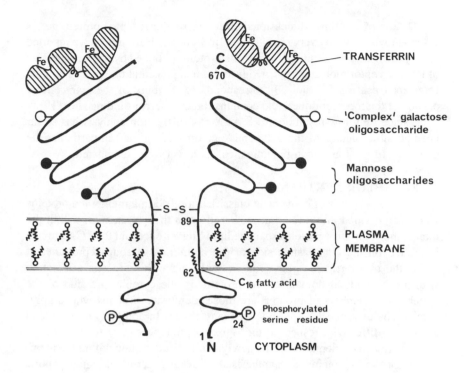

FIGURE 1. A schematic representation of the human transferrin receptor.

covalent structure of each monomer is completed by way of two further posttranslational modifications. The first of these is the attachment of a fatty acid, probably palmitate (C_{16}), to the hydrophobic intramembranous region of the polypeptide. The second modification, and one that is possibly optional, is the phosphorylation of serine residue 24 in the short hydrophilic cytoplasmic tail of the receptor.

Within the same species, transferrin receptors from different cell types appear to be chemically very similar, if not identical. Human placental and reticulocyte transferrin receptors have been found to be structurally indistinguishable with respect to molecular weight and proteolytic digestion patterns.[44] However, the techniques used to determine these physical characteristics are unlikely to reveal small structural differences, if these do indeed exist. Recently, Cotner et al.[45] have examined the structure and expression of transferrin receptors from different tissues using a variety of monoclonal antibodies. Their results suggest that whilst all transferrin receptors within a single species appear to be derived from the same gene, receptors from different cell types do not necessarily express the same range of antigenic epitopes. The structural explanation for this apparent receptor heterogeneity has yet to be elucidated, but a likely possibility is at the level of posttranslational modification — glycosylation or phosphorylation.

Details of the three-dimensional structure of the receptor protein are as yet unknown. It is only very recently that Borhani and Harrison[85] have reported the crystallisation of a soluble form of the protein, obtained by tryptic digestion of intact receptor molecules purified from human placental tissue. The soluble fragment (residues 121 to 760) corresponds to the bulk of the extracellular portion of the receptor dimer, and contains the transferrin-binding sites. However, since only low-resolution (3.8 Å) X-ray diffraction analysis has so far been possible, details of the polypeptide chain folding, and in particular the geometry of the transferrin-binding sites, have yet to be elucidated.

E. RECEPTOR SYNTHESIS

For the purposes of convenient classification, plasma membrane proteins have been divided into three groups, based upon their orientation within the membrane.[46] Group 1 proteins span the lipid bilayer once and their C-terminus is located on the cytoplasmic side of the membrane. Group 2 proteins, of which the transferrin receptor is an example, have the opposite orientation with the N-terminal domain of the protein on the cytoplasmic side of the membrane. Members of group 3 are those membrane proteins whose polypeptide chains cross the lipid bilayer many times. In addition, group 1 and 2 proteins differ with respect to the signal peptide necessary for the correct translocation and orientation of the newly synthesised protein within the membrane. Group 1 proteins are synthesised with an N-terminal signal peptide which is subsequently cleaved from the protein once membrane insertion has occurred. Group 2 proteins, such as the transferrin receptor, are synthesised without a cleavable signal peptide. In the case of the human transferrin receptor, an internal sequence corresponding to the transmembrane segment (residues 62 to 89) functions as a signal peptide.[47] During the process of protein synthesis, this section of the polypeptide chain becomes inserted initially into the membrane of the rough endoplasmic reticulum (RER). The insertion occurs in such a way that the flanking N-terminal part of the newly synthesised chain becomes orientated facing the cytoplasmic side of the RER membrane. As polypeptide chain assembly continues, the C-terminal domain remains on the noncytoplasmic side of the RER membrane, such that it will become later located on the exterior surface of the cell membrane.

Zerial et al.[47] have shown that deletion of the base sequence within the receptor gene that codes for the transmembrane region completely abolishes the capacity for membrane insertion.

Much of the posttranslational modification of the newly synthesised receptor occurs within the RER and Golgi system before the molecule arrives at the plasma membrane.[87] The three oligosaccharide chains are all initially synthesised within the RER as the high-mannose type. Two remain essentially unaltered during further passage through the Golgi system, whereas the third chain becomes extensively modified into a "complex" type with many galactose residues. The functional significance of the oligosaccharide chains has yet to be fully elucidated, but there is some evidence that whilst they are essential for transferrin binding to the receptor on the reticulocyte membrane, this may not be true for other cells with transferrin receptors.[48] For example, human leukaemic cells treated with tunicamycin in order to inhibit oligosaccharide synthesis express transferrin receptors for which the binding affinity for transferrin is reduced, but not completely abolished.[49] The covalent attachment of a molecule of palmitic acid to each receptor monomer occurs within the vesicles of the Golgi system. However, because of the relatively slow rate of acyl group turnover,[50] it is unlikely that the fatty acid plays a direct role in either receptor processing or membrane insertion. The final posttranslational modification of the receptor is the phosphorylation of serine residue-24 within the cytoplasmic tail of the molecule. The addition of the phosphate group, using ATP as the preferred phosphate donor, occurs once the receptor has been inserted in the membrane. Various catalysts have been proposed for this reaction, including protein kinase C, cyclic AMP-dependent kinase, and a multifunctional Ca^{2+}/calmodulin-dependent kinase.[51] Since phosphorylation occurs not only in isolated membranes, but also with the purified receptor alone, it has even been suggested that kinase activity may be part of the receptor itself.[8] The role of phosphorylation-dephosphorylation in the process of receptor cycling is still a matter of active research and controversy. It will be discussed in a later section of this chapter when the intracellular iron cycle is considered.

F. TRANSFERRIN-BINDING CHARACTERISTICS OF THE RECEPTOR

Transferrin receptors, particularly those present on the membranes of cells with a high requirement for iron, such as the haemoglobin-synthesising red cell precursors (reticulocytes), have a very high affinity for diferric transferrin. At the pH of blood plasma (7.4), binding constants in the range 10^7 to 10^9 M^{-1} have been reported.[3,4,10,19,20] Affinity constants of this order of magnitude more than account for the very efficient uptake of the normal levels of diferric transferrin found in human plasma. Despite a few early reports suggesting that the affinity of the receptor for diferric transferrin and apotransferrin were the same,[52] it is now generally agreed that at pH 7.4 the receptor affinity for apotransferrin is much lower than for diferric transferrin, with the affinity for both monoferric species being intermediate between these two extremes. The physiological effect of these differing affinities at pH 7.4 is such that diferric transferrin possesses a significant functional advantage with respect to its iron-donating ability. At the normal level of diferric transferrin found in human plasma (4×10^{-6} M), neither the apo nor the monoferric species will significantly compete with the diferric molecule for the receptor-binding sites. The net result is that *in vivo*, transferrin receptors on the reticulocyte membrane will be almost entirely saturated with diferric transferrin.

The different binding affinities of the receptor for apo and diferric transferrin at pH 7.4 can be seen to have a physiological advantage. The same is also true, but for different reasons, when the affinities at acid pH are compared.

At pH 5.5, apotransferrin forms a very stable complex with the receptor, the affinity constant being much greater than that at pH 7.4. On the other hand, diferric transferrin forms a weaker complex with the receptor at pH 5.5 than at pH 7.4. This differential effect of pH on receptor binding has an important role to play in the intracellular iron cycle. Although this aspect of iron metabolism will be discussed in greater detail in a later section of this chapter, a brief outline at this stage seems in order.

At the pH of blood plasma (7.4), diferric transferrin binds to the reticulocyte with a high affinity. The transferrin-receptor complex becomes internalised (the endocytotic arm of the cycle) into an acidic endosomal vesicle. The internal pH of the cytoplasmic endosome (5.5) brings about the release of the two atoms of iron from the diferric transferrin molecule for onward passage to iron-requiring systems within the cell, such as haemoglobin synthesis, whilst at the same time the low pH stabilises the complex between the receptor and the residual apotransferrin. The exocytotic arm of the cycle returns this complex to the cell membrane. Once the complex has become fused back into the membrane, the external alkaline pH to which it is now exposed (7.4) brings about the rapid dissociation of the receptor-apotransferrin complex. Apotransferrin returns to the plasma in order to acquire two further atoms of ferric iron, whilst the receptor recycles back to the membrane, in an intact state, where it can bind another molecule of diferric transferrin.

The affinity for diferric transferrin of the receptor from different tissues of the same organism appears to be constant, and the same is also true for the receptor at different stages of red cell maturation. It would seem therefore that the possible structural heterogeneity of the receptor, referred to in the previous section, has little or no effect on the value of the binding constant.

G. THE RECEPTOR GENE

In 1982 two independent groups[53,54] located the structural gene locus for the human transferrin receptor on chromosome 3. Within a year, the position of the gene had been narrowed down to the region q22-ter.[55] As has already been mentioned in an earlier chapter, this places the gene for the transferrin receptor in proximity to the genes for the members of the siderophilin family — serum transferrin, lactoferrin, and melanoma antigen p97. The receptor cDNA has been cloned and sequenced, and from these results the primary structure of the protein was deduced.[43] Transferrin receptor mRNA is unusual in having a particularly long 3'-untranslated region containing 2650 nucleotides. This long stretch of nucleotides houses many regulatory elements that control the stability of the mRNA molecule. These will be described in more detail in the next section.

It is interesting to note the very close proximity on chromosome 3 of the genes for transferrin and the transferrin receptor. Although the two proteins are quite different in structure and function, it has been reported that a number of very short regions in both the nucleotide and amino acid sequences of transferrin share considerable sequence homology with the complementary (antisense) nucleotide and deduced amino acid sequence of the transferrin receptor.[56] In each case the regions of homology are located in receptor sequences external to the plasma membrane, in parts of the receptor molecule that might qualify as ligand (transferrin)-binding sites.

Kuhn et al.[56] and McClelland et al.[57] have cloned and sequenced the entire genomic sequence encoding the human transferrin-receptor gene. A stretch of 31 kB of DNA encodes the receptor. Since the protein monomer contains only 760 amino acids, requiring a minimum of 2.28 kB of DNA, an entire genomic sequence of 31 kB implies that the gene contains a very large proportion (92%) of noncoding intron sequences. Hybridisation studies have revealed that the gene contains at least 12 exons. In addition to the entire coding sequence, a number of regions of DNA immediately adjacent to the receptor gene have been cloned and sequenced. One particular clone comprising all of exon 1 together with the 12-kB nucleotide sequence upstream (5') from the mRNA-transcription start site has been studied in considerable detail with a view to identifying possible regulatory elements.[58]

H. CONTROL OF SYNTHESIS OF THE TRANSFERRIN RECEPTOR

Iron is acquired by proliferating eukaryotic cells through the receptor-mediated endocytosis of the iron-carrying protein transferrin. With the possible exception of liver cells, this mechanism is probably the only route by which iron, at least at normal physiological levels, enters most cells. When iron demands are increased, cells respond by expressing greater numbers of transferrin receptors on their plasma membranes. Likewise, when the cellular iron demands for iron are fully satisfied, the number of membrane transferrin receptors is reduced in order to avoid iron overload, which, if left unchecked, would invariably lead to cell damage by the free radicals produced from iron/dioxygen interactions. With such a central role to play in the control of iron entry, the expression of transferrin receptors on the cell membrane is, as might be expected, highly regulated.

The total number of transferrin receptors located within the cell membrane at any particular time is regulated at two different levels. The first, or short-term control mechanism, alters the proportional distribution of receptor molecules between the membrane and the cytoplasm of the cell. Under normal circumstances only about one third of the transferrin receptors of a cell are found to be present within the plasma membrane. The trafficking or cycling of receptors between the cytoplasm and the membrane, and the factors that regulate this process will be described in the next section. The second, or long-term mechanism, is the regulation of receptor synthesis.

In simple terms, protein synthesis is controlled either at the level of transcription (DNA to mRNA) or at the level of translation (mRNA to protein). For most eukaryotic proteins, control at the site of transcription is the normal rule. This works on the principle that, due to the inherent instability of mRNA, protein synthesis is regulated by controlling the rate at which mRNA molecules

TABLE 1
The Effect of Intracellular Iron Concentration on the Level of Stable Tf-Receptor mRNA, the Rate of Tf-Receptor Synthesis, and the Rate of Iron Uptake

	Low iron	High iron
Tf-receptor mRNA level	↑	↓
Tf-receptor synthesis	↑	↓
Iron uptake	↑	↓

are synthesised from the DNA template within the nucleus. Regulatory factors function by interacting with nucleotide sequences adjacent to the structural gene, stimulating or repressing mRNA synthesis. The example of transferrin, for which a long 5' promoter region regulates mRNA transcription in response to iron, hormones, and a range of nuclear proteins, has already been discussed in the previous chapter. In contrast, the major site for the regulation of expression of the transferrin receptor is at the level of translation, by controlling the storage and stability of receptor mRNA molecules already present within the cytoplasm.[58] Whilst this is unusual for eukaryotic proteins, it is by no means unique.[59] Other examples of proteins where translational (post-transcriptional) control through the regulation of mRNA stability has been demonstrated include ribonucleotide reductase, casein, heat-shock house-keeping proteins, chlorophyll-binding proteins, and ferritin — the iron-storage protein.[58]

The most important regulator of receptor synthesis is the level of intra-cellular iron. Alterations in the level of cell iron directly modify the levels of mature mRNA in the cytoplasm, rather than affect the rate at which the mRNA is transcribed from nuclear DNA (Table 1). When iron is in excess, the stability of the transferrin receptor mRNA within the cytoplasm decreases. Conversely, when iron levels are low, receptor mRNA molecules are stabilised, more receptor protein is synthesised, and iron uptake is thereby increased. The mechanisms by which iron regulates the stability of the receptor mRNA are not completely understood. There is evidence that within the exceptionally long 3'-untranslated region of the receptor mRNA molecule, there exist at least five copies of short nucleotide sequences that function as iron-response elements (IREs).[58] When intracellular levels of iron are high, iron binds, either directly or through a regulatory protein, to the IREs. This in turn destabilises the mRNA, leading to the premature degradation of the molecule. Conversely, when intracellular levels of iron are low, the IREs within the 3'-untranslated region of the mRNA remain vacant, and this stabilises the molecule. There is evidence that stabilisation of receptor mRNA in the absence of iron is due, in part, to specific stem-loop secondary structures within the 3'-untranslated region of the polynucleotide.[60] What is even more interesting is the recent discovery that the putative IREs within the 3'-

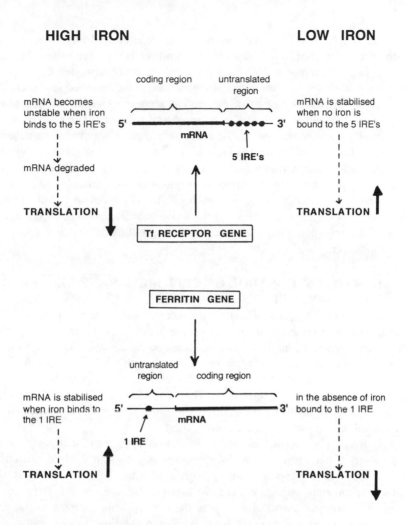

FIGURE 2. The comparative effects of high and low iron concentrations on the synthesis of the transferrin receptor and the synthesis of ferritin.

untranslated region of the transferrin receptor mRNA are also present, albeit as a single copy, within the 5'-untranslated region of the mRNA for ferritin.[58] The location of a common structural motif at opposite noncoding ends of two different mRNA molecules may be related to the different effects that iron has on the synthesis of the two proteins (Figure 2). High intracellular levels of iron stimulate ferritin synthesis whilst depressing the synthesis of the transferrin receptor. The use of a common regulatory nucleotide sequence in ferritin and transferrin receptor mRNA is the first example of concerted regulation of eukaryote mRNAs.

Whilst the evidence in favour of translational control of transferrin-receptor synthesis is considerable, the possibility that transcriptional control also has a role to play cannot be discarded. Rao et al.[61] have shown that intracellular levels of iron, at least in leukaemic cells, can exert a small effect on the rate of receptor mRNA transcription. However, although the 5′-promoter region of the transferrin-receptor gene has been cloned and sequenced,[62] no evidence could be found of nucleotide sequences within the promoter region of the receptor gene that were analogous to the IREs in the promoter region of the transferrin gene. The receptor promoter was found to contain the usual TATA box, as well as GC-rich regions, and a possible binding site for the nuclear transcription factor Sp1. There are some similarities of nucleotide sequence within the promoter regions of the transferrin and transferrin-receptor genes. These have been suggested as possible recognition sites for premitotic signals responsible for the well-established, coordinated expression of these two genes in proliferating of differentiating cells such as activated T lymphocytes.[63]

I. SHORT-TERM CONTROL OF CELL MEMBRANE RECEPTOR LEVELS — REGULATION OF RECEPTOR CYCLING

Long-term regulation of transferrin-receptor expression is mediated, in the most part, by the action of iron on the stability of the receptor mRNA (posttranscriptional control). However, there is considerable evidence to suggest that cells can respond far more rapidly than this long-term mechanism would allow, by acutely altering the distribution of receptors between the cytoplasm and the cell membrane. This short-term regulation of receptor expression is mediated by the action of hormones, growth factors, tumour-promoting agents, and even transferrin itself.

In its simplest form, the intracellular iron cycle can be thought of as consisting of two arms. The endocytotic arm begins with the internalisation of the membrane receptor, usually with a molecule of diferric transferrin attached, and ends with the release of iron from the receptor-transferrin complex. The exocytotic arm of the cycle then returns this complex to the cell membrane, where the receptor fuses back into the lipid bilayer whilst the apotransferrin is released into the extracellular fluid. The overall process is referred to as receptor cycling and takes between 3 and 15 minutes to complete, depending upon the cell type and experimental conditions. Without at this stage defining the individual steps involved in the process, the cycle can be considered as being controlled by two first-order rate constants, one for the endocytotic arm (k_{endo}), and the other for the exocytotic arm (k_{exo}). Even without altering the absolute number of receptors in the cell, any change in either or both of these rate constants will lead to an alteration in the distribution of receptors between the membrane and the cytoplasm. For example, if the value of k_{exo} is increased, then receptor exocytosis will be enhanced and the appearance of more receptors on the cell membrane will lead to an increase in the uptake of transferrin-bound iron.

When the cycle was first investigated it was thought that only those membrane receptors to which transferrin was bound would be capable of being endocytosed.[64,65] However, it has now been conclusively shown that in the case of most cells that have been examined, the transferrin receptor does internalise even in the absence of bound transferrin.[66-69] This implies that receptors, without transferrin attached, cycle between the membrane and the cytoplasm at a basal rate determined by the ratio of the two rate constants. During the last few years, a considerable amount of research has been directed towards elucidating the mechanisms by which this cycle is controlled, as well as identifying the signals that regulate the process.

Although the binding of transferrin to the membrane receptor is not essential in order to trigger the endocytotic process, transferrin does have the effect of increasing the rate of receptor cycling. This is achieved by effecting an increase in both rate constants and also by diverting the transferrin-receptor complex to an alternative intracellular pathway with more rapid kinetics for exocytosis.[69]

In addition to diferric transferrin, a number of hormones, peptide growth factors, and tumour-promoting agents have been shown to exert an influence on the distribution of transferrin receptors between cytoplasm and cell membrane. Induction of cell division is associated with a wide range of diverse biochemical events, one of which is often a significant increase in the number of transferrin receptors on the cell membrane. In most examples, the time between exposure of cells to a particular mitogen and the appearance of increased numbers of transferrin receptors on the cell membrane is so short (5 minutes) that it cannot be accounted for by increased receptor synthesis. The most likely explanation for this acute response is a rapid translocation of receptors from the cytoplasm to the cell membrane.[70] Mitogenic agents that have been shown to promote this movement include epidermal growth factor,[70] insulin-like growth factor-1,[71] platelet-derived growth factor,[72] and interleukin-1.[72] The process has been found to be calcium/calmodulin dependent,[72,73] implicating the involvement of the calcium-requiring enzyme protein kinase C.[74] Many growth factors are thought to work by stimulating the activity of protein kinase C, and since this enzyme catalyses the phosphorylation of membrane proteins, much interest has recently been devoted to the possibility that phosphorylation of the transferrin receptor might be important in the regulation of receptor cycling. The site of receptor phosphorylation is the serine residue at position 24 within the cytoplasmic tail of the protein. Davis and Meisner[74] have shown by site-directed mutagenisis of human transferrin receptor cDNA that substitution of serine-24 by threonine or alanine does not prevent the receptor either from binding transferrin or from participating in the normal endocytosis-exocytosis cycle. They concluded that the regulation of receptor cycling by protein kinase C must therefore be independent of receptor phosphorylation at serine-24. Nevertheless, an indirect role for protein kinase C in the regulation of receptor cycling is supported by many experimental observations. Factors that are known to stimulate protein kinase C activity frequently result in a rapid redistribution of transferrin receptors. These include, in addition to the growth factors already listed, diacyl glycerols[74] and the phorbol esters[65,74] — a group of powerful tumour-promoting agents of plant origin. The effects of these agents often vary amongst different cell types. For example, whilst phorbol esters induce a rapid increase in the number of transferrin receptors in the cell membranes of human fibroblasts,[74] they have been found to induce an equally rapid internalisation, and therefore decrease, in the number of membrane receptors in human K562 erythroleukaemic cells.[65]

The peptide hormone insulin has been shown to affect the distribution of transferrin receptors, particularly in adipose tissue. Insulin elicits a rapid translocation of intracellular transferrin receptors to the plasma membrane of adipocytes, resulting in a twofold increase in the number of receptors on the cell membrane, which in turn leads to a significant rise in the rate of uptake of iron-loaded transferrin.[75] Insulin was thought to have exerted this effect by increasing the rate constant for receptor externalisation (k_{exo}). An alternative mechanism to explain the mode of action of insulin has recently been proposed by Alvarez et al.[76] These workers showed that the posttranslational acylation of the transferrin receptor involves the attachment of palmitic acid to cysteine residues 62 and 67. Palmitoylation of the receptor was found to be associated with an inhibition of the rate of receptor endocytosis. Insulin stimulates palmitoylation and thereby indirectly decreases the rate of receptor endocytosis, leading to a greater number of receptors being expressed on the cell membrane.

III. THE TRANSFERRIN-IRON CYCLE IN ERYTHROID CELLS

Immature erythroid cells in the bone marrow (normoblasts) and the circulation (reticulocytes) have demands for iron that, under most circumstances, exceed those of any other tissue. Normoblasts can achieve rates of iron uptake in the region of 500,000 atoms per cell per minute. The flow of the iron traffic is essentially unidirectional, namely cellular uptake and incorporation into haemoglobin. Reticulocytes can be isolated in large numbers and purified comparatively easily. For these reasons, most of the early studies on the mechanism of cellular iron uptake from transferrin utilised immature red cells.[2,77] The picture that has emerged as a result of research carried out over the last 30 years is a process of transferrin-bound iron uptake by reticulocytes that is usually referred to as the transferrin cell cycle, or the endocytotic iron cycle. It has been the subject of many excellent review articles,[8,10,17,35,78,79] and the brief synopsis that follows describes only those aspects of the erythroid iron cycle for which there is sound evidence and general agreement.

The cycle is initiated by the binding of transferrin, preferentially in the diferric form, to vacant transferrin receptors distributed over the entire surface of the reticulocyte cell membrane. Within 4 to 5 minutes of this initial binding event, the transferrin-receptor complexes have migrated laterally across the membrane to become concentrated and clustered into clathrin-coated pits.

Invagination of the pits results in the internalisation of the transferrin-receptor complex into a membrane-bounded intracellular compartment, variously referred to as a receptosome, endocytotic vesicle, or endosome.

Up to this stage in the process, the mechanism of the receptor-ligand internalisation does not differ significantly from that of most other macromolecules. It is, however, during the next few steps in the transferrin cycle that differences become apparent. For most internalised macromolecules, the ultimate fate of the endosome containing the receptor-ligand complex is to be directed to the proteolytic machinery within the lysosome. At this site, either or both of the components of the complex are rapidly degraded. For example, in the case of the epidermal growth factor (EGF), both EGF and its receptor are targeted for destruction within the lysosome. On the other hand, for some macromolecules such as low-density lipoproteins (LDLs), whilst the ligand is destined for destruction within the lysosome, the earlier dissociation of the receptor-ligand complex within a prelysosomal compartment allows the receptor to escape back to the cell membrane. In complete contrast, the entire complex of transferrin and its receptor manages to elude the proteolytic machinery of the lysosome, returning to the cell membrane intact, relieved only of its burden of iron.

Soon after the endosomes containing the transferrin-receptor complexes have migrated into the cytoplasm away from the cell membrane, they are relieved of their clathrin coats. The pH of the interior of the endosome is then rapidly reduced from 7.4 to about 5.5 by the action of an ATP-dependent proton pump. This acidification benefits the transferrin receptor complex in a number of ways. It induces a reversible conformation-transition of the receptor, leading to self-association, and thereby affording protection against proteolytic attack. Acidification also promotes the release of the iron bound to the molecule of transferrin. However, even at a pH of 5.5, total release of the transferrin-bound iron would be a process taking many hours to complete. Since the molecule of transferrin spends only a few minutes within the cell cytoplasm during the course of the iron cycle, clearly there is more to the release of the iron than simple proton attack. Small-molecular-weight iron chelators, already present within the cytoplasm, are thought to facilitate the process of iron release and to assist in the onward transit of the iron to the mitochondria (for haem synthesis) or to ferritin (for iron storage). The acidified environment of the endosome now contains the residual receptor-apotransferrin complex. For most receptor-ligand complexes, the acid pH would result in an uncoupling of the complex, and for this reason the endosomal compartment following acidification is frequently referred to as the compartment for uncoupling ligand and receptor (CURL). However, in the case of the apotransferrin-receptor complex, whereas at the alkaline pH of blood plasma this complex would rapidly dissociate, at pH 5.5 the association between the receptor and the iron-free apotransferrin is stabilised and the complex remains intact.

The endocytotic arm of the cycle is now complete. During the remainder of the journey of the receptor-apotransferrin complex through the cell, the vesicle is directed back to and fuses with the plasma membrane. Following exocytosis, the complex still bound to the membrane encounters the extracellular pH of 7.4. This induces the apotransferrin to spontaneously dissociate from the receptor, become released from the membrane, and then return to the extracellular fluid in order to sequester further atoms of ferric iron. Meanwhile, the vacant receptor, still attached to the membrane, can return for another intracellular voyage. This intracellular cycle may be repeated as many as 300 times before the receptor becomes finally degraded beyond the stage of further repair.

A schematic representation of the intracellular iron cycle, as thought to occur at least in erythroid cells, is shown in Figure 3.

Of the many characteristics of the receptor-transferrin interaction, the one that is probably the most significant in assisting the functioning of the cycle is the high affinity of the receptor for iron-loaded transferrin at pH 7.4, and the high affinity of the receptor for iron-free apotransferrin at the acidic pH of the endosome. There still remain many aspects of this proposed cycle that require further elucidation. Not least amongst these is the question of how the transferrin-receptor complex within the endosome escapes from being directed to the lysosome, where it would inevitably be degraded. Clearly, a mechanism for sorting the endosomes occurs within the cell cytoplasm. This must involve a highly specific process of signalling to ensure that endosomes, rich in receptor-apotransferrin complexes, are diverted away from the lysosome pathway and on to an exocytotic route back to the cell membrane. There is some evidence that recycling may occur through the Golgi system acting as a sorting station as well as a site for the repair of damaged molecules of both the transferrin and its receptor.

IV. THE UPTAKE OF IRON BY NONERYTHROID CELLS AND THE CONTRIBUTION OF THE TRANSFERRIN-IRON CYCLE

The receptor-mediated endocytosis (RME) model for the uptake of transferrin-bound iron via a plasma membrane transferrin receptor is now generally accepted as being the mechanism by which erythroid cells acquire most, if not all, of the iron these cells require for haemoglobin synthesis. Once the general principle of the endocytotic iron cycle had been established, mainly from work on reticulocytes, it was assumed that a similar mechanism would be operative in all other cells and tissues, particularly since transferrin receptors had been identified on the plasma membranes of most other nonerythroid cells. However, the recent the accumulation of a considerable amount of experimental evidence suggests that in many nonerythroid tissues, particularly the liver, the RME model alone does not account for how these cells

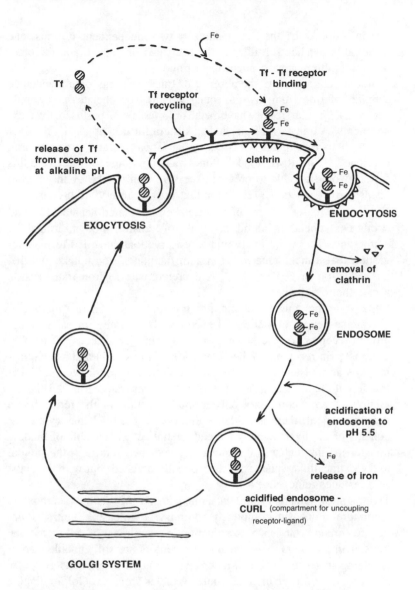

FIGURE 3.   A schematic representation of a suggested route for the receptor-mediated uptake of transferrin-bound iron by human reticulocytes — the transferrin cell cycle.

obtain all, or even part, of their iron requirements. Many of the experimental results that have led to the suggestion that alternative mechanisms for iron uptake exist in nonerythroid cells have been extensively discussed in a number of recent review articles.[10,17,35,79] These include the following:

1.   The uptake of iron by hepatocytes continues to increase even when the extracellular concentration of diferric transferrin is far in excess of the amount required to saturate all of the transferrin receptors. This implies

that iron uptake by the liver occurs by two independent systems, one a saturable mechanism utilising the transferrin receptor, and the other a nonsaturable receptor-independent route.

2.   Cultured cells grown in the absence of transferrin can obtain adequate supplies of iron from low-molecular-weight iron chelates and simple iron salts. Similar results have been reported from perfused liver experiments. A transferrin-independent system for iron uptake by the liver should help to explain why this organ is particularly prone to iron overload. If the RME model alone was functional in the liver, this system would be able to prevent excessive iron uptake by the mechanisms of receptor down-regulation that operate in erythroid cells.

3.   Hypoxia increases the rate of iron uptake by isolated hepatocytes, and strong Fe^{2+} chelators inhibit the uptake of transferrin-bound iron at the membrane. These and many related observations have led to the suggestion that a membrane redox system facilitates iron uptake and that the reduction of Fe^{3+} to Fe^{2+} is a prerequisite to iron translocation across the membrane.

4.   Hepatocyte membranes contain a high-affinity receptor that binds glycoproteins devoid of sialic acid residues. The number of asialoglycoprotein receptors on the hepatocyte membrane far exceeds the number of transferrin receptors. When a mixture of transferrin and asialotransferrin is administered to an animal, asialotransferrin delivers a higher fraction of the injected iron to the liver than does transferrin.[80] Although asialotransferrin comprises only a small fraction of the total plasma transferrin pool, there is evidence that one of the nonhepatocyte components of the liver, namely the endothelial cell, is capable of binding transferrin, internalising the molecule, and then returning the protein to the extracellular space with the iron still attached, but with the sialic acid residues removed.[30,81]

5.   Treatment of human erythroleukaemic cells (K562) with the carboxylic ionophore monensin completely inhibits the release of intracellular transferrin, and causes a 50% reduction in the number of cell membrane transferrin receptors. The remaining receptors are still capable of participating in an iron cycle. Monensin is thought to exert its effect by blocking the transfer of intracellular vesicles from the Golgi complex to the cell membrane. These results have been interpreted as indicating that some cells have two distinct transferrin-recycling pathways. One pathway is monensin-sensitive and represents transferrin-receptor recycling through the Golgi system, whilst an alternative monensin-resistant route bypasses the Golgi complex on the way back to the cell membrane.

It is clear from these and many other observations that there is not, as yet, a consensus view regarding the mechanisms of iron uptake by nonerythroid cells. At least five essentially different models have been proposed, and some of these do not involve the participation of the transferrin receptor, or even transferrin itself. A detailed discussion of each model is outside the scope of this book, but the schemes are listed below with appropriate references:

1. **Transferrin receptor-mediated endocytosis** — the RME model that operates in erythroid cells
2. **Absorption/fluid-phase endocytosis** (receptor independent) of transferrin-bound iron and small molecular iron chelates[82]
3. **Redox-mediated plasma membrane model** — with transferrin receptor-associated NADH reductase activity catalysing the reduction of ferric ions[83]
4. **The ferritin receptor model** — hepatocyte uptake of ferritin via a ferritin receptor; the ferritin being supplied by the Kupffer cells of the liver following the digestion of effete red cells[84]
5. **Asialoglycoprotein receptor** uptake of asialotransferrin by hepatocytes[30]

As a final comment on this subject, it seems appropriate to quote from a recent review by Theil and Ainsen[35] in which the authors concluded a section entitled, "Are Transferrin and its Receptor Essential for Physiological Uptake?" with the following remarks:

"The constellation of studies cited point to a mechanism of transferrin iron uptake by hepatocytes that does not entail participation of transferrin receptors. In the light of all that is known and appreciated today, flaws and discrepancies in the arguments can be discerned, but the question of receptor-independent uptake in nonerythroid cells is important and merits continuing examination. To assume that what is true of the highly specialised erythroid cell is true of all cells would be a mistake, and the last word in cellular uptake of iron from transferrin has yet to be uttered."

REFERENCES

1. **Martin, A. W., Heubers, E., Heubers, H., Webb, J., and Finch, C. A.,** A monosited transferrin from a representative deuterostome, *Blood,* 64, 1048, 1984.
2. **Jandl, J. H. and Katz, J. H.,** The plasma to cell cycle of transferrin, *J. Clin. Invest.,* 42, 314, 1963.
3. **Newman, R., Schneider, C., Sutherland, R., Vodenlich, L., and Greaves, M.,** The transferrin receptor, *Trends Biochem. Sci.,* 7. 397, 1982.
4. **Young, S. and Bomford, A.,** Transferrin and cellular iron exchange, *Clin. Sci.,* 67, 273, 1984.
5. **Bomford, A. B.,** Transferrin and its receptor: their roles in cell function, *Hepatology,* 5, 870, 1985.

6. **May, W. S.,** Transferrin receptor: its biological significance, *J. Membr. Biol.,* 88, 205, 1985.
7. **Irie, S.,** Transferrin-mediated cellular iron uptake, *Am. J. Med. Sci.,* 293, 103, 1987.
8. **Heubers, H. and Finch, C. A.,** The physiology of transferrin and transferrin receptors, *Physiol. Rev.,* 67, 520, 1987.
9. **Morgan, E. H.,** Role of transferrin receptors and endocytosis in iron uptake by hepatic and erythroid cells, *Ann. N.Y. Acad. Sci.,* 526, 65, 1988.
10. **Thorstensen, K. and Romslo, I.,** The role of transferrin in the mechanism of cellular iron uptake, *Biochem. J.,* 271, 1, 1990.
11. **Katz, J. H.,** Iron and protein kinetics studied by means of doubly-labelled human crystalline transferrin, *J. Clin. Invest.,* 40, 2143, 1961.
12. **Cavill, I. and Ricketts, C.,** The kinetics of iron metabolism, in *Iron in Biochemistry and Medicine,* A. Jacobs and M. Worwood, Eds., Academic Press, London, 1974, chap. 18.
13. **Sutherland, R., Delia, D., Schreider, C., Newman, R., Kemshead, J., and Greaves, M.,** Ubiquitous cell-surface glycoprotein on tumour cell is proliferation-associated receptor for transferrin, *Proc. Natl. Acad. Sci. U.S.A.,* 78, 4515, 1980.
14. **Trowbridge, I. S. and Lopez, F.,** Monoclonal antibody to transferrin receptor blocks transferrin binding and inhibits tumour cell growth in vitro, *Proc. Natl. Acad. Sci. U.S.A.,* 79, 1175, 1982.
15. **Trowbridge, I. S. and Newman, R. A.,** Monoclonal antibodies to transferrin receptor: probes for receptor structure and function, in *Receptors and Recognition, Series B,* Vol. 17, Chapman and Hall, London, 1984, 235.
16. **Panaccio, M., Zalcberg, J. R., Thompson, C. H., Leyden, M. J., and McKensie, A.,** Heterogeneity of the human transferrin receptor and use of anti-transferrin-receptor antibodies to detect tumour in vivo, *Immun. Cell Biol.,* 65, 461, 1987.
17. **de Jong, G., van Dijk, J. P., and van Eijk, H. G.,** The biology of transferrin, *Clin. Chim. Acta,* 190, 1, 1990.
18. **Shumak, K. H. and Rachkewitch, R. A.,** Transferrin receptors on human reticulocytes: variation in site number in haemotologic disorders, *Am. J. Haematol.,* 16, 23, 1984.
19. **Testa, U.,** Transferrin receptors: structure and function, *Curr. Top. Haematol.,* 5, 127, 1985.
20. **Trowbridge, I. S., Newman, R. A., Domingo, D. L., and Sauvage, C.,** Transferrin receptors: structure and function, *Biochem. Pharmacol.,* 33, 925, 1984.
21. **Morgan, E. H. and Baker, E.,** Role of transferrin receptor and endocytosis in iron uptake by hepatic and erythroid cells, *Ann. N.Y. Acad. Sci.,* 256, 65, 1988.
22. **Soda, R. and Tavassoli, M.,** Liver endothelium and not hepatocytes or Kupffer cells have transferrin receptors, *Blood,* 63, 270, 1984.
23. **Kishmoto, T. and Tavassoli, M.,** Endothelial binding of transferrin in fractionated liver cell suspensions, *Biochem. Biophys. Acta,* 846, 14, 1985.
24. **van Berkel, T. J. C., Dekker, C. J., Kruijt, J., and van Eijk, H. G.,** The interaction in vivo of transferrin and asialotransferrin with liver cells, *Biochem. J.,* 243, 715, 1987.
25. **Galbraith, R. M. and Galbraith, G. M.,** Expression of transferrin receptors on mitogen-stimulated human peripheral blood lymphocytes: relation to cellular activity and related metabolic events, *Immunology,* 44, 703, 1981.
26. **Faulk, W. P., Hsi, B. L., and Stevens, P. J.,** Transferrin and transferrin receptors in carcinoma of the breast, *Lancet,* 2, 390, 1980.
27. **Tei, I., Makino, Y., Kadofuku, T., Kanamaru, I., and Konno, K.,** Increase in transferrin receptors in regenerating liver cells after partial hepatectomy, *Biochem. Biophys. Res. Commun.,* 121, 717, 1984.
28. **Leibman, A. and Ainsen, P.,** Transferrin receptors of the rabbit reticulocyte, *Biochemistry,* 16, 1268, 1977.
29. **Vogel, W., Bomford, A., Young, S., and Williams, R.,** Heterogeneous distribution of transferrin receptors on parenchymal and nonparenchymal cells: biochemical and morphological evidence, *Blood,* 69, 264, 1987.

30. **Tavasolli, M.,** The role of liver endothelium in the transfer of iron from transferrin to the hepatocyte, *Ann. N.Y. Acad. Sci.,* 526, 83, 1988.

31. **Rudolph, J. R., Regoeczi, E., and Southward, S.,** Quantification of rat hepatocyte transferrin receptors with poly- and monoclonal antibodies and protein A, *Histochemistry,* 88, 187, 1983.

32. **Klausner, R. D., Harford, J., and Renswoude, J.,** Rapid internalisation of the transferrin receptor in K 562 cells is triggered by ligand binding or the treatment with phorbol esters, *Proc. Natl. Acad. Sci. U.S.A.,* 81, 3005, 1984.

33. **Watts, C.,** Rapid endocytosis of the transferrin receptor in the absence of bound transferrin, *J. Cell Biol.,* 100, 633, 1985.

34. **Willingham, M. C. and Pastan, I.,** Ultrastructural immunochemical localisation of transferrin receptor using a monoclonal antibody in human KB cells, *J. Histochem. Cytochem.,* 33, 59, 1985.

35. **Theil, E. C. and Ainsen, P.,** The storage and transport of iron in animal cells, in *Iron Transport in Microbes, Plants and Animals,* G. Winkelmann, D. van der Helm, and J. B. Neilands, Eds., VCH Publishers, Weinheim, West Germany, 1987, chap. 26.

36. **Omary, M. B. and Trowbridge, I. S.,** Biosynthesis of the human transferrin receptor in cultured cells, *J. Biol. Chem.,* 256, 12888, 1981.

37. **Iacopetta, B. J., Morgan, E. H., and Yeoh, G. C. T.,** Transferrin receptors and iron uptake during erythroid cell development, *Biochim. Biophys. Acta,* 687, 204, 1982.

38. **Leibman, A. and Ainsen, P.,** Transferrin receptor of the rabbit reticulocyte, *Biochemistry,* 16, 1268, 1977.

39. **Hu, H. Y. and Ainsen, P.,** Molecular characteristics of the transferrin-receptor complex of rabbit reticulocytes, *J. Supramol. Struct.,* 8, 349, 1978.

40. **Wada, H. G., Hass, P. E., and Sussman, H. H.,** Transferrin receptor in human placental brush border membranes, *J. Biol. Chem.,* 254, 12629, 1979.

41. **Seligman, P. A., Schleicher, R. B., and Allen, R. H.,** Isolation and characterisation of the human transferrin receptor from human placenta, *J. Biol. Chem.,* 254, 9943, 1979.

42. **van Driel, I. R., Stearne, P. A., Grego, B., Simpson, R. J., and Godling, J. W.,** The receptor for transferrin on murine myeloma cells: one-step purification based on its physiology, and partial amino acid sequence, *J. Immunol.,* 133, 3220, 1984.

43. **Schneider, C., Owen, M. J., Banville, D., and Williams, J. G.,** Primary structure of transferrin receptor deduced from the mRNA sequence, *Nature (London),* 311, 675, 1984.

44. **Enns, C. A. and Sussman, H. H.,** Similarities between the transferrin receptor proteins on human reticulocytes and human placentae, *J. Biol. Chem.,* 256, 12620, 1981.

45. **Cotner, T., Das Gupta, A., Papayannopoulou, T., and Stamatoyannopoulos, C.,** Characterisation of a novel form of transferrin receptor expressed on normal erythroid progenitors, *Blood,* 73, 214, 1989.

46. **Wickner, W. T. and Lodish, H. F.,** Multiple mechanisms of protein insertion into and across membranes, *Science,* 230, 400, 1985.

47. **Zerial, M., Melancon, P., Schneider, C., and Garoff, H.,** The transmembrane segment of the human transferrin receptor functions as a signal peptide, *EMBO J.,* 5, 1543, 1986.

48. **Steiner, M.,** Identification of the binding sites for transferrin in reticulocytes, *Biochem. Biophys. Res. Commun.,* 94, 861, 1980.

49. **Hunt, C. R., Reigler, R., and Davis, A. A.,** Changes in glycosylation alter the affinity of the human transferrin receptor for its ligand, *J. Biol. Chem.,* 264, 9643, 1989.

50. **Adam, M. A., Rodriguez, A., Turbide, C., Larrick, J., Meighen, E., and Johnstone, R. M.,** In vitro acylation of the transferrin receptor, *J. Biol. Chem.,* 259, 15460, 1984.

51. **Grasso, J. A., Bruno, M., Yates, A. A., Wei, L., and Epstein, P. M.,** Calmodulin dependence of transferrin receptor recycling in rat reticulocytes, *Biochem. J.,* 266, 261, 1990.

52. **Ward, J. H., Kushner, J. P., and Kaplan, J.,** Preference of transferrin receptors for diferric transferrin, in *Structure and Function of Iron Storage and Transport Proteins,* I. Urushizaki, P. Ainsen, I. Listowsky, and J. W. Drysdale, Eds., Elsevier, Amsterdam, 1983, 341.

53. **Enns, C. A., Soumalaninen, H., Gebhardt, J., Schroder, J., and Sussman, H.,** Human transferrin receptor: expression of the receptor is assigned to chromosome 3, *Proc. Natl. Acad. Sci. U.S.A.,* 79, 3241, 1982.

54. **Goodfellow, P., Banting, G., Sutherland, R., Greaves, H., Solomon, E., and Povey, S.,** Expression of human transferrin receptor is controlled by a gene on chromosome 3: assignment using species specificity of a monoclonal antibody, *Somatic Cell Genet.,* 8, 197, 1982.

55. **Bost, K. L., Smith, E. M., and Blalock, J. E.,** Regions of complimentarity between the messenger RNAs for epidermal growth factor, transferrin, interleukin-2 and their respective receptors, *Biochem. Biophys. Res. Commun.,* 128, 1373, 1985.

56. **Kuhn, L. C., McClelland, A., and Ruddle, F. H.,** Gene transfer, expression and molecular cloning of the human transferrin receptor gene, *Cell,* 37, 95, 1984.

57. **McClelland, A., Kuhn, L. C., and Ruddle, F. H.,** The human transferrin receptor gene: genomic organisation and the complete primary structure deduced from a cDNA sequence, *Cell,* 39, 267, 1984.

58. **Theil, E. C.,** Regulation of ferritin and transferrin receptor mRNAs, *J. Biol. Chem.,* 265, 4771, 1990.

59. **Raglow, R.,** Regulation of messenger RNA turnover in eukaryotes, *Trends Biochem. Sci.,* 12, 358, 1987.

60. **Mullner, E. W. and Kuhn, L. C.,** A stem-loop in the 3' untranslated region mediates iron-dependent regulation of transferrin receptor mRNA stability in the cytoplasm, *Cell,* 53, 815, 1988.

61. **Rao, K., Harford, J. B., Rouault, T., McClelland, A., Ruddle, F. H., and Klausner, R. D.,** Transcriptional regulation by iron of the gene for the human transferrin receptor, *Mol. Cell. Biol.,* 6, 236, 1986.

62. **Casey, J. L., Di Jeso, B., Rao, K., Rouault, T. A., Klausner, R. D., and Harford, J. B.,** The promoter region of the human transferrin receptor gene, *Ann. N.Y. Acad. Sci.,* 526, 54, 1988.

63. **Bowman, B. H., Yang, F., and Adrian, G. S.,** Transferrin: evolution and genetic regulation of expression, *Adv. Genet.,* 25, 1, 1988.

64. **Karin, M. and Mintz, B.,** Receptor-mediated endocytosis of transferrin in developmentally totipotent mouse teratocarcinoma stem cells, *J. Biol. Chem.,* 256, 3245, 1981.

65. **Klausner, R. D., Harford, J., and van Renswoude, J.,** Rapid internalisation of the transferrin receptor in K562 cells is triggered by ligand binding or treatment with a phorbol ester, *Proc. Natl. Acad. Sci. U.S.A.,* 81, 3005, 1984.

66. **Watts, C.,** Rapid endocytosis of the transferrin receptor in the absence of bound transferrin, *J. Cell. Biol.,* 100, 633, 1985.

67. **Stein, B. S. and Sussman, H. H.,** Demonstration of two distinct transferrin receptor recycling pathways and transferrin-receptor internalisation in K562 cells, *J. Biol. Chem.,* 261, 10319, 1986.

68. **Ajoika, R. S. and Kaplan, J.,** Intracellular pools of transferrin receptors result from constitutive internalisation of unoccupied receptors, *Proc. Natl. Acad. Sci. U.S.A.,* 83, 6445, 1986.

69. **Girones, N. and Davis, R. J.,** Comparison of the kinetics of cycling of the transferrin receptor on the presence or absence of bound diferric transferrin, *Biochem. J.,* 264, 35, 1989.

70. **Wiley, H. S. and Kaplan, J.,** Epidermal growth factor rapidly induces a redistribution of transferrin receptor pools in human fibroblasts, *Proc. Natl. Acad. Sci. U.S.A.,* 81, 7456, 1984.

71. **Davis, R. J., Faucher, M., Racaniello, L. K., Carruthers, A., and Czech, M. P.,** Insulin-like growth factor-1 and epidermal growth factor regulate the expression of transferrin receptors at the cell surface by distinct mechanisms, *J. Biol. Chem.,* 262, 13126, 1987.

72. **Ward, D. V. and Kaplan, J.,** Mitogenic agents induce redistribution of transferrin receptors from internal pools to the cell surface, *Biochem. J.,* 238, 721, 1986.

73. **Grasso, J. A., Bruno, M., Yates, A. A., Wei, L., and Epstein, P. M.,** Calmodulin dependence of transferrin receptor recycling in rat reticulocytes, *Biochem. J.,* 266, 261, 1990.

74. **Davis, R. J. and Meisner, H.,** Regulation of transferrin recycling by protein kinase C is independent of receptor phosphorylation at serine 24 in Swiss 3T3 fibroblasts, *J. Biol. Chem.,* 262, 16041, 1987.

75. **Tanner, L. I. and Lienhard, G. E.,** Insulin elicits a redistribution of transferrin receptors in 3T3-L1 adipocytes through an increase in the rate constant for receptor externalization, *J. Biol. Chem.,* 262, 8975, 1987.

76. **Alvarez, E., Girones, N., and Davis, R. J.,** Inhibition of the receptor-mediated endocytosis of diferric transferrin is associated with the covalent modification of the transferrin receptor with palmitic acid, *J. Biol. Chem.,* 265, 16644, 1990.

77. **Morgan, E. M. and Appleton, T. C.,** Autoradiographic localisation of labelled transferrin in rat reticulocytes, *Nature (London),* 223, 1371, 1969.

78. **May, W. S.,** Transferrin receptor: its biological significance, *J. Membr. Biol.,* 88, 205, 1985.

79. **Crichton, R. R. and Charloteaux-Wauters, M.,** Iron transport and storage, *Eur. J. Biochem.,* 164, 485, 1987.

80. **van Berkel, T. J. C., Dekker, C. J., Kruigt, J., and van Eijk, H. G.,** The interaction in vivo of transferrin and asialotransferrin with liver cells, *Biochem. J.,* 243, 715, 1987.

81. **Tavassoli, M.,** Desialation of transferrin by liver endothelium: evidence for two cellular pathways for transferrin metabolism, *Trans. Assoc. Am. Physicians,* 99, 219, 1986.

82. **Sibille, J.-C., Octave, J.-N., Scheider, Y., Trouet, A., and Crichton, R. R.,** Transferrin protein and iron uptake by cultured hepatocytes, *FEBS Lett.,* 150, 365, 1982.

83. **Thorstensen, K. and Romslo, T.,** Uptake of iron from transferrin by isolated rat hepatocytes. A redox-mediated plasma membrane process?, *J. Biol. Chem.,* 263, 8844, 1988.

84. **Sibille, J.-C., Ciriolo, M., Kondo, H., Crichton, R. R., and Ainsen, P.,** Subcellular localisation of ferritin and iron taken up by rat hepatocytes, *Biochem. J.,* 262, 685, 1989.

85. **Borhani, D. W. and Harrison, S. C.,** Crystallization and X-ray diffraction studies of a soluble form of the human transferrin receptor, *J. Mol. Biol.,* 218, 685, 1991.

86. **Do, S., Enns, C. A., and Cummings, R. D.,** Human transferrin receptor contains O-linked oligosaccharides, *J. Biol. Chem.,* 265, 114, 1990.

87. **Enns, C. A., Clinton, E. M., Reckow, C. L., Root, B. J., Do, S., and Cook, C.,** Acquisition of the functional properties of the transferrin receptor during its biosynthesis, *J. Biol. Chem.,* 266, 13272, 1991.

Chapter 8

GENETIC VARIATION OF HUMAN TRANSFERRIN

I. INTRODUCTION

In 1949, Pauling et al.[1] demonstrated by the use of a simple electrophoretic technique that the inherited disease sickle cell anaemia was associated with the appearance in the red cells of affected individuals of a structurally abnormal form of haemoglobin, HbS. The abnormal or mutant form of haemoglobin could be distinguished from normal haemoglobin (HbA) on the basis of an altered electrophoretic mobility. This was to be an historically important observation in the field of human biology and genetics for two reasons. First, it demonstrated that the disease of sickle cell anaemia, which at that time (1949) had just been shown to be an inherited condition obeying Mendel's laws of genetics,[2] was a disorder with a molecular basis. Second, this was the first clear demonstration of the inheritance of a genetically abnormal or variant form of a human protein. The year 1949 can be considered as the year in which the subject of human biochemical genetics — the study of the extent to which individuals differ one from another on the basis of the structure of their gene products — was finally launched. A further 8 years was to elapse before Ingram[3] discovered the molecular difference between normal haemoglobin (HbA) and sickle cell haemoglobin (HbS), the substitution of a glutamic acid residue at position 6 in the β chain by a residue of valine. Nevertheless, in the intervening years (1949 to 1957), considerable advances were to be made in our understanding of the extent to which human proteins exhibited genetic variation, and human serum transferrin was to play a significant part in this story.

Soon after the discovery of the electrophoretically abnormal form of haemoglobin associated with sickle cell anaemia (HbS), a number of other inherited abnormalities of haemoglobin structure were detected by means of simple electrophoretic techniques. These included the variants HbC, HbD, and HbE. At the time, biologists might have been excused for imagining that the gene for human haemoglobin was the exception, rather than the rule, in being particularly or even uniquely susceptible to mutation. With the benefit of hindsight it is now possible to speculate how this misconception might have arisen. Haemoglobin is found in very high concentrations within human red cells, and has the additional advantage, not shared by many other human proteins, of being a coloured molecule. In order to detect mutations that result in an alteration in the overall charge on the molecule, simple electrophoretic methods are all that are normally required. There is no necessity to locate where the molecule has migrated in the electric field using any form of stain, since haemoglobin has a red colour.

Most other proteins in human cells and tissue fluids are both colourless and present at concentrations far less than that of haemoglobin. Therefore, in order to answer the question, "Do human proteins, other than haemoglobin, exhibit electrophoretically abnormal phenotypes?", biochemical geneticists in the early 1950s had to devise methods to detect where colourless proteins had migrated after electrophoresis. The first protein stains to be used for this purpose, such as, for example, Amido Black, were both nonspecific and of a relatively low sensitivity.

Human plasma is a fluid containing many hundreds of different proteins, but only a few are present at sufficiently high concentrations so as to enable their detection, after electrophoresis, by these nonspecific protein stains. The first example of a human protein, other than haemoglobin, to be shown to exhibit inherited electrophoretic variation, was the plasma protein haptoglobin, in 1955.[4,5] This discovery was soon followed in 1957 by two further examples — albumin[6] and **transferrin**.[7]

The discovery of genetic variation of human serum transferrin in the late 1950s made an important and significant contribution to the early stages in the development of the subject of human biochemical genetics. In addition, much has been learnt subsequently from the study of the genetic variation of both human and animal (Chapter 9) transferrin that has contributed significantly to our understanding of the biological role and mechanism of action of this iron-carrying protein. The vast majority of the 50 or more different genetic variants of human transferrin that have been discovered over the last 34 years (1957 to 1991) have been detected by means of electrophoresis of human plasma samples. The history of their discovery, for technical reasons to be explained shortly, conveniently falls into two sections. When human plasma is subjected to electrophoresis at an alkaline pH, using as a supporting medium either starch, agarose, or polyacrylamide, transferrin migrates towards the anode in the β-globulin fraction. Using this technique, a large number of different electrophoretic variants have been detected in human populations. In most cases the frequency of the variant phenotypes is comparatively low, and therefore in any population there is an obvious and common homozygous genotype. This is exemplified phenotypically as a single electrophoretically migrating protein band which, for reasons to be described later, is referred to as the Tf C phenotype. The variant electrophoretic phenotypes are most often observed in individuals who, on later family analysis, are found to be of a heterozygous genotype — with one normal, or common, transferrin allele (Tf^C) and one variant allele. The products of the variant alleles detected by electrophoresis at alkaline pH have been subdivided into two groups. Those with a faster (more anodal) mobility than Tf C are referred to as the Tf B variants, whilst those with a slower mobility than Tf C have been designated as the Tf D variants. The discovery, frequency, population distribution, and chemical characterisation of more than 35 different transferrin alleles, discovered during the period from 1957 to 1991, will be discussed in the next section.

Always implicit in these studies, certainly until 1978, was the conclusion that the common transferrin phenotype — Tf C — characterised by a single migrating protein band represented a single, homogeneous genotype. A chance discovery in 1978 clearly showed that this simple interpretation was not correct. This arose as a result of the application of an alternative method for the separation of plasma proteins. Electrophoresis of plasma at a single, usually alkaline pH is only capable of resolving complex mixtures of proteins when the individual components differ significantly, one from another, with respect to their overall charge. For this reason, until 1978 the common Tf C phenotype was considered to be a single variant possessed by most individuals. However, using the technique of isoelectric focussing (IEF) in a narrow pH range, Kuhnl and Spielmann[8] and Thymann[9] independently discovered a considerable degree of genetic heterogeneity within the Tf C phenotype. Since then, as many as 13 different alleles have been described, the products of which can be distinguished, one from another, by means of IEF, but not by using the more conventional electrophoretic techniques at a single alkaline pH. The subject of the genetic variation of human serum transferrin, as revealed by IEF, is commonly referred to as Tf C subtyping. It should be emphasised, however, that there is no inherent difference, at least in genetic terms, between the transferrin variation detected by these two electrophoretic procedures. However, since Tf C subtyping has, over the last 10 years, attracted considerable interest from forensic scientists, population geneticists, and clinicians, the subject will be discussed in more detail in a separate section, later in this chapter.

II. GENETIC VARIATION OF HUMAN TRANSFERRIN DETECTED BY ELECTROPHORESIS AT AN ALKALINE pH

A. HISTORICAL INTRODUCTION

In the early 1950s, electrophoresis of plasma proteins was usually carried out with filter paper as the supporting medium. The resolution that paper electrophoresis could achieve appears relatively crude when compared with the results that can be obtained using present-day electrophoretic techniques. Even with the introduction of starch gel electrophoresis by Smithies[4] in 1955, the number of protein components that could be resolved from a sample of human plasma was comparatively few — albumin, $\alpha 1$- and $\alpha 2$-globulins, β-globulin, and γ-globulin. In 1956, Smithies and Poulik[10] combined the two techniques of paper and starch gel electrophoresis by developing a two-dimensional procedure for the separation of plasma proteins. This method was found to be capable of resolving the proteins of human plasma into at least 20 fractions. In particular, the β-globulin fraction was shown to contain at least four separate components, designated bands A, B, C, and E. Protein C, whose identity at the time was unknown, is quantitatively the most predominant of the β-globulins.

In the following year, 1957, Smithies[7] reported the discovery of a small number of plasma samples in which the β-globulin electrophoretic pattern was clearly different from that found in the vast majority of human plasmas. An additional β-globulin band, with a slower anodal mobility than protein C, was detected in the plasma of two Negroes from New York (out of 47 tested) and five Australian aborigines (out of 21 tested). The abnormal β-globulin band was designated D, and in each of the seven samples, bands C and D appeared to be present in approximately equal concentrations. In a further report the following year (1958), Horsfall and Smithies[11] extended the study to other population groups, as well as examining plasma samples from other members of the aboriginal families in which the unusual β-globulin CD phenotype had originally been found. Amongst several hundred plasma samples, largely from people of European ancestry, β-globulin D was not observed. Amongst the aboriginal families, however, several further examples of the variant CD phenotype were found, and in addition, one individual was found in which the normal β-globulin C band was totally absent and the D variant protein was present at a high concentration. Fortunately, this particular individual with the rare D phenotype was married with six children. Her husband was of the common C phenotype, and all the children were found to have the variant CD phenotype in which β-globulins C and D were present in the plasma at approximately equal concentrations. Smithies[7] had previously postulated, on the basis of the racial differences in the occurrence of the CD variant phenotype, that human β-globulin might be exhibiting genetic variation. The results from this one aboriginal family provided the first genetic evidence in support of this theory. Accordingly, Horsfall and Smithies[11] proposed that human β-globulin was under the control of two codominant alleles at a single autosomal gene locus, and that the genotype β^C/β^C resulted in the presence of the β-globulin C band in plasma, and the absence of D (the common C phenotype). The heterozygous combination of alleles, β^C/β^D, would lead to the appearance of both proteins in the plasma, since the alleles were codominant. This would be expressed as the variant CD phenotype. Finally, the very rare D phenotype in which only the D band was present would be the expression of the homozygous genotype β^D/β^D.

Within a few months, Smithies[12] published a further report in the summer of 1958 presenting the results of an electrophoretic survey of the plasma samples from 425 Canadian blood donors at Toronto General Hospital. No examples of the CD or D phenotypes were found, and 420 of those tested had the common C phenotype. In the plasma of the remaining five individuals, band C was detected at about half the normal concentration. However, in addition, the β-globulin B band, a minor component of all plasmas that migrated more anodally than C, was found in these five people at significantly higher concentrations, such that the C and B bands appeared with approximately equal staining intensity. From the results of subsequent family studies, Smithies concluded that he had discovered a third allele (β^B) at the gene locus for human β-globulin.

It is possible to summarise the experimental observations reported by Smithies as follows:

"Human plasma contains a number of proteins migrating in the β-globulin region. The most predominant member of this group is β-globulin C, a protein that in most people migrates as a single electrophoretic band. This common phenotype (C) is genetically controlled by two identical alleles — β^C, at an autosomal gene locus. In Negro and aboriginal populations a variant allele (β^D) is present at a low gene frequency. The product of this rare allele is the β-globulin protein D, which has a slower anodal mobility than C. In a Canadian population, a second variant allele has been detected — β^B, the product of which is a plasma β-globulin band with a faster anodal mobility than C. This has been designated β-globulin B.''

Towards the end of 1958, one further report on the subject of human β-globulin genetic variation was published by Harris et al.[13] This group analysed plasma samples from 153 Africans from Gambia, and 139 English people, using starch gel electrophoresis and the two-dimensional procedure of Smithies.

In the Gambian samples, whilst most of the individuals were found to have the common C phenotype, four unrelated people had a variant electrophoretic pattern in the β-globulin region, with an additional, slower migrating band. Three of the variant phenotypes appeared to be identical and were thought to correspond to the CD phenotype previously described by Smithies. However, in the fourth sample the extra D band had a distinctly slower electrophoretic mobility. Harris deduced that this was the product of a new rare variant allele of the D family. The β-globulin variant reported by Smithies in the Negro and aboriginal population, and then discovered by Harris in three individuals from Gambia, was redesignated β-globulin D_1. The new variant discovered by Harris in the fourth Gambian sample was designated D_2.

Amongst the 139 English people tested, Harris found no examples of either the βCD_1 or the βCD_2 variant phenotypes. The common C phenotype was found in 137 of the samples. The two remaining samples both had a variant phenotype, in each case associated with the appearance of an extra, more anodally migrating B band in addition to the normal C band. The two phenotypes were not, however, identical. One appeared to be identical to the variant pattern discovered by Smithies in the Canadian survey, and this was designated the β-globulin CB_1 phenotype. In the second variant discovered by Harris, the new B band did not migrate as far towards the anodal pole as did that of the B_1 variant. This new variant was designated β-globulin CB_2. By combining his results with those of Smithies, Harris concluded that a whole series of β-globulin variant phenotypes could occur as a result of the presence in human populations of five alternative alleles at the β-globulin gene locus — the common allele β^C, and four rare alleles β^{B1}, β^{B2}, β^{D1}, and β^{D2}. Harris further suggested that the situation with regard to the human β-globulin gene locus might prove to be analogous to that found with respect to the many genetically determined variants of human haemoglobin that had so far (1958) been described. Figure 1 depicts the six electrophoretic phenotypes of human β-globulin that had been discovered by the end of 1958.

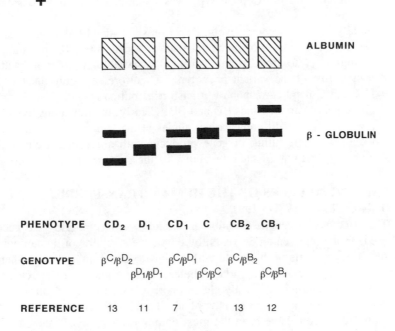

FIGURE 1. A diagram showing the six variant electrophoretic phenotypes of human serum β-globulin that had been discovered by the end of 1958.

The identity of the β-globulin component of human plasma exhibiting this genetic variation remained a mystery for a further 6 months. Then, in the summer of 1959, Smithies and co-workers[14,15] published the results from a series of experiments, concluding that the β-globulin molecule that they had been studying for the past 2 years was the iron-binding and iron-transport protein **transferrin**.

The evidence upon which this conclusion was based can be summarised as follows:

1. From the average iron-binding capacity of normal human plasma, the molecular weight of transferrin, and the fact that transferrin can bind two atoms of iron, it was calculated that the concentration of transferrin in plasma should be in the region of 2.5 mg/mL. By scanning the stained electrophoretic gels with a photoelectric reflectometer, it was estimated that the concentration of β-globulin C in plasma of the βC phenotype was between 2.2 and 2.8 mg/mL.

2. The electrophoretic mobility of pure human transferrin was found to be identical to that of the β-globulin C protein.

3. Orally administered radioactive iron (^{59}Fe) was found to bind almost exclusively to the β-globulin C protein when the plasma from an

individual with the C phenotype was examined by two-dimensional electrophoresis.

4.   Finally, and most conclusively, ^{59}Fe iron salts added to human plasma was found, by means of starch gel electrophoresis and subsequent autoradiography, to bind to the genetically variable β-globulin bands, irrespective of the variant phenotype. Therefore, not only did the β-globulin C band correspond to transferrin, but so also did the electrophoretically variant bands βD and βB. Clearly, the mutations that had given rise to the different variant alleles at the human transferrin gene locus, whilst resulting in gene products with altered electrophoretic mobility, had not affected the ability of the proteins to bind iron.

B. VARIANT ALLELES OF THE HUMAN TRANSFERRIN B AND D GROUPS, 1959 TO 1991

The discovery of genetic variation of human transferrin in 1957 has been followed, in the intervening 34 years, by extensive sampling of human populations in many parts of the world with a view to determining the number, range, and frequency of the variant alleles. The techniques of starch gel electrophoresis, and more recently electrophoresis in a variety of alternative supporting media (agar, agarose, and polyacrylamide) with improved powers of protein resolution, have been the most commonly employed methods. It is not possible to estimate with any accuracy the total number of individuals that have been screened to date (1991). In a comprehensive review by Mourant et al.[16] of the papers published up to the end of 1972, the total stood at 94,665. Almost certainly over the last 20 years this number has increased by at least a factor of 10. The actual number (and this of course only takes into account the results of surveys that have been published) is likely to be well in excess of 1 million, particularly with the renewed interest in genetic variation of human transferrin that followed the discovery of the Tf C subtypes in 1978.[8,9]

The presence of a variant allele at the transferrin gene locus, either within a family or a larger population group, has usually been discovered when the product of the variant allele is a molecule of transferrin electrophoretically distinguishable from the product of the common Tf[C] allele. Such a variant allele can only be classified as new, or unique, when the gene product can be distinguished, not only from that of the common C allele, but also from all the other variant alleles previously described. Ultimately, as the chemical structures (amino acid substitutions) of the different transferrin variants are elucidated, it will be possible to be more confident when reporting the discovery of a "new" variant allele. Unfortunately, at the present time, the structural analysis of the human transferrin variants lags well behind the situation that exists in the case of the human haemoglobin variants, where the amino acid substitutions of more than 500 different variants are known. Therefore, electrophoretic comparison remains the principal method available for distinguishing between the human transferrin variants.

For this reason it is difficult to be precise about the number of different variant alleles of human transferrin that have been discovered to date (1991).

In a recent review on this topic in 1988, Farhud et al.[17] found evidence in the published literature of 35 different variant alleles. Their gene products were either of the B or D (fast or slow) electrophoretic subgroups. Since then at least two further variants have been detected and partially characterised, taking the total number of different alleles at the human transferrin gene locus to 38, including the common Tf^C allele.

The nomenclature that has been used to describe the different variants of human transferrin (detected after electrophoresis at alkaline pH) has undergone a number of modifications over the years. It has been agreed that the gene products of variant alleles with an electrophoretic migration more anodal (faster) than Tf C should be referred to as the B variants. Likewise, variants with a mobility less anodal (slower) than Tf C have been designated the D variants. As the first few variants were discovered during the period from 1957 to 1960, numerical subscripts were used in order to distinguish the different variant alleles. The lower the number, the more anodal the mobility. For a time this system proved adequate, with the variants described up to 1961 being as follows: B_0, B_1, B_2, B_3, **C**, D_1, D_2, and D_3, in order of decreasing anodal mobility. However, as the flow of newly discovered variants increased in the 1960s it soon became apparent that this system of nomenclature could not be continued. For example, in 1961 Parker and Bearn[18] described a new variant of human transferrin within the population of the Navajo Indians. Since the mobility of the variant was intermediate between that of Tf D_0 and Tf D_1, it was called Tf D_{0-1}. As further examples of a similar situation arose, transferrin variants began to take on the names of the places or populations in which they had first been detected ($B_{SEATTLE}$ and $D_{INDONESIA}$). Some recently reported variants have been given, as a temporary designation, the name of the family in which they were found (B_{SHAW}). Clearly, this mixed form of labelling will become even more confusing in the future and will need to be resolved. It is, however, a problem that is not unique to transferrin variation.

The discovery of the B and D variants of human transferrin has been reviewed at regular intervals over the last 34 years in an attempt to keep pace with the appearance in the literature of reports of new variants — Giblett (1962),[19] Kirk (1968),[20] Giblett (1969),[21] Buettner-Janusch (1970),[22] Walter (1975),[23] Mourant et al. (1976),[16] Cooper (1978),[24] Gaensslen (1983),[25] Kamboh and Ferrell (1987),[26] and Farhud et al. (1988).[17]

Many of these reviews have attempted to arrange, in the form of a diagram, the transferrin variants on a scale of relative electrophoretic mobility. This type of scheme provides a basis for comparing newly discovered variants with older ones. Until such time as the variant proteins have been structurally analysed (amino acid substitution) or better still, the mutant alleles have been cloned and sequenced (nucleotide base substitution), the method of electrophoretic comparison remains the most reliable index of transferrin variant characterisation.

As will be discussed later in this chapter, most of the variant transferrin alleles occur at very low frequencies (<0.01) in human populations. For this reason they have usually been first discovered in individuals who are genetically heterozygous, with one normal Tf^C allele and one Tf^{variant} allele present at the transferrin gene locus of diploid cells. The phenotypic expression of the heterozygous genotype results in the appearance in the blood plasma of two electrophoretically distinguishable bands — Tf C and either Tf B$_{variant}$ or Tf D$_{variant}$. In most cases the two transferrin proteins have been found to be present in approximately equal proportions. In order to reduce the complexity of the diagram, only the relative mobilities of the single allele products are shown in Figure 2. In effect, this is how the homozygous phenotype would appear electrophoretically. However, it is only in the case of the more frequently occurring variant alleles that the homozygote phenotypes have been detected in families or populations. The electrophoretically distinguishable gene products of 38 transferrin alleles are depicted in Figure 2. In theory, this genetic diversity could generate a maximum of 666 different human transferrin phenotypes. The fact that only about 50 of these possible phenotypes have ever been discovered is evidence of the low frequency at which most of the variant alleles occur within the population.

C. THE STRUCTURE AND PROPERTIES OF THE TRANSFERRIN B AND D VARIANTS

When one considers that transferrin is the fourth most abundant protein in human plasma — being present at a concentration of 2.5 g/L — it seems surprising that so few of the genetically determined variant forms have been isolated, purified, and characterised with respect to their amino acid substitutions. A 20-mL sample of plasma from a heterozygous phenotype might be expected to yield between 10 and 20 mg of the variant protein. If this amount of a genetic variant of human haemoglobin were to be available, it would be more than sufficient material in order to carry out peptide mapping, amino acid analysis, and sequence determination of the globin chain. Transferrin, however, with its molecular weight of about 80,000, is nearly five times larger than globin. Since digestion of transferrin with the proteolytic enzyme trypsin can produce as many as 84 unique peptides, the problems associated with two-dimensional peptide mapping are that much more difficult. An alternative approach has been to carry out an initial cleavage of the protein with cyanogen bromide. With only nine methionine residues present in human transferrin, this procedure yields a maximum of ten peptides. Nevertheless, these peptides still need to be separated and further digested with a range of proteolytic enzymes.

Until recently, only three genetic variants of transferrin had been studied in sufficient detail to enable the amino acid substitutions to be determined, and the last of these was published as long ago as 1967 (Table 1). All three (B$_2$, D$_1$, and D$_{CHI}$) are examples of variants where the mutant alleles occur at a comparatively high frequency within particular populations. In addition, they have apparently normal characteristics with respect to iron binding and release. Most of the other transferrin variants that have been purified

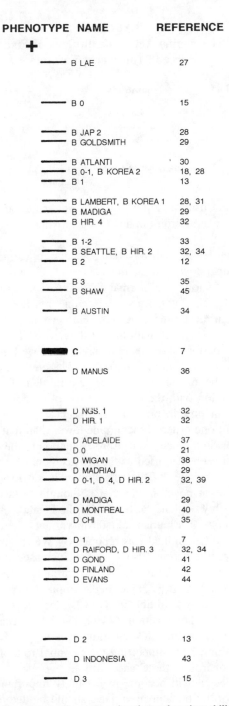

FIGURE 2. A diagram showing the comparative electrophoretic mobilities of the gene products of 38 human transferrin alleles.

TABLE 1
The Amino Acid Substitutions of Five
Human Transferrin Variants

Variant	Substitution	Ref.
D_1	$277^{\text{Aspartic acid}\rightarrow\text{Glycine}}$	48, 49
D_{CHI}	$300^{\text{Histidine}\rightarrow\text{Arginine}}$	50
B_2	$652^{\text{Glycine}\rightarrow\text{Glutamic acid}}$	51
D_{EVANS}	$394^{\text{Glycine}\rightarrow\text{Arginine}}$	44, 46, 47
B_{SHAW}	$378 \text{ or } 381^{\text{Isoleucine}\rightarrow\text{Aspartic acid}}$	45

sufficiently to permit iron binding and release studies to be carried out, have also been shown to exhibit iron-binding characteristics indistinguishable from those of the common Tf C type.[26]

In 1982, Evans et al.[44] discovered a new rare variant of the human transferrin D group (slow) during the course of a survey of 5000 serum samples. Whilst this variant had normal characteristics of iron uptake, it was found that one of the iron atoms, namely the one attached to the C-site, was particularly labile in the presence of urea. Furthermore, the iron-free C-site of the variant, when compared with that of the normal Tf C transferrin, was less stable to both thermal and urea denaturation, as well as being unable to bind copper, zinc, or aluminium.[46] A further characteristic of the Tf D_{EVANS} variant that clearly distinguishes the molecule from that of normal transferrin (Tf C) is its interaction with the transferrin receptor of human lymphocytes *in vitro*. The variant protein binds to the receptors of these cells with an association constant one order of magnitude lower than that of normal transferrin.[47] This results in a much reduced iron donation to the cells. The amino acid difference has been identified as the replacement of glycine at position 394 by an arginine residue.[48] This substitution is sufficiently close to the aspartic acid residue at position 393 that is thought to be involved in iron binding, as to possibly explain the lability of the C-site iron in this variant.

The fifth example of a human transferrin variant where the amino acid substitution has been determined was reported by Welch and Langmead[45] in 1990. Interestingly, this variant also shows an increased lability of the iron attached to the C-site, but, unlike the Evans variant, the one described by Welch and Langmead[45] (Tf B_{SHAW}) has an electrophoretic mobility faster than Tf C. The amino acid substitution in Tf B_{SHAW} is the replacement of the isoleucine residue at either position 378 or 381 by an asparagine residue. Again, like the Evans variant, this substitution is very close to the aspartic acid residue at position 392, supporting the essential role of this amino acid in the the binding of iron to the C-site.

In future studies, it will become increasingly important that the amino acid substitutions of the transferrin variants should be determined. Not only will this provide a means of distinguishing variant phenotypes that are electrophoretically very similar, but it will also provide valuable information as to the relative importance of different amino acids in the process of iron binding and release, and also that of receptor recognition. Increasingly nowadays, these data are more likely to be obtained from the analysis of the nucleotide sequences of the cloned variant genes.

D. THE SILENT (Tf⁰) ALLELE AND CONGENITAL ATRANSFERRINAEMIA

Of the 300 or more gene loci that have so far been found to exhibit genetic variation in human populations, the transferrin gene locus would be unusual, possibly even unique, if amongst the variant phenotypes there were not found to be present examples of a silent or null allele, Tf^0. Transferrin appears to be essential for the delivery of iron, at least at normal physiological levels, to most tissues, with the possible exception of the liver. One can therefore predict that the consequences for the homozygous genotype (Tf^0/Tf^0) are likely to be very serious, if not life-threatening. For this reason alone it might be expected that the frequency of the silent allele would be extremely low, resulting from a strong negative selective pressure. The ultimate phenotypic expression of the homozygous genotype (Tf^0/Tf^0) would be the failure to deliver transferrin-bound iron to the intracellular sites for utilisation and storage, coupled with an inability to redistribute the iron from iron stores. The pathway leading from the transferrin gene within the nucleus to the appearance in cells of the iron-loaded protein is long and complex, and subject to careful regulation at many stages. The details of the process have been described in previous chapters. It is possible to imagine many steps in the pathway where genetically controlled disorders could occur, resulting in either partial or complete atransferrinaemia (Figure 3). At the molecular level, the genetic defects likely to result in the phenotypic expression of atransferrinaemia could range from the complete deletion of the transferrin gene to single-base changes in coding (exon), noncoding (intron), or adjacent promoter regions of the gene. If the example of the human haemoglobin gene is in any way analogous, all of these mutations are possible.

The first reported case of congenital atransferrinaemia was by Heilmeyer et al.[53] in 1961. Subsequently, other investigators have described similar examples of this rare genetic disorder.[54-58] These very rare cases share many clinical and biochemical features, including iron-deficient, microcytic, and hypochromic anaemia, lack of response to the administration of iron; low red cell count; low serum iron level; trace amounts of transferrin in the plasma, often less than 3 mg/100 mL (normal range 180 to 320 mg/100 mL); excessive deposition of iron (haemosiderosis) within the liver, pancreas, adrenal gland, and cardiac muscle; and finally, very low or absent iron stores in the bone marrow. The genetic basis of this disorder has been confirmed by family studies as an autosomal recessive. Both parents of the affected individual, whilst having near normal red cell indices, invariably exhibit a mild hypotransferrinaemia, with about 50% of the normal level of plasma transferrin. Whilst a long-term clinical assessment of very few of the heterozygotes has

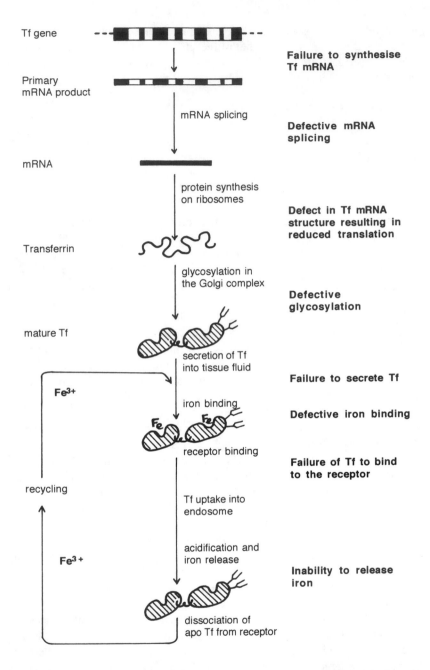

FIGURE 3.   Some of the possible sites where mutations could give rise to partial or complete atransferrinaemia.

been possible, there are indications that they are liable to become mildly siderotic later in life.

The most severe of the clinical consequences of congenital atransferrinaemia result from the excessive accumulation of the iron within the liver, pancreas, and at a later stage, cardiac muscle. This suggests that in the absence of transferrin, alternative iron-carrying molecules within the plasma are capable of transporting and delivering dietary iron to the liver and pancreas, but presumably not to the cells of the bone marrow. A number of possible candidates have been suggested, and these include citrate, carbonate, ascorbate, amino acids, carbohydrates, and to a lesser extent, plasma proteins such as albumin.[59,60]

A similar disorder of hereditary hypotransferrinaemia with haemosiderosis has been described in mice.[61] Again, the pattern of inheritance is a Mendelian autosomal recessive, and the affected animals, which would otherwise have a very short life-span, can be kept alive by frequent intravenous injections of purified transferrin.

The frequency of congenital atransferrinaemia in human populations is extremely rare, so much so that it is not possible to accurately estimate its incidence. Therefore, the carrier or heterozygous genotype (Tf^C/Tf^0) must be present within the population at large, unless one postulates that all cases of atransferrinaemia have arisen as a consequence of new mutations in the parental germ cell lines. Even assuming a homozygote frequency of as little as 1 in 10^7, it is possible to calculate from the Hardy-Weinberg equation that the frequency of the heterozygote would be in the order of 1 in 1500. This phenotype is unlikely to be detected during the course of an electrophoretic survey of plasma samples. The normal range of plasma transferrin concentration is between 180 and 320 mg/100 mL, so a 50% reduction in the heterozygote will still result in an intensely staining protein band.

Situations where the presence of the silent allele has been indicated have often been in family studies, particularly in cases of disputed parentage. Although the B and D groups of the electrophoretic variants of human transferrin, because of their low frequency, are of little value in such cases, the same is not true for the highly polymorphic alleles of transferrin that can only be detected by IEF (to be discussed in a later section). The gene products of the two most common subtype alleles, Tf^{C1} and Tf^{C2}, have found many useful forensic applications, including paternity testing. There have been occasional reports in the literature of transferrin subtyping results which, at first sight, would imply that a woman could not be the biological mother of her child. Such an example would be where the mother's phenotype appears to be Tf C_2, whereas that of her child is Tf C_1. Normally the C_2 phenotype would be interpreted as the expression of the homozygous genotype Tf^{C2}/Tf^{C2}, such that a mother would have to pass a Tf^{C2} allele to all of her children. Clearly, in the example quoted, this has not happened, and therefore a maternal exclusion is indicated. However, if all other genetic tests fail to confirm a maternal exclusion, the presence of a silent Tf^0 allele could be invoked in order to explain the anomalous transferrin phenotypes. The genotypes of the mother and child in the example quoted would be redesignated Tf^{C2}/Tf^{C0} and Tf^{C1}/Tf^{C0}, respectively, and therefore allow the mother to pass the silent allele to the child. In those situations where the presence of a silent Tf^0 allele within a family has been postulated, additional confirmation has often been obtained following careful measurements of the serum transferrin levels, usually by sensitive immunological procedures.

Even when the few isolated reports of the silent transferrin allele found during the course of family studies are added to the handful of clinical examples of atransferrinaemia, it is still evident that the frequency of the Tf^0 within human populations is extremely low. However, not all cases of hypotransferrinaemia have a genetic basis. Decreased levels of plasma transferrin are frequently associated with a wide range of acquired diseases, including portal cirrhosis of the liver, chronic infection, neoplasia, and some renal disorders.[62] This aspect of transferrin chemistry and pathophysiology will be discussed in Chapter 10.

E. THE FREQUENCY OF THE B AND D VARIANT TRANSFERRIN ALLELES AND THEIR WORLDWIDE DISTRIBUTION

Genetically determined variant phenotypes of human serum transferrin have been found in nearly every population so far tested. Of the 37 different B and D variant alleles that have been described, the vast majority have been found to occur as rare alleles, at a very low frequency, often being confined to a single family or small population group. However, three of the variant alleles have been detected at sufficiently high frequencies so as to permit their classification as examples of genetic polymorphism. The term polymorphism was coined by Ford[63] in 1940 to describe "the occurrence together in the same locality of two or more discontinuous forms of a species in such a proportion that the rarest of them cannot be maintained by recurrent mutation." In the context of the extensive, genetically determined enzyme and protein diversity that is now evident in all human populations, Harris[64] in 1970 suggested that the term polymorphism should be used to describe situations where, "at a given gene locus two or more alleles occur in a population, each with frequencies greater than 0.01." Although the distinction between rare alleles (< 0.01) and polymorphic alleles (> 0.01) appears to be entirely arbitrary, it is still a useful definition, widely employed by biochemical geneticists. For a gene locus where a single variant allele occurs at a frequency of 0.01 and therefore the normal or common allele has a frequency of 0.99, the incidence of the heterozygous variant phenotype will be in the order of 1 in 50 of the population (2%).

The three variant alleles at the human transferrin gene locus that have been found at frequencies greater than 0.01 in a number of human populations are Tf^{D1}, Tf^{DCHI}, and Tf^{B0-1}. A fourth variant whose frequency approaches that of a polymorphic allele is Tf^{B2}.

Tf^{D1} — This variant allele occurs widely in Africa, south of the Sahara, with the variant phenotype CD_1 being found at frequencies ranging from 1 to 15%. Similar frequencies are found amongst the American Negro population. In addition, the D_1 allele occurs at even higher frequencies amongst the aboriginal population of Australia and the Melanesian populations of New Guinea, Fiji, and the New Hebrides. It has been confirmed that the D_1 variants of the African and aboriginal populations have the same amino acid substitution.[65] Reports of the D_1 allele in other parts of the world, albeit at much lower frequencies, include Finland, Sweden, Germany, Greece, and Greenland (Eskimos). It remains to be confirmed, by amino acid analysis, whether these are indeed examples of the same D_1 variant as present in Africa and Australia.

Tf^{DCHI} — This variant, which has an electrophoretic mobility only slightly faster than D_1, is found amongst the populations of south and southeast Asia — China, Japan, Cambodia, Vietnam, and India. In addition, the same variant appears to be present in the Indian populations of most Central American countries and some of the South American tribes. One further group where the incidence of the CD_{CHI} phenotype has been found at a frequency of nearly 2% is amongst the Lapps in Finland. Kirk[20] has suggested that the Tf^{DCHI} allele is of Mongoloid origin, supporting other anthropological evidence that the Mongoloid dispersion took place from North Asia, in both easterly and westerly directions.

Tf^{B0-1} — This variant allele, absent from Africa and most of Europe, is principally confined to the Indian tribes of North and Central America. A particularly high frequency of the CB_{0-1} phenotype is found amongst the Navajo Indians (7%). There is a suggestion that the Tf^{B0-1} allele might also be of Mongoloid origin, since the same variant phenotype has been found amongst the Lapps in Finland.

Tf^{B2} — Although not quite reaching a true polymorphic frequency, this is the most frequently occurring variant allele in the caucasian populations of Europe and North America.

The worldwide distribution of the polymorphic and rare alleles at the human transferrin gene locus has been the subject of a number of reviews over the last 25 years.[16,20,25,26] Table 2 is an attempt to combine much of this published data in order to compare the distribution of the B and D variant alleles throughout the major geographical regions of the world.

TABLE 2
The Population Distribution of Tf B and Tf D Variants[16,20,25,26]

	Phenotype numbers							Gene frequencies

Europe

Finland

n	C	CB_{0-1}	CB_2	CB_1	CD_{CHI}	CD_{FIN}	CD_1	
4,939	4,716	69	19	18	90	6	21	$C = 0.978$
								$D_{CHI} = 0.0091$
								$B_{0-1} = 0.007$
								$D_1 = 0.0021$
								$B_2 = 0.0019$
								$B_1 = 0.0018$
								$D_{FIN} = 0.0006$

Sweden

n	C	CB_1	CB_{1-2}	CD_1	
3,755	3,714	7	30	4	$C = 0.9946$
					$B_{1-2} = 0.004$
					$B_1 = 0.00093$
					$D_1 = 0.00053$

West Germany

n	C	CB_1	CB_2	CD_1	
4,669	4,614	1	41	13	$C = 0.9952$
					$B_2 = 0.0033$
					$D_1 = 0.0014$
					$B_1 = 0.00011$

Norway

n	C	CB_{1-2}	CB_2	
950	941	2	7	$C = 0.9952$
				$B_2 = 0.0037$
				$B_{1-2} = 0.0011$

Hungary

n	C	CB_0	CB_{0-1}	
1,007	1,002	1	4	$C = 0.9975$
				$B_{0-1} - 0.002$
				$B_0 = 0.005$

Greece

n	C	CB_2	CB_{1-2}	CD_1	CD_{CHI}	$CB_{ATLANTI}$	
3,345	3,332	3	1	7	1	1	$C = 0.998$
							$D_1 = 0.0011$
							$B_2 = 0.00045$
							$B_{1-2} = 0.00015$
							$D_{CHI} = 0.00015$
							$B_{ATLANTI} = 0.00015$

Asia

India

n	C	D_{CHI}	
1,186	1,177	9	$C = 0.9962$
			$D_{CHI} = 0.0038$

Ceylon

n	C	CB_2	CD_{CHI}	$D_{CHI}D_{CHI}$	
462	453	1	7	1	$C = 0.989$
					$D_{CHI} = 0.0097$
					$B_2 = 0.0011$

TABLE 2 (continued)
The Population Distribution of Tf B and Tf D Variants[16,20,25,26]

Phenotype numbers					Gene frequencies

Asia

Bhutan

n	C	CD_{CHI}			
152	149	3			C = 0.990 D_{CHI} = 0.0099

Cambodia, Laos, and Vietnam

n	C	CD_{CHI}			
1,007	926	81			C = 0.96 D_{CHI} = 0.04

Philippines

n	C	CD_{CHI}			
928	910	18			C = 0.9903 D_{CHI} = 0.0097

China (including Hong Kong and Taiwan)

n	C	CD_{CHI}			
1,027	963	64			C = 0.9688 D_{CHI} = 0.0312

Japan

n	C	CD_{CHI}			
1,519	1,489	30			C = 0.9901 D_{CHI} = 0.0099

Malaya

n	C	CD_{CHI}	$D_{CHI}D_{CHI}$		
538	517	20	1		C = 0.98 D_{CHI} = 0.02

Thailand

n	C	CD_{CHI}	$D_{CHI}D_{CHI}$		
472	439	32	1		C = 0.964 D_{CHI} = 0.036

Africa

Ethiopia

n	C	CD_1			
626	624	2			C = 0.9984 D_1 = 0.0016

Liberia

n	C	CD_1	CB_2		
332	308	23	1		C = 0.963 D_1 = 0.035 B_2 = 0.0015

Senegal

n	C	CD_1	D_1D_1	CB_2	
1,199	1,123	74	1	1	C = 0.967 D_1 = 0.032 B_2 = 0.0004

Gambia

n	C	CD_1			
1,009	966	43			C = 0.979 D_1 = 0.021

Nigeria

n	C	CD_1	D_1D_1		
369	325	43	1		C = 0.939 D_1 = 0.061

TABLE 2 (continued)
The Population Distribution of Tf B and Tf D Variants[16,20,25,26]

	Phenotype numbers				Gene frequencies

Africa

Congo (Bantu)

n	C	CD_1	D_1D_1		
755	704	50	1		C = 0.966
					D_1 = 0.034

Central African Republic (Pigmies)

n	C	CD_1	D_1D_1		
160	122	32	6		C = 0.862
					D_1 = 0.138

Uganda

n	C	CD_1			
300	290	10			C = 0.983
					D_1 = 0.017

South Africa (Bushmen)

n	C	CD_1	D_1D_1		C = 0.945
238	213	24	1		D_1 = 0.055

South Africa (Bantu)

n	C	CD_1	D_1D_1		
1,490	1,413	76	1		C = 0.974
					D_1 = 0.026

North America

Whites

n	C	CB_1	CB_2	CD_1	
10,878	10,744	2	109	23	C = 0.994
					B_2 = 0.005
					D_1 = 0.0011
					B_1 = 0.00009

Negroes

n	C	CD_1	D_1D_1		
1,615	1,482	132	1		C = 0.959
					D_1 = 0.041

Navajo Indians

n	C	CB_2	CB_{0-1}		
230	213	1	16		C = 0.963
					B_{0-1} = 0.035
					B_2 = 0.002

Eskimoes (Alaska, Greenland, and Canada)

n	C	CB_2	CD_1		
1,785	1,780	1	4		C = 0.9986
					D_1 = 0.0011
					B_2 = 0.00028

Central America (Indians)

Mexico

n	C	CD_{CHI}	CB_{0-1}		
3,197	3,151	23	23		C = 0.9928
					D_{CHI} = 0.0036
					B_{0-1} = 0.0036

TABLE 2 (continued)
The Population Distribution of Tf B and Tf D Variants[16,20,25,26]

	Phenotype numbers				Gene frequencies
Central America (Indians)					
Guatemala					
n	C	CD_{CHI}	$CB_?$		
559	536	22	1		C = 0.979
					D_{CHI} = 0.0196
					$B_?$ = 0.0009
Honduras					
n	C	CD_{CHI}	$D_{CHI}D_{CHI}$		
706	661	43	2		C = 0.967
					D_{CHI} = 0.033
Panama					
n	C	CD_{CHI}			
452	428	24			C = 0.973
					D_{CHI} = 0.027
Nicaragua					
n	C	CD_{CHI}	$D_{CHI}D_{CHI}$		
441	407	30	4		C = 0.957
					D_{CHI} = 0.043
South America (Indians)					
Argentina					
n	C	CB_1			
971	966	5			C = 0.9974
					B_1 = 0.0026
Bolivia					
n	C				
1,071	1,071				C = 1.0000
Brazil					
n	C	CB_2	CD_{CHI}		
1,365	1,363	1	1		C = 0.99926
					B_2 = 0.00037
					D_{CHI} = 0.00037
Ecuador					
n	C	CD_{CHI}			
723	674	49			C = 0.966
					D_{CHI} = 0.034
French Guiana					
n	C	CD_{CHI}	$D_{CHI}D_{CHI}$	CB_2	
570	380	151	16	23	C = 0.819
					D_{CHI} = 0.161
					B_2 = 0.020
Peru					
n	C	CD_{CHI}			
913	909	4			C = 0.9978
					D_{CHI} = 0.0022
Paraguay					
n	C				
561	561				C = 1.0000
Venezuela (mixed tribes)					
n	C	CD_{CHI}	$D_{CHI}D_{CHI}$		
1,662	1,496	131	35		C = 0.939
					D_{CHI} = 0.061

TABLE 2 (continued)
The Population Distribution of Tf B and Tf D Variants[16,20,25,26]

	Phenotype numbers				Gene frequencies
South America (Indians)					
Venezuela (Pariri and Yupa tribes)					
n	C	CD_{CHI}	$D_{CHI}D_{CHI}$		
160	55	65	30		C = 0.610
					D_{CHI} = 0.390
Venezuela (Yanomama tribe)					
n	C				
429	429				C = 1.0000
Australia					
Aborigines					
n	C	CD_1	D_1D_1	CB_1	
2,225	1,701	457	57	10	C = 0.870
					D_1 = 0.128
					B_1 = 0.0022
Melanesia					
New Britain					
n	C	CD_1	D_1D_1	CB_{LAE}	
865	647	186	26	6	C = 0.859
					D_1 = 0.138
					B_{LAE} = 0.0035
New Guinea					
n	C	CD_1	D_1D_1	CB_{LAE}	
6,252	4,710	1,389	135	18	C = 0.863
					D_1 = 0.133
					B_{LAE} = 0.014
Polynesia and Micronesia					
Various islands including Caroline, Gilbert, Marshall, Cook, Ellice, Tonga, Tokelau, and Solomon					
n	C	CD_1	CB_2		
1,869	1,860	8	1		C = 0.09976
					D_1 = 0.0021
					B_2 = 0.00027

III. TRANSFERRIN C SUBTYPES AS REVEALED BY ISOELECTRIC FOCUSSING

A. HISTORICAL INTRODUCTION

By the middle of the 1970s, the genetic variation of human serum transferrin, as revealed by plasma protein electrophoresis at an alkaline pH, was well established. More than 25 variant alleles had been discovered, the products of which could be distinguished from the common Tf^C allele by virtue of their faster (B group) or slower (D group) electrophoretic mobilities. With one or two exceptions, most of the variant alleles had been found to occur at very low frequencies in human populations. Even in the case of variant alleles found at frequencies in excess of 0.01 (polymorphic variants) in certain population groups (D_1, D_{CHI}, and B_{0-1}), the incidence of the most commonly occurring variant phenotypes (heterozygotes) was sufficiently low such as to make human transferrin polymorphism a useful additional marker in anthropological studies, but of little practical use in the field of medicolegal science. The transferrin system was occasionally used in cases of disputed paternity,[25] but, particularly in European populations, the exclusion probabilities are extremely low (about 1%).

This situation was to change dramatically towards the end of the 1970s with the application of the technique of isoelectric focussing (IEF) in polyacrylamide gels to the task of resolving complex protein mixtues. In IEF, amphoteric substances are separated in an electric field, across which there is both a voltage and a pH gradient. During the course of the electrophoresis, proteins migrate according to their net charge, until they reach that part of the pH gradient that is equal to their isoelectic point (pI). At this point the proteins cease to migrate under the influence of the voltage gradient, since they have now acquired a net charge of zero. They remain focussed within a discrete region of the gel. The resolution of IEF far exceeds that of conventional electrophoresis at a single pH. By selecting the appropriate and often narrow-range pH gradient, proteins with differences in pI of as little as 0.02 pH units can often be separated.

In 1977, Kuhnl and Spielmann[66] reported the discovery of a new, genetically determined polymorphic system within the human plasma proteins. This had been revealed by the use of IEF of plasma samples in a pH gradient from 3.5 to 9.5. The unidentified protein exhibited five different phenotypic patterns amongst the 515 individuals tested. Since the protein had been detected after electrophoresis, not only with a sensitive protein stain, but also by virtue of its apparent specific reaction with an antiserum to the human plasma protein, haptoglobin, the polymorphic system was designated "Hp[a]".

In the following year (1978), Thymann[9] reinvestigated this new system, using a much narrower pH range in the focussing gels (pH 4 to 6.5). The region of the gradient where the proteins in question were found to focus was around pH 5.8, which is quite different from the pI of human haptoglobin. Furthermore, an immunological reaction with antihaptoglobin antiserum was not obtained. Instead, Thymann demonstrated conclusively, both by using pure human transferrin as a reference and also by employing an anti-human transferrin antibody to detect the proteins by immunoprecipitation, that the plasma protein exhibiting the new polymorphism was transferrin. The transferrin polymorphism revealed by IEF did not correspond to any of the already known transferrin phenotypes. Thymann tested 132 individuals from the Danish population and discovered three polymorphic phenotypes, tentatively designated Tf 1, Tf 2-1, and Tf 2. All but three of the individuals had the common Tf C phenotype when tested by conventional electrophoresis at pH 8.5. Thyman concluded from these observations that this "new" polymorphism might be the result of genetic subtypes within the Tf C phenotype that remain hidden during plasma protein electrophoresis at pH 8.5, only becoming exposed as a result of the greater resolving power afforded by the technique of IEF.

In the same year (1978), Kuhnl and Spielmann[8] also reported that their earlier discovery of a genetic polymorphism of the "Hp^a" system was indeed a genetic variation within the Tf C phenotype, only observed when plasma samples were subjected to IEF. Family studies confirmed the autosomal co-dominant inheritance of two common alleles (Tf_1^C and Tf_2^C) within a German population, occurring at gene frequencies of 0.81 and 0.19, respectively. The heterozygous genotype is phenotypically expressed (Tf C2-1) by the appearance of two transferrin bands separated by less than 0.1 pH units within the pH gradient.

A year later, Kuhnl and Spielmann[67] discovered a third variant allele within the Tf C phenotype (Tf^{C3}), thereby increasing the number of commonly occurring Tf C subtypes to six instead of the one Tf C phenotype that could be detected by conventional electrophoretic techniques (Figure 4). The product of the Tf^{C3} allele has a pI intermediate between that of C_1 and C_2, requiring a very narrow pH gradient within the gels in order to be clearly distinguished from C_1.

Genetic polymorphism within the Tf C phenotype has been found in all populations so far tested.[26] The most common of the Tf C subtypes, Tf C1, has been found to occur at frequencies ranging from as low as 42% in some of the tribes of Northern India[69] to as high as 90% in the Micronesian islands of the Pacific Ocean.[70] It became clear from the IEF results being reported towards the end of the 1970s that transferrin exhibited a range and degree of genetic polymorphism within human populations hitherto unsuspected. Interestingly, and at about the same time, the greater resolving power of the IEF technique led to the discovery of an increased number of phenotypes (subtypes) within two other well-established polymorphic systems in human populations: the red cell enzyme phosphoglucomutase-1,[71] and the plasma protein vitamin D-binding globulin (Gc).[72]

B. TRANSFERRIN C SUBTYPES 1978 TO 1991; THE VARIANT ALLELES AND THEIR WORLDWIDE DISTRIBUTION

Following the discovery of genetic microheterogeneity within the Tf C phenotype in 1978, the technique of plasma protein IEF has been used to carry our extensive population surveys in order to ascertain the range and incidence of genetic variation (Tf C subtypes) at the human transferrin gene locus. By 1987, more than 30,000 individuals from 122 population groups had been tested and reported, and the results available at that time were comprehensively reviewed by Kamboh and Ferrell.[26] At least 13 different alleles within the C phenotype have been discovered, the products of which

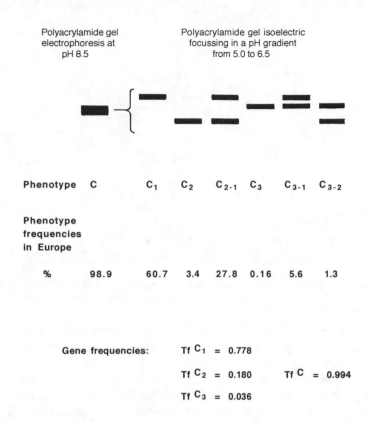

FIGURE 4. A diagram showing the electrophoretic mobilities of the six common Tf C subtypes of human serum transferrin as revealed by isoelectric focussing, and the approximate phenotype frequencies in a European population.

are distinguishable, one from another, by the use of narrow pH gradients in an IEF field (Figure 5). The variant C alleles have been numbered in a sequence that corresponds approximately to their order of discovery. Four of the variant alleles reach polymorphic frequencies (> 0.01) in one or more major population groups:

Tf^{C1} This is by far and away the most common allele, reaching frequencies of between 0.80 and 0.95 amongst Negro, Polynesian, and aboriginal communities. In Europe and amongst North American whites, the C_1 allele frequency is usually between 0.75 and 0.78. In most Asian populations, lower frequencies are encountered (0.65 to 0.70).

Tf^{C2} The distribution of C_2 gene frequencies is in most cases reciprocal to that of C_1. The lowest values are found amongst American Indians, aboriginals, and Polynesians (0.01 to 0.03). In Europe the frequency increases to between 0.13 and 0.19, whilst in Asia the highest values are found (0.15 to 0.34).

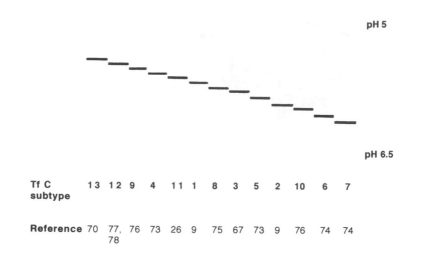

Tf C subtype	13	12	9	4	11	1	8	3	5	2	10	6	7
Reference	70	77, 78	76	73	26	9	75	67	73	9	76	74	74

FIGURE 5. A diagram showing the comparative electrophoretic mobilities, by isoelectric focussing in a pH range from 5 to 6.5, of the gene products of 13 Tf C subtype alleles.

Tf^{C3} The C$_3$ allele is widely distributed in European (0.04 to 0.07) and Asian (0.01 to 0.04) populations. Apart from sporadic reports of C$_3$ in some American Negro and Indian populations, East Asians, and certain Pacific Island communities, the allele appears to be absent from all other populations. Since many of the early surveys will have been carried out using IEF techniques in which the resolution of C3 from C1 is likely to have been poor, some of the negative results could warrant repeat examination.

Tf^{C4} The C$_4$ allele appears to be confined to populations of the New World. It was originally discovered amongst the Indians of Brazil (0.02), and subsequently found to be present at even higher frequencies (0.18) in many of the tribes of North American Indians.

Most of the remaining Tf^C alleles (5 to 13) are rare and confined to restricted ethnic groups or geographical locations.[26]

The interpretation of the human transferrin phenotypes after IEF is far more difficult than that following conventional electrophoresis at a single alkaline pH. The cause of the problem is the ability of IEF to resolve mixtures of proteins with very similar isoelectric points. In human plasma, molecules of transferrin can differ structurally, one from another, in ways other than the single amino acid changes brought about by genetic variation. The degree of iron saturation, as well as an extensive heterogeneity within the two oligosaccharide chains, particularly the number of sialic acid residues, can combine to produce a large family of isotransferrins within a single plasma sample. It has been calculated[80] that for an individual genetically heterozygous for the C$_1$ and C$_2$ alleles, and taking into account that a molecule of transferrin can carry between zero and eight residues of sialic acid, ahd furthermore can exist in four molecular forms with respect to iron binding (apoTf, Fe–Tf, Tf–Fe, and diferric Tf), the maximum number of possible isotransferrins likely to focus between pH 5 and pH 6.5 is **72**. Fortunately, many of these isotransferrins, particularly in freshly drawn plasma, are likely to be present at insignificant concentrations. Nevertheless, it is usual to saturate the plasma with iron prior to IEF in order to reduce the number of transferrin bands.

C. MEDICOLEGAL APPLICATIONS

The discovery that human transferrin can be subtyped by electrofocussing techniques, and that at least three of the alleles are reasonably well distributed amongst most populations, has greatly enhanced the value of the transferrin system as a useful marker in forensic science.[25] In paternity cases involving people of European origin, the probability of exclusion is increased from 1 to 15% when the transferrin C subtypes are determined. In the case of black Americans, when Tf C subtypes are added to the already existing polymorphism of the Tf^{D1} allele, the probability of exclusion increases from 5 to 19%. Because of the problems associated with the potentially large number of isotransferrins that could be present in biological fluids, the use of Tf C subtyping in dried stains of blood, saliva, and seminal fluid has found little application in case work.

IV. HUMAN TRANSFERRIN VARIANTS AND THEIR ADAPTIVE SIGNIFICANCE

The gene locus for human transferrin exhibits extensive genetic variation in all populations. The frequency of the variant alleles ranges from being extremely rare (for example, Tf^0, Tf^{BSHAW}, and Tf^{DEVANS}) to highly polymorphic (Tf^{C2} and Tf^{C3}). The question has been asked of the human transferrin gene locus, as indeed it has of many other polymorphic gene loci, ''Are all the variant alleles selectively neutral, or do some confer an adaptive advantage or disadvantage on the individual?'' In many cases the selective disadvantage of a variant allele at a particular human gene locus (for example, the haemoglobin sickle cell gene) is obvious, and in this example it is only by virtue of the selective advantage of the allele in the heterozygous genotype (resistance to falciparum malaria) that the frequency of the deleterious gene is maintained at such a high level in certain populations — balanced polymorphism in action. In other situations where a balanced polymorphism has not been found to exist, the most usual explanation for the maintenance of the deleterious variant allele within the population is the event of recurrent mutation. Most of the variant (mutant) alleles that have been discovered at human gene loci are probably selectively neutral. If they do confer any differential biological advantage or disadvantage, these are likely to be so small and subtle as to remain undetected. The problem was summarised very clearly in 1978 by Clarke in Mourant's[81] book, *Blood Groups and Diseases,* when he wrote, ''Continuous variability is often accepted as a natural phenomenon, but discrete characters, such as those constituting genetic polymorphic systems, excite curiosity and seem to cry out for a meaning. Population geneticists, anthropologists, and medical men all seek to identify factors that keep the morphs in balance.'' An indirect approach to the study of these small differences has been to compare the frequency of phenotypes found in a group of individuals with a particular disease, with a control group of healthy people. Studies of this kind have shown the association between many polymorphic alleles and a wide range of clinical disorders. Examples include the association of gastric cancer with blood group A, peptic ulcer with blood group O, nodular non-toxic goitre with the inherited inability to taste phenylthiocarbamide, and ankylosing spondylitis with the HLA antigen B27. These and many other examples were extensively reviewed by Mourant et al.[81] in 1978, but at that time none of the associations involved variant alleles at the human transferrin gene locus.

Only one of the variant alleles of the human transferrin gene has an obvious effect on biological fitness, and this is the silent or null allele, Tf^0. Since the frequency of this extremely deleterious allele is so low in all populations, one must conclude that there is no selective advantage for the heterozygous genotype.

A search for selective effects at any given gene locus necessarily involves a consideration of all points in the life cycle at which two genotypes could react differently and thereby cause differences in the production of progeny. Throughout the life cycle of mammals, stages at which selection might occur include the following:

1.   *Prezygotic selection* — a deviation from the expected combining frequency of gametes, thereby affecting the relative proportion of zygotes of different genotypes
2.   *Zygotic selection* — differential development of the embryo in the uterus
3.   *Embryonic selection* — differential implantation of the embryo
4.   *Prenatal selection* — differential survival of the implanted foetus
5.   *Postnatal selection* — differential survival to adolescence as a reaction to infection, etc.
6.   *Adult selection* — differential maturation, affecting the length of the fertile life and the quantity and quality of the gametes

There is considerable evidence — much of which was obtained during the period from 1960 to 1970 — that in some species of animals that exhibit transferrin polymorphism, selection at the transferrin gene locus occurs at early stages in the life cycle (stages 1 to 4). These include the well-documented examples of intrauterine selection in cattle[82] and prezygotic selection in deer mice.[83] These and other examples of selection operating in animals other than man will be discussed in more detail in Chapter 9.

In the case of human transferrin, most of the early studies on the possible adaptive significance of the variants, particularly members of the B and D groups, were carried out using a direct approach, by comparing the iron-binding properties of the different phenotypes. Most of the B and D variants that have been studied in any detail have been found to exhibit similar, if not identical properties to the common Tf C phenotype. Judged on these criteria alone, the variant alleles appear to be selectively neutral. The only exceptions have been the rare electrophoretic variants Tf[DEVANS] and Tf[BSHAW], both of which have normal characteristics of iron binding, but exhibit an increased lability of the iron attached to the C-site.[44,45] However, despite these phenotypic differences, individuals heterozygous for either of these variant alleles do not appear to be clinically affected (anaemic).

With the discovery of the transferrin C subtypes in 1978, and with the realisation that at least three of the Tf C alleles (C_1, C_2, and C_3) occur at polymorphic frequencies in most human populations, interest in the possible adaptive significance of variant transferrin alleles was reawakened. In 1985, Eckfeldt et al.[84] measured the concentration of iron, the iron-binding capacity, the percent iron saturation, and the immunologically determined concentration of transferrin in blood samples from 168 healthy blood donors. The population tested included examples of all six of the common Tf C phenotypes (1, 2-1, 2, 3-1, 3-2, and 3). No significant differences were found between any of the six phenotypes. However, when the concentrations of plasma transferrin were measured by an immunological technique, the level was found to be slightly higher in individuals with the Tf C 1 phenotype, when compared to the Tf C 2-1 and Tf C 2 phenotypes. The difference was small, and not found to be statistically significant. Wong and Sahan[85] have subsequently confirmed this observation, but in their study the difference in iron-binding capacity between the three phenotypes was found to be statistically significant (C 1, 70.4 μm/L; C 2, 60.4 μm/L). However, bearing in mind that the plasma content of transferrin is rarely more than 35% saturated with iron, the large residual capacity for binding iron is likely to make any small differences in transferrin concentrations between the three Tf C phenotypes of little biological or clinical significance.

Since the direct approach for identifying possible selective differences between the variant transferrin phenotypes has been relatively uninformative, many workers have sought to employ the more indirect methods, by comparing the frequencies of the variant phenotypes in particular disease groups with those of a control population. The rationale behind this approach to the problem appears, at first sight, to be straightforward:

1. Select a group of patients with a particular pathological condition.
2. Determine the frequency of the transferrin phenotypes within the group.
3. Determine the frequency of the transferrin phenotypes within a control group of healthy individuals, or refer to the published literature.
4. Compare the results and look for significant differences in phenotype, genotype, and gene frequencies between the two groups.

Geneticists and statisticians alike have pointed out that the design of such experiments has to be carried out with extreme care, otherwise the results could easily be misinterpreted.[81] Possible sources of error include the following:

1.   The number of individuals in the "disease group" must be sufficiently large so as to reduce the chances of sampling error.
2.   The disease in question should ideally be a single, clearly defined, and easily diagnosed pathological entity — for example, malignant neoplasms of the pylorus rather than a heterogeneous group of "cancers of the stomach".
3.   The control group has to be carefully selected in order to match the disease group for characteristics such as age, sex, and ethnic origin. The latter is particularly important for polymorphic gene loci, such as human transferrin, where the frequencies of the alleles vary considerably between different ethnic groups.

Notwithstanding these and many other problems associated with the proper design of such studies, a number of accounts have appeared in the literature, particularly during the last 10 years following the discovery of Tf C subtyping, reporting associations between certain transferrin phenotypes and a variety of pathological conditions, including cystic fibrosis,[86] occupational dermatosis,[87] spontaneous abortion,[88-90] neural tube defects,[89] birth weight,[91] premature delivery,[92] atopic dermatitis,[93] radiation-induced chromosomal damage,[94] rheumatoid arthritis,[95] multiple myeloma,[96] age,[97] and malaria.[98]

In many of these studies, particularly those carried out in the early part of the 1980s, the associations were found to be with the Tf^{C2} allele. However, the techniques of IEF available at that time would probably have been incapable of resolving the C 3 phenotype. Nowadays, with the technical advances that have occurred over the last few years, it is possible to unambiguously distinguish C 3 from both C 1 and C 2. For this reason it would be worthwhile to reexamine some of these earlier associations.

One such example that has already been reexamined is the association between human transferrin phenotypes and the incidence in recurrent spontaneous abortion. Transferrin genes have been found to be associated with fertility and spontaneous abortion in a number of nonhuman species, including cattle,[82] mice,[99] pigs,[100] and horses.[101] In 1980, Beckman et al.[88] reported an increased incidence of the human Tf^{C2} allele amongst Swedish women with a previous history of spontaneous abortion. In a more recent and extensive study by Weitkamp and Schacter,[89] using an IEF technique that, unlike the method used by Beckman et al. in 1980, was capable of clearly resolving the gene products of the three common alleles (Tf^{C1}, Tf^{C2}, and Tf^{C3}), a significantly higher frequency of the Tf^{C3} allele was found amongst couples in which the women had experienced three or more first-trimester spontaneous abortions. Such an association could be a function of the maternal genoytpe, the foetal genotype, or an interaction between the two. Weitkamp and Schacter[89] found no evidence to support the first of these explanations, since the increased frequency of C_3 was contributed equally by both parents. Unfortunately, the foetal transferrin phenotypes were not determined. Although there appears to be a differential effect of the human transferrin alleles on reproductive outcome, it remains to be established whether the effect is a direct one, or the influence of a gene closely linked to the transferrin locus.

In addition to providing data indicating an association between the transferrin C_3 allele and spontaneous abortion, Weitkamp and Schacter[89] also examined, from their control group, the segregation of the transferrin genotypes amongst 2000 healthy children born to 772 couples. The purpose of this part of the study was to determine whether differences in reproductive fitness existed between haploid sperm carrying C_1, C_2, or C_3 transferrin genes. It has previously been shown by Canham et al.[83] that the transmission of paternal transferrin genes in deer mice is profoundly influenced by the maternal transferrin genotype. Weitkamp and Schacter[89] have confirmed that an analogous situation exists in man, namely that the maternal transferrin genotype has an effect on the transmission ratio of the common transferrin alleles (C_1, C_2, and C_3) from heterozygous fathers to normal offspring ($p < 0.002$). This is an unusual example of the operation of selection in the human reproductive process. Evidence will be presented in the next chapter showing that in the case of certain animals, transferrin phenotypes are associated with differences in body weight and growth rates. In the human, however, there appears to be a lack of influence of maternal and foetal transferrin phenotypes on foetal growth and development.[102]

It is clear from these and other studies that much remains to be discovered about the adaptive significance of the human transferrin alleles. Even where positive associations have been well documented, little is known about how the process of selection is operating at the cellular level. It has to be remembered that transferrin, apart from being a vehicle for the transport of iron and one or two other metals, possibly has other important roles within the body, including antibacterial agent, growth factor, immunoregulator, and a means of protecting cells from the free radical-induced damage promoted by iron.

REFERENCES

1. **Pauling, L., Itano, H., Singer, S. J., and Wells, I. C.**, Sickle cell anaemia, a molecular disease, *Science*, 110, 543, 1949.
2. **Neel, J. V.**, The inheritance of sickle cell amaemia, *Science*, 110, 543, 1949.
3. **Ingram, V. M.**, Gene mutations in human haemoglobin: the chemical difference between normal and sickle cell haemoglobin, *Nature*, 180, 326, 1957.
4. **Smithies, O.**, Zone electrophoresis in starch gels: group variations in the serum protein of normal human adults, *Biochem. J.*, 61, 629, 1955.

5. **Smithies, O. and Walker, N. F.,** Genetic control of some serum proteins in normal humans, *Nature,* 176, 1265, 1955.

6. **Kneckel, M.,** Die Doppel-Albuminamie, eine neue erbliche Proteinanomalie, *Blut,* 3, 129, 1957.

7. **Smithies, O.,** Variations in human serum β-globulins, *Nature,* 180, 1482, 1957.

8. **Kuhnl, P. and Spielmann, W.,** Transferrin: evidence for two common subtypes of the Tf^C allele, *Hum. Genet.,* 43, 91, 1978.

9. **Thymann, M.,** Identification of a new serum protein polymorphism as transferrin, *Hum. Genet.,* 43, 225, 1978.

10. **Smithies, O. and Poulik, M. D.,** Two-dimensional electrophoresis of serum proteins, *Nature,* 179, 1033, 1956.

11. **Horsfall, W. R. and Smithies, O.,** Genetic control of some human serum β-globulins, *Science,* 128, 35, 1958.

12. **Smithies, O.,** Third allele at the β-globulin locus in humans, *Nature,* 181, 1203, 1958.

13. **Harris, H., Robson, E. B., and Siniscalco, M.,** β-Globulin variants in man, *Nature,* 182, 452, 1958.

14. **Smithies, O. and Hillier, O.,** The genetic control of transferrin in humans, *Biochem. J.,* 72, 121, 1959.

15. **Giblett, E. R., Hickman, C. G., and Smithies, O.,** Serum transferrin, *Nature,* 183, 1589, 1959.

16. **Mourant, A. E., Kopec, A. C., and Domaniewska-Sobczak, K.,** in *The Distribution of Human Blood Groups and Other Polymorphisms,* 2nd ed., Oxford University Press, London, 1976, 672.

17. **Farhud, D. D., Daneshmand, P., and Amirshani, P.,** A new transferrin variant from Iran (Tf B-Iran); review of 36 variant alleles, *Anthropol. Anz.,* 46, 357, 1988.

18. **Parker, W. C. and Bearn, A. G.,** Haptoglobin and transferrin gene frequencies in a Navajo population: a new transferrin variant, *Science,* 134, 106, 1961.

19. **Giblett, E. R.,** The plasma transferrins, in *Progress in Medical Genetics,* Vol. 2, A. G. Steinberg and A. G. Bearn, Eds., Grune & Stratton, New York, 1962, 34.

20. **Kirk, R. L.,** The world distribution of transferrin variants and some unsolved problems, *Acta Genet. Med. Gemellol.,* 17, 613, 1968.

21. **Giblett, E. R.,** in *Genetic Markers in Human Blood,* Blackwell Scientific, Oxford, 1969, chap. 3.

22. **Buettner-Janusch, J.,** Evolution of serum protein polymorphisms, *Annu. Rev. Genet.,* 4, 47, 1970.

23. **Walter, H.,** Transferrinsystem, in *Humangenetik. Ein kurzes Handbuch in funf Banden,* P. E. Becker, Ed., Georg Thieme Verlag, Stuttgart, 1975, 137.

24. **Cooper, D. W.,** in *The Biochemical Genetics of Man,* 2nd ed., B. J. H. Brock and O. Mayo, Eds., Academic Press, London, 1978, chap. 6.

25. **Gaensslen, R. E.,** in *Sourcebook in Forensic Serology, Immunology, and Biochemistry,* U.S. Department of Justice, Washington, DC, 1983, 589.

26. **Kamboh, M. I. and Ferrell, R. E.,** Human transferrin polymorphism, *Hum. Hered.,* 37, 65, 1987.

27. **Lai, L. Y. C.,** A new transferrin in New Guinea, *Nature,* 198, 589, 1963.

28. **Kirk, R. L., Matsumoto, H., and Katayama, K.,** Transferrin variants in Korea and Japan, *Jpn. J. Hum. Genet.,* 20, 470, 1978.

29. **Rao, P. R., Goud, J. D., and Rama Swamy, B.,** The occurrence of D$_{chi}$ and new D and B transferrin variants among caste groups of Andhra Pradesh (S. India), *Hum. Genet.,* 48, 235, 1979.

30. **Murray, R. F., Robinson, J. C., and Blumberg, B. S.,** A new transferrin variant from Greece, *Nature,* 204, 382, 1964.

31. **Barnett, D. R. and Bowman, B. H.,** A transferrin variant — B Lambert, *Acta Genet. (Basel),* 18, 573, 1968.

32. **Ferrell, R. E., Ueda, N., Satoh, C., Tanis, R. J., Neel, J. V., Hamilton, H. B., Inamizu, T., and Baba, K.,** The frequency in Japanese of 22 proteins. I. Albumin, ceruloplasmin, haptoglobin and transferrin, *Ann. Hum. Genet.,* 40, 407, 1977.

33. **Arends, T., Gallango, M. L., Parker, W. C., and Bearn, A. G.,** A new variant of human transferrin in a Venezuelan family, *Nature,* 196, 477, 1962.

34. **Sutton, H. E. and Jamieson, G. A.,** Transferrin, haptoglobin and ceruloplasmin, in *The Glycoproteins,* 2nd ed., A. Gottschalk, Ed., Elsevier, Amsterdam, 1972, 653.

35. **Parker, W. C. and Bearn, A. G.,** Haptoglobin and transferrin variants in human and primates: two new transferrin variants in Chinese and Japanese populations, *Ann. Hum. Genet.,* 25, 227, 1961.

36. **Malcolm, L. A., Woodfield, D. G., Blake, N. M., Kirk, R. L., and McDermid, E. M.,** The distribution of blood groups, serum proteins and enzyme groups on Manu Island (Admiralty Islands, New Guinea), *Hum. Hered.,* 22, 305, 1972.

37. **Cooper, D. W., Lander, H., and Kirk, R. L.,** D-Adelaide — a new transferrin variant in man, *Nature,* 204, 102, 1964.

38. **Glen-Bott, A. M., Harris, H., Robson, E. B., Bearn, A. G., and Parker, W. C.,** Transferrin D — Wigan, *Acta Genet. (Basel),* 14, 52, 1964.

39. **Harris, H., Penington, D. G., Robson, E. B., and Scriver, C. R.,** A further genetically determined transferrin variant in man, *Ann. Hum. Genet.,* 24, 327, 1960.

40. **Parker, W. C. and Bearn, A. G.,** Additional genetic variation of human serum transferrin, *Science,* 137, 854, 1962.

41. **Goud, J. D. and Rao, P. R.,** Transferrin, haptoglobin and group-specific types in tribal populations of Andhra Pradesh, *Hum. Hered.,* 30, 12, 1980.

42. **Seppala, M.,** Distribution of serum transferrin groups in Finland and their inheritance, *Ann. Med. Exp. Biol. Fenn.,* 43, 7, 1965.

43. **Lie-Injo Luen, E., Poey, N. G., and Mossberger, R. J.,** Haptoglobin, transferrin and haemoglobin in Indonesia, *Am. J. Hum. Genet.,* 20, 470, 1968.

44. **Evans, R. W., Williams, J., and Moreton, K.,** A varaint of transferrin with abnormal properties, *Biochem. J.,* 201, 19, 1982.

45. **Welch, S. and Langmead, L.,** A comparison of the structure and properties of normal human transferrin and a genetic variant of human transferrin, *Int. J. Biochem.,* 22, 275, 1990.

46. **Evans, R. W., Bomford, A., Clark, A. D., Garratt, R. C., Madden, A., and Young, S. P.,** Studies on a human transferrin variant, *Biochem. Soc. Trans.,* 12, 661, 1984.

47. **Young, S. P., Bomford, A., Madden, A. D., Garratt, R. C., Williams, R., and Evans, R. W.,** Abnormal in vitro function of a variant human transferrin, *Brit. J. Haematol.,* 56, 581, 1984.

48. **Evans, R. W., Meilak, A., Aitken, A., Patel, K. J., Wong, C., Garratt, R. C., and Chitnavis, B.,** Characterisation of the amino acid change in a transferrin variant, *Biochem. Soc. Trans.,* 16, 834, 1988.

49. **Wang, A. C. and Sutton, H. E.,** Human transferrin C and D_1, *Science,* 149, 435, 1965.

50. **Jeppson, J. O. and Sjoquist, J.,** in *Proceedings of the 14th Colloquium on Protides in Biological Fluids,* Elsevier, Amsterdam, 1966, 87.

51. **Wang, A. C., Sutton, H. E., and Howard, P. N.,** Human transferrin C and D_{CHI}, *Biochem. Genet.,* 1, 55, 1967.

52. **Wang, A. C., Sutton, H. E., and Riggs, A.,** A chemical difference between transferrin B_2 and C, *Am. J. Hum. Genet.,* 18, 454, 1966.

53. **Heilmeyer, L., Keller, W., Vivell, O., Keiderling, W., Betke, K., Wohler, F., and Schultze, H. E.,** Kongenitale Atransferrinamie bei einen sieben Jahre alten Kind, *Dtsch. Med. Wochenschr.,* 86, 1745, 1961.

54. **Heilmeyer, L.,** Die atransferrinemia, *Acta Haematol.,* 36, 40, 1966.

55. **Sakata, T.,** Case of congenital atransferrinaemia, *Shonika Shinryo,* 32, 1523, 1969.

56. **Cap, J., Lehotska, V., and Mayerova, A.,** Congenital atransferrinaemia in an eleven-month child, *Cesk. Pediatr.,* 23, 1020, 1968.

57. **Goya, N., Miyazaki, S., Kodate, S., and Ushio, B.,** A family of congenital atransferrinemia, _Blood,_ 40, 239, 1972.

58. **Gitlin, D. and Gitlin, J. D.,** Genetic alterations in the plasma proteins of man, in _The Plasma Proteins,_ Vol. 2, 2nd ed., Academic Press, New York, 1975, 321.

59. **Wright, T. L., Brissot, P., and Ma, W. L.,** Characterisation of the non-transferrin-bound iron clearance by the rat liver, _J. Biol. Chem.,_ 261, 10909, 1986.

60. **Brissot, P., Wright, T. L., Wa, W. L., and Weisiger, R. A.,** Efficient clearance of non-transferrin-bound iron by rat liver, _J. Clin. Invest.,_ 76, 1463, 1985.

61. **Bernstein, S. E.,** Hereditary hypotransferrinaemia with hemosiderosis, a murine disorder resembling human atransferrinaemia, _J. Lab. Clin. Med.,_ 110, 690, 1987.

62. **Heubers, H. A. and Finch, C. A.,** Transferrin: physiological behaviour and clinical implications, _Blood,_ 64, 763, 1984.

63. **Ford, E. B.,** in _The New Systematics,_ J. Huxley, Ed., Clarendon Press, Oxford, 1940, 493.

64. **Harris, H.,** in _The Principles of Human Biochemical Genetics,_ North-Holland, Amsterdam, 1970, 226.

65. **Wang, A-C. and Scott, I. D.,** Transferrin D_1: identity in Australian aborigines and American negroes, _Science,_ 156, 936, 1967.

66. **Kuhnl, P. and Spielmann, W.,** Hinweise auf einen weiteren Polymorphismus im Hp-system, 7th Inter. Congr. Soc. Forensic Haematogenetics, Hamburg, 1977.

67. **Kuhnl, P. and Spielmann, W.,** A third common allele in the transferrin system, Tf_3^C, detected by isoelectric focusing, _Hum. Genet.,_ 50, 193, 1979.

68. **Cortivo, P., Biasiolo, M., Crestani, C., Scorretti, C., and Benciolini, P.,** The polymorphism of transferrin by ultrathin-layer isoelectric focusing. Tf phenotypes and Tf C subtypes in the population of Padua, _For. Sci. Int.,_ 24, 65, 1984.

69. **Kamboh, M. I.,** Population genetic studies of PI, Tf, Gc and PGM 1. Subtypes amongst various caste groups in Northern India, _Acta Anthropogenet.,_ 8, 159, 1984.

70. **Kamboh, M. I. and Kirk, R. L.,** Distribution of transferrin (Tf) subtypes in Asian, Pacific and Australian Aboriginal populations: evidence for the existence of a new subtype allele Tf C6, _Hum. Hered.,_ 33, 237, 1983.

71. **Sutton, J. G. and Burgess, R.,** Genetic evidence for four common alleles at the phosphoglucomutase-1 locus (PGM_1) detectable by isoelectric focussing, _Vox Sang.,_ 34, 97, 1978.

72. **Constans, J., Vian, M., Cleve, H., Jaeger, G., Quilici, J. C., and Palisson, M. J.,** Analysis of the Gc polymorphism in human populations by isoelectric focussing on polyacrylamide gels. Demonstration of subtypes of the Gc^1 allele and of additional Gc variants, _Hum. Genet.,_ 41, 53, 1978.

73. **Constans, J., Kunhl, P., Viau, M., and Spielmann, W.,** A new procedure for the determination of transferrin C (TfC) subtypes by isoelectric focusing. Existence of two additional alleles, Tf4 and Tf5, _Hum. Genet.,_ 55, 111, 1980.

74. **Kuhnl, P., Constans, J., Viau, M., and Spielmann, W.,** Isoelectric focusing of the common transferrin C subtypes, _Electrophoresis,_ 2, 573, 1981.

75. **Dykes, D. D., Defurio, C. M., and Polesky, H. F.,** Transferrin (Tf) subtypes in US Amerindians, whites and blacks using thin layer agarose gels. Report on a new variant Tf_8^C, _Electrophoresis,_ 3, 162, 1982.

76. **Weidinger, S., Cleve, H., Schwarzfischer, F., Portel, W., Weser, J., and Gorg, A.,** Transferrin subtypes in Germany; further evidence for a Tf null allele, _Hum. Genet.,_ 66, 356, 1984.

77. **Walter, H., Strodtmann, H., Hilling, M., Singh, I. P., Bhasin, M. K., and Veeraju, P.,** Transferrin subtypes in six Indian population samples, _Hum. Hered.,_ 31, 152, 1981.

78. **Yuasa, I., Saneshige, Y., Okamoto, N., Ikawa, S., Hikita, T., Ikebuchi, K., Inoue, T., and Okada, K.,** Distribution of Hp, Tf, Gc and Pi polymorphisms in a Nepalese population, _Hum. Hered.,_ 33, 302, 1983.

79. **deJong, G., van Dijk, J. P., and van Eijk, H. G.,** The biology of transferrin, *Clin. Chim. Acta,* 190, 1, 1990.
80. **Dykes, D. D., Defurio, C. M., and Polesky, H. F.,** Isoelectric focussing for Tf subtypes in paternity testing, *Am. J. Clin. Pathol.,* 79, 725, 1983.
81. **Mourant, A. E., Kopec, A. C., and Domaniewska-Sobczak, K.,** in *Blood Groups and Diseases. A Study of Association of Diseases with Blood Groups and Other Polymorphisms,* Oxford University Press, New York, 1978.
82. **Ashton, G. C. and Fallon, G. R.,** β-Globulin type, fertility and embryonic mortality in cattle, *J. Reprod. Fertil.,* 3, 93, 1962.
83. **Canham, R. P., Birdsall, D. A., and Cameron, D. G.,** Disturbed segregation at the transferrin locus of the deer mouse, *Genet. Res.,* 16, 355, 1970.
84. **Eckfeldt, J. H., Dykes, D. D., Dahl, I. I., Skare, C. M., and Polesky, H. F.,** Lack of influence of the TfC genotypes on iron, iron-binding capacity, percentage saturation, and immunologically determined transferrin in blood donor sera, *Clin. Chim. Acta,* 145, 101, 1985.
85. **Wong, C. T. and Saha, N.,** Effects of transferrin genetic phenotype on total iron-binding capacity, *Acta Haematol.,* 75, 215, 1986.
86. **Pascali, V. L.,** Transferrin subtypes in cystic fibrosis, *Eur. J. Paediatr.,* 143, 133, 1984.
87. **Beckman, L.,** Transferrin C subtypes and occupational photodermatosis of the face, *Hum. Hered.,* 35, 89, 1985.
88. **Beckman, G., Beckman, L., and Sikstrom, C.,** Transferrin C subtypes and spontaneous abortion, *Hum. Hered.,* 30, 316, 1980.
89. **Weitkamp, M. D. and Schacter, B. Z.,** Transferrin and HLA; spontaneous abortion, neural tube defects, and natural selection, *N. Engl. J. Med.,* 313, 925, 1985.
90. **Saha, N.,** Transferrin subtypes and spontaneous abortion in a Chinese population, *Hum. Hered.,* 40, 141, 1990.
91. **Beckman, L.,** Relationship between transferrin C 2 and birth weight, *Hum. Hered.,* 37, 319, 1987.
92. **Auconi, P., Biagini, R., Colarizi, P., and Pascali, V.,** Transferrin C subtypes in extremely premature newborn infants, *Pediatr. Res.,* 16, 1022, 1982.
93. **Cislo, M.,** Examination of the correlation between transferrin C and atopic dermatitis, *Przegl. Dermatol.,* 76, 386, 1989.
94. **Beckman, L.,** Transferrin C 2 and radiation-induced chromosomal damage, *Hum. Hered.,* 38, 56, 1988.
95. **Rantapaa-Dahlquist, S.,** Transferrin C subtypes and rheumatoid arthritis, *Hum. Hered.,* 35, 279, 1985.
96. **Mitchell, R. J.,** Haptoglobin groups and transferrin subtypes in multiple myeloma, *Hum. Hered.,* 38, 117, 1988.
97. **Beckman, L.,** Decrease in transferrin C 2 frequency with age, *Hum. Hered.,* 36, 254, 1986.
98. **Pollack, S.,** Transferrin polymorphism and malaria, *Am. J. Med. Genet.,* 20, 403, 1985.
99. **Ashton, G. C. and Dennis, M. N.,** Selection at the transferrin locus in mice, *Genetics,* 67, 253, 1971.
100. **Imlah, P.,** Evidence for the Tf locus being associated with an early lethal factor in a strain of pigs, *Anim. Blood Groups Biochem. Genet.,* 1, 5, 1970.
101. **Weitkamp, L. R., MacCluer, J. W., and Guttormsen, S. A.,** Genetics of standard bred stallion reproductive performance, *J. Reprod. Fertil.,* 32, 135, 1982.
102. **Wong, C. T. and Saha, N.,** Lack of influence of maternal and fetal transferrin phenotypes on normal fetal growth, *Biol. Neonate,* 59, 156, 1991.

Chapter 9

ANIMAL TRANSFERRINS — STRUCTURE, PROPERTIES, AND GENETIC VARIATION

I. ANIMAL TRANSFERRINS — OCCURRENCE, STRUCTURE, AND PROPERTIES

The occurrence of transferrin-like proteins within the animal kingdom has already been discussed in Chapter 4 and summarised in Figure 1 of that chapter. Although an iron-binding protein has been found within the haemolymph of certain members of the phylum Arthropoda (crabs, spiders, and moths), the presence of a true transferrin protein, with iron-transport properties, seems to be confined to the phylum Chordata. Transferrin has been found in the blood plasma of all vertebrates in which it has been sought. Whilst much of our present day knowledge concerning the structure and function of transferrin has come from work carried out on the protein isolated from human plasma, there have been many important contributions to the subject arising from the study of other vertebrate transferrins, particularly chicken ovotransferrin and rabbit plasma transferrin.

All vertebrate transferrins are glycoproteins with molecular weights ranging from 61,000 to 87,000, and with a capacity to bind a maximum of two atoms of iron. Transferrins from many species have been purified and extensively characterised. The structure and properties of the protein from more than 30 species have been reported in the literature, with examples from all of the major vertebrate classes: fish, amphibians, reptiles, birds, and mammals. Transferrins from different species have been compared with one another, often to assist taxonomic classification, with respect to a wide range of chemical, physical, and biological properties. These have included molecular weight, amino acid composition, content and structure of the oligosaccharide chains, iron-binding characteristics, plasma concentration and turnover, electrophoretic mobility, antigenic determinants, and the ability of transferrin and transferrin receptors of different species to interact with each other. The results of these studies, as well as appearing in the literature as single reports, have also been the subject of many review articles.[1-14]

It is a difficult if not impossible task to adequately summarise the results from the many hundreds of publications that have appeared in the literature over the last 40 years. Nevertheless, it is possible to draw a number of general conclusions. All vertebrate transferrins follow a common structural pattern — a large monomeric glycoprotein consisting of two globular lobes, each containing an iron-binding site. Since the amino acid composition, and therefore by implication the amino acid sequence, can vary considerably between transferrins from different species, it has to be concluded that this large molecule can tolerate significant changes in primary structure whilst still retaining the ability to bind and transport iron. The transferrin gene has undergone a large amount of mutation during the process of evolution. One particularly significant event was the duplication of the transferrin gene occurring before the divergence of the urochordate and vertebrate lines. With the exception of the transferrin synthesised by the primitive urochordate *Pyura stolonifera*,[15] the size of the transferrin molecule has remained fairly constant throughout the phylum Chordata. Such differences as have been found are likely to be due as much to variation in oligosaccharide structure as they are to differences in amino acid content.

Comparisons of the chemical and physical properties of the transferrins from different species have frequently been used in order to study phylogenetic relationships. One approach has been to measure the magnitude of antigenic differences between transferrins by quantitative microcomplement fixation. Mao and Dessauer[16] compared the antigenic properties of transferrin from 32 species of natricine snakes. Their results indicate that transferrin structures differ markedly amongst species, appearing to offer a sensitive "clock" for timing the divergence of evolutionary lines. The evolutionary lines leading to the present day natricine genera originated during the Miocene period. *Natrix* has undergone extensive speciation since then, and the majority of structural changes in the transferrins of resulting species seem to have been nonadaptive and selectively neutral.

A similar biochemical approach has been used to study the evolution of the flightless birds such as the ratites (ostrich, rhea, cassowary, emu, kiwi, and tinamou)[17] and the penguins.[18] Quantitative immunological comparison of transferrins indicates that all the ratites are allied phylogenetically and are of a monophyletic origin relative to other birds, whereas the penguins are more closely related to the flying aquatic birds. Furthermore, by comparing the immunological characteristics of the transferrins from representatives of all 27 orders of the class Aves, Prager et al.[19] have shown that transferrin has evolved far more slowly in birds than in any other vertebrate.[19] This finding is supported by evidence from other proteins, including albumin, lysozyme, and cytochrome *c*.

II. GENETIC VARIATION OF ANIMAL TRANSFERRINS

The first report of genetic variation of an animal transferrin appeared in the journal *Nature* in November 1957. Ashton[20] published evidence showing

TABLE 1
Some Examples of Animals (Phylum Chordata; Subphylum Vertebrata, Superclass Gnathostomata) in which Plasma Transferrin Has Been Shown to Exhibit Genetic Variation

Class	Order	
Actinopterygii		Carp,[25,26,29] herring,[30] plaice,[31] cod,[32] tuna,[33] trout,[34] jaraquis,[35] bass,[36] halibut,[37] spot,[38] flounder,[39] hake,[40] salmon,[41] haddock,[24] paradise fish[42]
Amphibia		Toad,[43-45] frog[46-49]
Reptilia		Snake,[1] lizard[50]
Aves		Chicken,[51-56] pigeon,[62,63,65,67,68] dove,[63,64] goose,[59,60] magpie,[71] quail,[57,58] pheasant,[69] partridge,[54] gull,[70,71] crow,[71] duck,[61] scoter,[71] blackbird[54]
Mammalia	Primates	Man (Chap. 8), lemur,[73] orangutan,[77] baboon,[75,85] gibbon,[77] marmoset,[74] macaque,[76,79-84,86] chimpanzee[77,78]
	Rodentia	Mouse,[90-96] rat[97,98] vole,[107] ground squirrel,[103-106] deer mouse,[99] mastomys[102]
	Lagomorpha	Rabbit[115,116]
	Carnivora	Wolf,[123] dog,[120] cat,[124] fox,[126] seal[127]
	Perrisodactyla	Horse[129,130]
	Artiodactyla	Sheep,[140-149] goat,[134,138] pig,[150,151] cow,[171-175] fallow deer,[162] red deer,[161] reindeer,[164,166] water buffalo[167-170]

an inherited phenotypic variation within the β_2-globulin (transferrin) fraction of cattle plasma, as demonstrated by starch gel electrophoresis. It was a month later before Smithies[21] first reported genetic variation of human serum transferrin. By the end of 1958, two further examples of vertebrate transferrin polymorphism had been discovered — in sheep[22] and goats.[23]

In the period from 1958 to the present day, a considerable number of vertebrate genera and species have been examined in order to determine whether the transferrin exhibits genetic polymorphism. It is difficult to estimate precisely the total number of different species that have been tested, since negative results are rarely published. Transferrin polymorphism has been described in more than 70 vertebrate species, and a selection of examples is given in Table 1. There is little reason to suppose that if a sufficient number of animals from a given species were to be examined, the probability of discovering genetic variation of the plasma transferrin, whether rare or polymorphic, would be extremely high. This conclusion is based on the observation, previously discussed, that transferrin appears to be able to tolerate a wide range of selectively neutral (nonadaptive) mutations without compromising its biological functions.

In some species there is good evidence that the process of selection is operating both for and against certain of the variant transferrin alleles, and that it is the balance between these opposing forces that maintains the allele at polymorphic frequencies within that species. In other cases, transferrin polymorphism has proved to be a valuable tool with which to study phylogenetic relationships with other species, or patterns of migration within the same species. There are even examples of animals, such as the horse, where transferrin polymorphism has been applied to problems of pedigree analysis and paternity testing. In the remaining part of this chapter, a selection of the vertebrate species in which genetic variation of plasma transferrin has been demonstrated (Table 1) will be described and discussed in more detail.

A. CLASS: ACTINOPTERYGII (BONY FISH)

Transferrin polymorphism has been described in many species of both freshwater and seawater fish, including carp,[25,26,29] herring,[30] plaice,[31] cod,[32] tuna,[33] trout,[34] jaraquis,[35] bass,[36] halibut,[37] spot,[38] flounder,[39] hake,[40] salmon,[41] haddock,[24] and paradise fish.[42] The results from many of these studies have been used for a number of practical applications, including delineation of individual fish populations, establishing taxonomic and phylogenetic relationships, identifying instances of cross breeding, and monitoring the migration and spawning patterns of fish populations. The extent of genetic variation at the transferrin gene locus of teleost fish can be realised by considering the results of a survey reported by Turner and Jamieson[24] in 1987. Blood specimens from 63 species of teleost fish in 30 taxonomic families were examined. In more than half of the species, transferrin was found to exhibit extensive polymorphism, with the products of four or more variant alleles being identified by starch gel electrophoresis in each case. The most extreme example of transferrin polymorphism was found in the haddock, where as many as 21 variant alleles were discovered.

1. Carp

A three-allele transferrin polymorphism in the carp (*Cyprinus carpis*) was first reported by Creysell et al.[25] with a fourth variant allele being reported later by Valenta and Kalal.[26] There seemed to be nothing unusual about carp plasma transferrin until a report published in 1973 indicated that up to four distinct transferrin proteins could be detected in the plasma of any one individual carp.[27] From these observations, Reichenbach-Klinke[27] suggested that these proteins were the product of four transferrin alleles within an individual fish, this being genetically possible, since the carp is a tetraploid species in which duplicated gene loci (four alleles) had already been shown to be operative with respect to a number of enzymes. Valenta et al.[29] subsequently reexamined the situation with respect to transferrin polymorphism in the carp, discovering a total of seven variant alleles. However, analysis of the transferrin phenotypes of 688 offspring indicated unambiguously that only a single transferrin gene locus is active in the carp, despite this species being one of the few members of the Cyprinid family that is tetraploid. The heterogeneity of carp plasma transferrin that led Reichenbach-Klinke[27] to propose a duplicated gene locus cannot be attributed to variable numbers of sialic acid residues, since carp transferrin is unusual in having a particularly low carbohydrate content and no sialic acid.[29]

2. Tuna

Transferrin polymorphism has been described in three tuna species: skipjack tuna (*Katsuwonus pelamis*), southern bluefin tuna (*Thunnus maccoyi*), and yellowfin tuna (*T. albacares*).[33] Three variant alleles have been detected, and there is evidence that a mechanism of differential selection operates to maintain the transferrin polymorphism in randomly mating populations. Whilst there appears to be an excessive number of newborn with one particular phenotype (Tf 2-3), this is balanced within the tuna population by a reduction in the life-span of those fish with the Tf 2-3 phenotype.

B. CLASS: AMPHIBIA
1. Toad

In 1966, Guttman discovered that plasma transferrin exhibited a most extreme form of polymorphism within two species of African toads, *Bufo regularis* and *B. rangeri*.[43] Amongst 67 *B. regularis* from 13 localities, a total of 32 different transferrin phenotypes were detected by means of starch gel electrophoresis. In a smaller sample of 15 *B. rangeri*, six transferrin phenotypes were discovered. The phenotypic variation within the toad populations was confirmed as being due to the inheritance of codominant alleles at an autosomal gene locus.[44] As many as 29 different variant transferrin alleles appeared to be present within the small group of two closely related toad species. Guttman suggested that, as a consequence of interspecies hybridisation, the introduction of genes from the gene pool of one species into the gene pool of the other (introgression), might account for some of this extreme variability. In a later study, Guttman and Wilson[45] described a similar situation of extensive transferrin polymorphism within a population of American toads (*B. americanus*).[45] In this case, amongst the 185 animals tested, 13 transferrin alleles were present in 36 different phenotypic combinations. In addition, it was noted that within the *B. americanus* population there was a significant deficiency in the number of heterozygotes found, when compared with the number predicted by the Hardy-Weinberg equilibrium. Guttman proposed a number of possible explanations to account for the extreme polymorphism at the transferrin gene locus:

1. Introgression
2. Balanced selection — hybrid vigour
3. Disease resistance

To account for the heterozygote deficiency, evidence for a "null" or "silent" transferrin allele within the toad population was sought for, but not found. Guttman concluded that only two possible mechanisms remained to explain the heterozygote deficiency:

1. Inbreeding
2. Selection against heterozygotes (negative heterosis)

The second of the two explanations was favoured, supported by evidence that negative heterosis occurred either seasonally or within certain age groups in natural populations of toads.

2. Frog

A similar degree of transferrin polymorphism, although not quite as extensive as that found in the toad, has been reported by Gartside and Watson[46] in the tree frog, *Litoria ewingi*. A survey of transferrin variation in 33 populations (661 frogs) throughout southeastern Australia and Tasmania revealed the presence of nine variant transferrin alleles. In most cases (640), the phenotypes appeared electrophoretically as either single (homozygous) or double (heterozygous) transferrin bands. Codominant inheritance at an autosomal gene locus was confirmed by *in vitro* hybridisation experiments. In the remaining 21 frogs, three- and four-banded transferrin patterns were detected. These anomalous phenotypes could have been the result of posttranslational modifications, such as the loss of sialic acid residues or variable degrees of iron binding. An alternative explanation, proposed by Gartside and Watson,[46] was that of gene duplication, such that the animals in question had inherited three or even four transferrin alleles. No genetic evidence was provided to support this hypothesis.

In contrast to the tree frog, Dunlap[47] has reported that amongst two species of leopard frog, *Rana pipiens* and *R. blairi,* the transferrin is monomorphic. However, the transferrin from these two species differs in electrophoretic mobility, and both proteins are detected in interspecies hybrids. Although Dunlap failed to detect genetic variation of transferrin in either *R. pipiens* or *R. blairi,* this may have been peculiar to the particular frog populations that were sampled. In an earlier report, transferrin polymorphism was found during the course of a survey of both *R. pipiens* and a third species of leopard frog, *R. berlanderi.*[48] Transferrin has also been found to be highly polymorphic in two species of North American cricket frogs, *Acris crepitans* and *A. gryllus.*[49]

C. CLASS: REPTILIA
1. Snake

During the course of an extensive comparative study of transferrins from more than 150 species of reptiles and amphibians, Dessauer et al.[1] discovered a marked phenotypic variation, both within geographically limited populations and between populations from different areas, in most species of colubrid snakes that were studied. Transferrin polymorphism is particularly common amongst species of the genera *Natrix* (grass snakes), *Thamnophis* (garter snakes), *Coluber* (black snakes), and *Lampropeltis* (king snakes).

2. Lizard

Transferrin polymorphism amongst closely related species of lizard from the genus *Anolis* has been used to confirm and supplement taxonomic conclusions derived from more traditional criteria.[50] Eight species of the *Roquet* group of anolid lizards that are widely distributed throughout the Lesser

Antilles islands of the Caribbean were found to exhibit seven different plasma transferrin phenotypes.

D. CLASS: AVES
1. Chicken

Genetic variation of plasma transferrin in the domestic fowl (*Gallus gallus*) was first reported by Ogden et al.[51] in 1962. From the results obtained from amongst the offspring of tested matings, it was deduced that the phenotypic variation was due to the presence of two alternative codominant alleles (Tf[a] and Tf[b]) at an autosomal gene locus. Subsequently, a number of additional variant alleles have been described.[52-55]

The discovery of genetic variation of chicken transferrin occurred at a time when the molecular and genetic relationship between the iron-binding proteins present in chicken egg white (conalbumin), chicken egg yolk (transferrin), and chicken serum (transferrin) was still a matter of controversy. It was known at that time (1962) that whilst the transferrin of chicken egg yolk and chicken serum appeared to be indistinguishable electrophoretically, the same was not true when conalbumin and serum transferrin were compared. These two molecules, whilst having very similar molecular weights, amino acid compositions, and iron-binding characteristics, could be clearly distinguished by virtue of their isoelectric points. It was suggested by Williams[56] that conalbumin and transferrin were glycoproteins differing only in their carbohydrate composition. This implied that the protein components of both molecules were identical, and therefore controlled by the same gene locus. The confirmation of this hypothesis came with the demonstration that the genetically determined transferrin phenotypes of hen serum were matched by an equivalent phenotypic variation in the conalbumin electrophoretic patterns.[51] By studying the electrophoretic polymorphism of transferrin resulting from the three most common alleles, it has been shown conclusively that chicken serum transferrin, chicken egg yolk transferrin, chicken egg white conalbumin (also known as ovotransferrin), and a fourth iron-binding protein found in the seminal plasma of male birds, are all genetically determined by the same autosomal gene locus.[55] This single gene locus exhibits genetic polymorphism, and the frequency of the variant alleles differs considerably amongst various breeds of domestic chicken.[55]

2. Quail

Transferrin polymorphism in the Japanese quail *Cortunix cortunix japonicus* is controlled by an autosomal gene locus at which two alternative codominant alleles (Tf[B] and Tf[C]) have been detected in domestic populations of the bird.[57] The three electrophoretic phenotyes found in quail serum (B, BC, and C) are matched by similar phenotypic variations in the conalbumin present in the egg white. It has recently been found that within a large population of commercially bred birds, the Tf[C] allele was absent.[58]

3. Goose

Three transferrin and three equivalent conalbumin phenotypes have been detected in the domestic goose, *Anser anser*.[59] On the basis of family studies, it was shown that the transferrin polymorphism is determined by two codominant alleles (Tf^A and Tf^B). However, whereas in the chicken the allele frequencies differ considerably between breeds, this has not been found to be the case in domestic geese.[60]

4. Duck

Transferrin polymorphism amongst breeding colonies of the eider duck — *Somateria mollisima* from Scotland, Holland, and Iceland — was discovered when three distinct electrophoretic phenotypes of conalbumin (ovotransferrin) were reported by Milne and Robertson.[61] Significant differences in the frequency of the two transferrin alleles (Tf^a and Tf^b) within the bird colonies has provided evidence of reproductive isolation in situations where this had not previously been suspected.

5. Pigeon

Genetic variation of transferrin in the feral rock dove (pigeon), *Columba livia,* was first described by Mueller et al.[62] Two commonly occurring alleles (Tf^A and Tf^D) account for the presence of three electrophoretically distinguishable phenotypes. A similar degree of transferrin polymorphism has been found in many closely related members of the Columbidae family. These include the wood pigeon (*C. palumbus*),[63] the speckled pigeon (*Columbus guinea*),[62] the red-collared dove (*Streptopelia tranquebarica*),[64] and the barbary dove (*S. risoria*).[63] However, in a survey of collared doves (*S. decaoctoa*) from a number of areas in Ireland, transferrin was found to be monomorphic.[63] Since this particular species had only recently been introduced into the country, it would seem likely that this is an example of a ''founder effect''.

In all pigeon populations that have been studied, the frequencies of the two transferrin alleles have been found to be close to 0.5. The fact that only two alleles occur and that the observed genotype frequencies agree closely with those predicted by the Hardy-Weinberg equilibrium has led to the suggestion that powerful selective pressures may be operating in order to maintain this polymorphism. Frelinger[65] has suggested that the transferrin polymorphism in pigeon populations is maintained by differences in fertility amongst female birds. This conclusion was based on the discovery that the ovotransferrin from heterozygous (Tf AB) females inhibits microbial growth far better than the ovotransferrin from either of the homozygous phenotypes. As a result, heterozygous females hatch a larger percentage of their eggs. The increased antimicrobial protection afforded to the offspring of heterozygous females extends beyond the time of hatching, since squabs (unfledged pigeons) continue to express the maternal transferrin phenotype for at least 14 days after hatching. It is only at a later stage in the life of the fledgling birds that their own transferrin phenotype becomes fully expressed.[66]

An additional difference between the pigeon transferrin phenotypes that may have an effect on selective pressure has been shown by Brown and Sharp.[67] Adult birds of the transferrin A phenotype have significantly lower levels of blood glutathione than either the AB or B phenotypes. Since glutathione is thought to have an important role to play in providing protection against free radical damage, the lower levels of glutathione associated with the transferrin A phenotype might possibly qualify as a selective disadvantage.

In an attempt to provide evidence to explain the molecular basis of the possible adaptive difference between transferrin phenotypes, Frelinger[68] determined the chemical difference between the A and B forms of pigeon transferrin. A single amino acid change (asparagine in A replaced by serine in B) was found, but it has yet to be established how, if at all, this affects the biological functions of the molecule.

E. CLASS: MAMMALIA
1. Order: Primates

Transferrin polymorphism, involving two or more codominant alleles, is common in both of the primate suborders Prosimii and Anthropoidea.[72]

The transferrin phenotypes of prosimian primates are particularly complex, none more so than those of lemurs.[73] The number of variant alleles (22) found within a relatively small population sample suggests that transferrin polymorphism may be a characteristic that appeared at an early stage in primate evolution.[72]

Amongst the anthropoid primates, genetic variation at the transferrin gene locus has been discovered in species from each of the three superfamilies, Ceboidea (New World monkeys: marmosets),[74] Cercopithecoidea (Old World monkeys: baboons[75] and macaques),[76] and Hominoidea (Apes: gibbons,[77] orangutans,[77] chimpanzees,[78] and man).

a. Macaques (Genus Macaca)

Of the many different species of macaques, the rhesus monkey (*Macaca mulatta*) has been the most extensively studied with respect to transferrin polymorphism. Transferrin heterogeneity was first reported in 1960 by a number of independent groups (reviewed by Lai),[76] and from these early reports it soon became apparent that the range and extent of genetic variation at the transferrin gene locus of *M. mulatta* was extremely large. Goodman and Poulik,[79] for example, discovered 16 different transferrin phenotypes within a sample of just 77 rhesus monkeys from a region on the Nepal-India border. To account for this observation, the presence of eight variant transferrin alleles within the colony was postulated, although at the time the family data necessary to confirm the pattern of inheritance were not available. Subsequent surveys have revealed at least two further variant alleles at the transferrin gene locus of rhesus monkeys,[80,81] bringing the total to ten. Since in most rhesus populations that have been studied all of the ten alleles occur at frequencies greater than 0.01, the number of different phenotypes likely to be present, even within a small group of animals, is very large. Brown et al.[82] have described a colony of only 38 monkeys in which examples of 16 phenotypes were found to be present.

M. mulatta inhabits a geographical range encompassing a large portion of Asia. The extensive dispersal of the species has led to genetic differentiation throughout the range. This is well exemplified by the differences in frequency of the transferrin alleles that have been found in rhesus colonies at a variety of locations.[81] The adaptive significance, if any, of the different transferrin phenotypes is an intriguing question that has yet to be resolved. There have been some reports suggesting that not all of the phenotypes are of equal biological fitness. Smith and Small[83] have examined the influence of the most common allele (Tf^C) on rates of survival, infant growth, and fertility. Male infants with no C allele were found to experience slower growth rates than those with either one or two C alleles. However, amongst the female infants, animals heterozygous for the Tf C allele had the highest growth rates, but these same animals on reaching sexual maturity experienced a lower fertility and higher incidence of abortions and stillbirths. On the basis of these observations, Smith and Small[83] suggested that opposing directions of selection at different stages in the life cycle of *M. mulatta* help to maintain a stable equilibrium at the transferrin locus.

A further difference between the phenotypes has been found in respect to the levels of blood glutathione.[84] Tf CC homozygotes have significantly lower levels of blood glutathione than any of the other transferrin phenotypes. A similar association between transferrin phenotypes and blood glutathione has already been described in an earlier section of this chapter (pigeon transferrin).

Transferrin polymorphism has been detected in most other species of the genus *Macaca*,[76] including *M. irus* (cynomolgus or crab-eating monkey), *M. nemestrina* (pig-tailed macaque), and *M. speciosa* (stump-tailed macaque), although in some situations polymorphism has been found in one part of the species range, but not in another.[85] However, by way of an exception, in the Japanese macaques (*M. fascuta fascuta* and *M. fascuta yakui*) transferrin monomorphism appears to be the rule.[76]

b. Chimpanzee (Genus Pan)

Boyer and Young[87] in 1960 described seven β-globulin (transferrin) phenotypes in the sera from 25 chimpanzees, *Pan troglodytes* (a species previously designated as *P. satyrus*). The inheritance of the phenotypes was not determined, but the authors suggested a possible explanation — four codominant alleles (A, B, C, and D) at an autosomal gene locus. Goodman et al.[88] later confirmed these observations, finding the same seven phenotypes in a colony of 75 chimpanzees.[88] In a subsequent analysis of the familial relationships of these animals, Goodman and Riopelle[89] confirmed the mechanism of inheritance originally proposed by Boyer and Young.[87]

Chimpanzees have a broad geographical distribution, extending thousands of miles through the rain forests of central Africa, from the Atlantic coast of The Gambia to the mountains of Tanzania. Within this area, chimpanzee morphology varies considerably and at least four races of *P. troglodytes* are recognised.[78] Goodman et al.[78] have shown that the frequency of the variant transferrin alleles differs significantly amongst these four groups.[78]

2. Order: Rodentia

a. Mouse

Whilst for most vertebrates that have been examined transferrin polymorphism appears to be the rule, a curious situation occurs in the house mouse (*Mus musculus*). Natural populations do not exhibit transferrin polymorphism,[90,91] whereas in the inbred strains of laboratory mice, two alternative codominant alleles (Tf^a and Tf^b) have been detected at the transferrin gene locus.[92] In most strains of laboratory mice, the Tf^b allele is predominant, if not exclusive. The Tf^a allele is confined to the CBA strain and its derivatives.

The striking contrast between natural and laboratory populations has been studied for evidence of selection at the transferrin locus.[94] Data on litter size, survival rate, sex ratio, and allele segregation from 13 generations of a laboratory mouse colony have provided evidence showing that the Tf^b allele has a significant selective advantage over the Tf^a allele under defined conditions. From these results it has been suggested that this might lead to the elimination of the Tf^a gene from the population, and could account in part for the absence of the gene from natural populations of the house mouse.[94]

An additional, although extremely rare variant at the mouse transferrin locus has been discovered in the form of a "silent" or "null" allele.[95] Animals homozygous for this allele suffer from a severe and almost invariably lethal form of hereditary hypotransferrinaemia. The molecular basis for this disorder has recently been identified as a mutation in the transferrin gene, resulting in defective splicing of the nuclear precursor mRNA, such that at least two large intron sequences are retained in the mRNA molecules that reach the cytoplasm.[96]

b. Rat

Genetically determined electrophoretic variation of serum transferrin in the black rat, *Rattus rattus*, was reported by Moriwaki et al.[97] in 1969. Family studies confirmed the inheritance of the three common phenotypes as being due to the presence of two codominant alleles (Tf^R and Tf^N) at an autosomal gene locus. In a later and more extensive study of rat colonies throughout Asia and Oceania, the same group discovered a further ten variant transferrin alleles.[98] The presence and frequency of the 12 transferrin alleles has been found to correlate well with the three cytotaxonomic groups into which rats from this part of the world have been divided on the basis of chromosome numbers: Asian rats (2N = 38), Oceanic rats (2N = 42), and a third intermediate group prevalent in Sri Lanka (2N = 30).

c. Deer Mouse

Rasmussen and Koehn[99] first reported the inheritance of electrophoretic variants of transferrin in *Peromyscus maniculatus* (deer mouse) populations from Arizona. Codominant alleles Tf^A, Tf^B, and Tf^C accounted for the six electrophoretic phenotypes that were observed within the population. Similar transferrin polymorphism has been found in other closely related *Peromyscus* species: *P. boyllii* (brush mouse), *P. critinus* (canyon mouse), *P. eremicus* (cactus mouse), and *P. polionotus* (oldfield mouse), as well as additional variant alleles (Tf^D and Tf^E).[99,100] Canham et al.[101] have described two alleles (Tf^J and Tf^M) in deer mice from western Canada, as well as evidence of a disturbed segregation at the transferrin gene locus. Amongst the offspring of matings between heterozygous (Tf JM) parents, Canham et al.[101] noted a significant deficiency in the numbers of both the Tf J and Tf JM phenotypes. It was suggested that selective penetration by facility, whereby Tf^M sperm (from JM males) fertilizes a majority of Tf^M ova (from JM females), provided the most satisfactory explanation for this observation.

d. Mastomys

Mastomys (*Praomys natalensis*) is a wild African rodent that is intermediate between the rat and the mouse in appearance, but differs from both with respect to the number of chromosomes (2N = 36). The animal has been extensively studied because of its high incidence of spontaneous tumours (stomach, thymus, kidney, prostate gland, and bone marrow).[102] Since genetic factors are thought to be involved, and also because of the possible role of transferrin as a mitotic signal, Ootsu et al.[102] examined the serum transferrin phenotypes of the species. Three electrophoretic phenotypes were discovered, and family studies confirmed the autosomal inheritance of two codominant alleles (Tf^K and Tf^M). However, no disturbance in the pattern of segregation of phenotypes amongst the offspring was detected, and it remains to be established whether there exists any association between transferrin phenotypes and the occurrence of spontaneous neoplasms in this species.

e. Squirrel

Ground squirrels (genus *Spermophilus*) are widely distributed throughout Eurasia and North America — a land mass separated by the Bering Strait between Siberia and Alaska, and usually referred to as the Holartic region. In times past, the Holartic land masses have been periodically united by a "Bering land bridge", resulting from the lowering of the world ocean level as a consequence of Pleistocene glaciations. The spread of animal species, particularly reindeer, wolf, moose, and squirrel across this land bridge has been well recognised. Nadler and co-workers[103-106] have studied the serum transferrin from many of the species of Holartic squirrels, discovering as many as 18 variant alleles. By mapping the distribution and frequency of these alleles, it has been possible to examine the evolutionary relationship amongst these many species. Five of the variant transferrin alleles are common to all Holartic squirrel species, a further six are confined to the North American species, and the remaining seven alleles serve to distinguish the Eurasian taxonomic groups.

f. Vole

Maurer[107] first demonstrated genetic variation of serum transferrin in the vole (genus *Microtus*) during the course of a survey of three closely related species — *M. pennsylvannicus* (meadow vole), *M. ochrogaster* (prairie vole), and *M. breweri* (beach vole). Six different transferrin alleles were identified (A to F), with codominant inheritance being confirmed by family studies. As a result of subsequent studies carried out by Tamarin and Krebs[108,110] and Gaines et al.,[109] there is now considerable evidence suggesting that the process of selection operates at the transferrin gene locus of this species. By following the fluctuations in the frequencies of the transferrin alleles in vole populations over periods of 2 to 3 years, these researchers have shown that transferrin genotypes have differential effects on a number of the parameters that contribute to biological fitness: growth rate, body weight, preimplantation mortality, postimplantation mortality, and reproductive potential.

3. Order: Lagomorpha
a. Rabbit

Transferrin has been reported to be genetically monomorphic in all breeds of domestic rabbit (*Oryctolagus cuniculus*) so far examined,[111-113] with any minor differences in electrophoretic mobility of serum transferrin being attributed to different degrees of iron binding or variations in the number of sialic acid residues (posttranslational modifications).[114]

Recently, however, evidence has been published showing that whilst transferrin monomorphism appears to be the rule amongst domestic rabbit breeds, the same is certainly not true amongst rabbit populations in the wild. Arana et al.[115] discovered three electrophoretically distinct transferrin phenotypes in the populations of wild rabbits from northeast and central Spain. The occurrence of two codominant alleles (Tf^A and Tf^B) was supported by population data, but not confirmed by family studies. Evidence for two additional alleles (Tf^C and Tf^D) has recently come from a survey of the wild rabbit population of Portugal.[116] The frequency of the Tf^A allele, which is the only gene detected up to now in domestic breeds, varies from 0.2 to 0.95 amongst different wild rabbit colonies sampled throughout mainland Portugal.

4. Order: Carnivora
a. Dog (and other Canidae)

Evidence for the occurrence of transferrin polymorphism in the domestic dog (*Canis familiaris*) was first reported in 1966 by Bernoco et al.[117] and by Braend.[118] Stevens and Townsley[119] later examined the serum transferrin phenotypes from 248 dogs (pure breeds and cross breeds), as well as the offspring from a number of matings. Their results confirmed the presence of six transferrin phenotypes, genetically controlled by three codominant alleles: Tf^A, Tf^B, and Tf^C. The B and C alleles made up more than 98% of the gene pool. Juneja et al.[120] subsequently extended this study, analysing serum samples from 1127 dogs belonging to 60 different breeds. The Tf^B and Tf^C alleles were found to be present in all breeds, but often at significantly different frequencies. Tf^A is a rare allele, being confined to only a small number of breeds. In addition, Juneja et al.[120] discovered two further transferrin alleles, each being present in a single breed only: Tf^D (cocker spaniel) and Tf^E (poodle).

In recent years there have been a number of studies on the electrophoretic variation of serum proteins and red cell enzymes in domestic dogs and related Canidae.[121,122] These studies have often been carried out in an attempt to clarify the taxonomic relationship between the many breeds of domestic dog, and also between dogs and their canine relatives, including the wolf, the jackal, the dingo, and the coyote. *C. familiaris* is one of the oldest domesticated animals, having been associated with man for more than 10,000 years. During this time, conscious and unconscious selection by man has moulded dogs into a bewildering variety of breeds, exhibiting a wide range of morphological characteristics. It is generally agreed that the domestic dog descended from the wolf (*C. lupus*), a suggestion that is supported by the discovery that the common transferrin phenotypes of the Alaskan wolf are indistinguishable from those of the dog.[123] However, both serum protein and red cell enzyme phenotypes, as well as chromosome numbers, indicate that the domestic dog is also closely related to other Canidae, particularly the coyote (*C. latrans*) and the jackal (*C. aureus*). Indeed, the sporadic occurrence of the rare Tf^A gene in some unrelated breeds of dog may be evidence of introgression from jackals into the gene pool of *C. familiaris*.[120]

b. Cat

Allan et al.[124] have described an electrophoretic variation of serum transferrin in the domestic cat, *Felis catus*. By means of starch gel electrophoresis and isoelectric focussing, seven distinct transferrin phenotypes were detected amongst the 36 animals that were tested. Family studies confirmed the genetic basis for this extensive transferrin polymorphism in the domestic cat — four codominant alleles at an autosomal gene locus.

c. Fox

Genetic polymorphism of the serum transferrin from the arctic fox (*Alopex lagopus*) was reported by Balbierz and Nicolajczuk[125] in 1972. More recently, Juneja et al.[126] tested the serum samples from families of arctic foxes, silver foxes (*Vulpes vulpes*), and arctic-silver hybrids. Two transferrin alleles (Tf^F and Tf^S) were found in the arctic foxes, and two (Tf^F and Tf^D) in the silver foxes. The F types of both fox species are indistinguishable electrophoretically.

d. Seal

Transferrin variation has been found within some species of seals (grey, harp, ringed, southern fur, and Weddel), but not amongst others (hooded, bearded, elephant, and harbour).[127] Kerley[128] has recently investigated the transferrin phenotypes of sympatric populations of two fur seal species,

Arctocephalus tropicalis and *A. gazella,* cohabiting the same small Antarctic island. The two colonies were found to be fixed for alternative transferrin alleles, indicating an absence of gene flow between the two biologically distinct species.

5. Order: Perrisodactyla
a. Horse

Genetically determined transferrin polymorphism in the horse, *Equus caballus,* was first described by Braend and Stormont[129] in 1964. During the course of a study of Shetland ponies and of thoroughbred, Arabian, and appaloosa horses, they identified six codominant autosomal alleles at the transferrin gene locus, generating a considerable degree of phenotypic variation. Since then, a further eight alleles have been described, bringing the total to 14 (D, F_1, F_2, H_1, H_2, J, M, O, R, D_2, D_3, F_3, G, and X).[130] This highly polymorphic system has proved to be extremely valuable in distinguishing horse breeds and is routinely used in equine paternity cases.

E. przewalskii is a close relative of the modern horse and is a species believed to be extinct in the wild. Herds of captive horses, derived from about 12 ancestors, are maintained in various zoological collections. Despite obvious morphological differences between *E. caballus* and *E. przewalskii,* as well as differences in the number of chromosomes, interspecies hybrids remain fertile. The suggestion that very little genetic divergence has taken place is supported by the discovery that the two species share many of the same variant transferrin alleles.[131]

Even in the serum of horses homozygous at the transferrin gene locus, a considerable degree of electrophoretic heterogeneity exists. Starch gel electrophoresis resolves the serum transferrin from Tf O homozygotes into nine bands.[132] Many of the individual components differ, one from another, in terms of their molecular weight, as well as the number, degree of branching, and chemical composition of the glycan chains.

Schmid and Braend[133] have recently reported the discovery of a silent allele at the horse transferrin gene locus. This was discovered, as indeed have many of the examples of silent alleles at the human transferrin gene locus, during the course of routine blood testing in a paternity case. Confirmation that the silent allele had been transmitted from a thoroughbred mare to five of her offspring was obtained from quantitative immunodiffusion studies.

6. Order: Artiodactyla
a. Goat

Transferrin polymorphism in the goat (genus *Capra*) was first recognised as long ago as 1958 by Ashton and McDougall[134] as a phenotypic variation in the β-globulin region of goat sera. Amongst 60 animals of the British Saanen breed, three electrophoretically distinct phenotypes were discovered, genetically controlled by two codominant alleles (A and B). Watanabe et al.[135,136] later demonstrated that the protein responsible for the variable β-globulin phenotypes of goat serum was transferrin. They noted considerable differences in the distribution of the three common transferrin phenotypes amongst different goat breeds from Japan, Germany, Switzerland, Italy, and Hungary. In addition, a third rare allele (Tf^C) was encountered in the native goats of Korea, Thailand, and the Philippines.[137] More recently, two further alleles have been described, bringing the total to five (A to E).[138] The Tf^A and Tf^B alleles are by far the most common, and amongst the domestic goat breeds in the U.S. (Alpine and Spanish) these are the only two alleles to have been encountered, albeit at significantly different frequencies in the two breeds.[139]

b. Sheep

Ashton[140] first described phenotypic differences in the β-globulin region of serum from domestic sheep (*Ovis aries*) in 1958. Amongst the 118 animals tested (mixed breeds), eight electrophoretic phenotypes were discovered. Although at that time insufficient mating data had been obtained, Ashton suggested that it seemed probable that the various phenotypes would prove to be inherited. Within six months, and as a result of testing a further 500 animals, Ashton[141] discovered a further six variant phenotypes, bringing the total to 14. Family data confirmed the inheritance of these variant phenotypes as being controlled by five codominant alleles at an autosomal gene locus. This was followed by the discovery that the serum protein within the β-globulin region that exhibited such an extensive genetic polymorphism in domestic sheep was the iron-binding protein transferrin.[142]

It is now well established that transferrin polymorphism occurs in all breeds of both domestic and wild sheep. At least 13 variant alleles have now been discovered (A, B, C, D, E, G, H, I, K, L, M, P, and Q) and their genetic control confirmed.[143-147] Further examples of additional variants have been detected in species of wild sheep from different parts of the world, including *O. canadensis* (bighorn sheep), *O. dalli* (dall sheep), *O. musimon* (mouflon), and *O. linnaeus* (wild Iranian sheep).[138,148,149]

Within domestic sheep breeds, the alleles most frequently encountered are those originally discovered by Ashton — A, B, C, D, and E. Despite differences in geographic sampling, individual sheep breeds generally exhibit greater similarity in transferrin gene frequencies than is observed amongst breeds,[143] and to this end, transferrin polymorphism has proved to be a useful genetic marker in parentage control and breed characterisation. As yet, there is no evidence to suggest that the extensive array of transferrin phenotypes found throughout domestic and wild sheep populations are anything other than selectively neutral. For example, no correlation has been found between transferrin phenotype and susceptibility to scrapie.[145]

c. Pig

Transferrin polymorphism in the domestic pig, *Sus scrofa,* was first described in 1960 by Ashton[150] and by Kristjansson.[151] Three phenotypes, controlled by two codominant alleles (A and B), were confirmed by family studies. Within a few years two further variant alleles (C and D) had been discovered,[152] albeit occurring at a very low gene frequency. It is now evident that transferrin polymorphism is extensive, not only within different breeds of the domestic pig, but also within the wild pig populations of Europe and Asia,[153-158] with at least seven different variant alleles having been discovered. The distribution and frequencies of the transferrin alleles have been used as a valuable genetic marker for studies on the phylogenetic relationships between wild and domestic pigs.[158] Evidence that selective pressures might be operating in order to maintain the transferrin polymorphism within the pig population was provided by Kristjansson[159] in 1964, with the discovery that there was a correlation between transferrin phenotype and reproductive fitness.

d. Deer

Genetically determined variation of the serum transferrin of red deer, *Cervus elaphus,* was first described in 1962 by Lowe and McDougall,[160] with three codominant alleles accounting for the six electrophoretic phenotypes. A fourth variant has recently been discovered amongst farmed red deer of Czechoslovakian origin.[161]

The closely related species, *C. dama* (fallow deer), is an ungulate that is widely distributed over most parts of Europe, both in the wild and in farm populations where fallow deer have become an economically important species. Transferrin polymorphism was first described by Herzog[162] in 1989, the variation being restricted to two codominant alleles at an autosomal locus.

In complete contrast to either the red deer or the fallow deer, the reindeer (*Rangifer tarandus*) exhibits extensive genetic variation at the transferrin gene locus. As many as 13 variant alleles have been reported to be present in the reindeer herds of the U.S.S.R.,[163] whilst 12 have been found in Norwegian reindeer.[164] The mechanisms responsible for the high degree of transferrin variation in both semidomestic and wild reindeer herds are poorly understood, although there is some evidence for balanced selection. Zhurkevich and Fomicheva[165] have described an association between certain phenotypes and susceptibility to bacterial infection, whilst Roed[166] has recently shown an association between some of the transferrin alleles and the body weights of reindeer calves.

e. Cattle

Genetically determined differences in the β-globulin region (transferrin) of cattle serum was first reported in 1957 by Ashton[171] and by Hickman and Smithies.[172] Five different electrophoretic phenotypes were discovered by Ashton during the course of a survey of more than 300 cattle from 12 breeds. Ashton proposed a mechanism to explain the inheritance of the five phenotypes, based upon a group of five closely linked genes. This complex genetic model seemed at the time the only way possible to explain the results that had been obtained from preliminary family studies. The situation was clarified a year later when a sixth transferrin phenotype was discovered.[173] It then became possible to explain the family data using a much simpler and more conventional model, namely a single autosomal gene locus at which three codominant alleles could be identified: Tf^A, Tf^D, and Tf^E. The various diploid combinations of these three alleles would result in six possible genotypes and phenotypes. Amongst the breeds tested by Ashton, the Tf^A (0.26 to 0.75) and Tf^D (0.26 to 0.68) alleles were found to be the most common. It was also noted that the frequency of the Tf^E allele, albeit rare, occurred more often in those breeds of cattle that originated from the climatically more severe parts of the British Isles. Ashton suggested that transferrin polymorphism in cattle might be associated with the characteristic of climate tolerance.

At least ten variant alleles have now been discovered at the transferrin gene locus of cattle, with Tf^A, Tf^{D1}, Tf^{D2}, and Tf^E being the four most frequently encountered. Many of the rare alleles appear to be confined to particular breeds, such as, for example, the Tf^J gene in the Korean and Japanese Brown cattle.[174] Two particular aspects of cattle transferrin are worthy of special mention. The first concerns the possible operation of a balanced polymorphism helping to maintain the frequency of the variant alleles, and the second relates to the peculiarly complex heterogeneity of cattle transferrin as shown by the multiple electrophoretic components of each homozygous phenotype.

Ashton[175] first noticed in 1959 that the proportion of the two possible phenotypes amongst the offspring from reciprocal matings (homozygote × heterozygote) involving the A and D alleles was influenced by the maternal genotype. Of 154 calves resulting from such matings, 97 had the same phenotype as the dam, whereas only 57 shared the same phenotype as the sire. Random association of the two alleles (A and D) at fertilization, and comparable foetal viability, should have resulted in an equal number of live-born calves with phenotypes identical to either the dam or the sire (72 of each). It appeared from these results that a cattle embryo with a transferrin genotype different from the mother was more susceptible to early foetal mortality than an embryo with the same genotype as the dam. Ashton calculated that within a population of cattle where the Tf^E allele was absent and the frequency of A and D were equal (0.5), only 83% of all conceptions would result in a viable offspring, assuming there was no other cause of prenatal death. He also noted that the estimated loss due to transferrin incompatibility (A and D alleles only) was in close agreement with the observed foetal loss (12%) in cattle herds, published by the Milk Marketing Board.

The situation with regard to the rarer Tf^E allele is quite different. In this case, where the mother's genotype includes the Tf^E allele, there is found to be a significant lack of the same gene in the offspring. There appears to be an antagonism between a Tf^E mother and her Tf^E embryo, resulting in a deficit of Tf^E offspring. In this context it is significant that the E allele is the least frequent of the three originally discovered by Ashton, being entirely absent from breeds of cattle in the southern areas of the British Isles (Jersey, Guernsey, and South Devon). If the Tf^E allele confers such a selective disadvantage, as appears to be the case, one might reasonably expect that it would be rapidly eliminated by the process of natural selection. The fact that this does not appear to have happened in cattle breeds in the north of the British Isles suggests that Tf^E must confer a counterbalancing advantage (climate tolerance?). If this is true, then the genetic variation of transferrin within cattle provides a good example of a balanced polymorphism.

The second characteristic of cattle transferrin that has received much attention over the last 10 years is the extensive electrophoretic heterogeneity displayed by the protein, even within the serum of homozygous animals. Most animal transferrins, even when fully saturated with iron, show some degree of structural heterogeneity when subjected to electrophoresis. Homozygous phenotypes often appear as one major protein band, with an additional one or two minor components being present within the plasma. In most instances, differences in the number of sialic acid residues (posttranslational modifications) have been found to be the primary cause. Cattle transferrins demonstrate a very extreme form of this heterogeneity, with homozygous phenotypes having as many as four major and six minor components. The molecular basis for the complex electrophoretic pattern of cattle transferrin has yet to be fully explained. Whilst it has been shown that some of the heterogeneity is indeed due to variation in sialic acid content,[176,177] this property alone does not explain all of the electrophoretic multiplicity. Hatton et al.[178] have suggested that sialic acid variability serves to mask an underlying heterogeneity, the cause of which is likely to reside within the polypeptide chain of the molecule. One such example has been the discovery by Maeda et al.[179] that some molecules of cattle serum transferrin possess an internal scission within the polypeptide chain, resulting in two fragments (70,000 and 6,000 kDa) that remain held together by the disulphide bridges. This structural modification results in an alteration in the net charge, and therefore electrophoretic mobility of the protein.

Genetic variants of cattle transferrin are one of the few examples, with the exception of humans, where the nature of the amino acid differences between the products of variant alleles has been sought. Maeda et al.[180] compared the structures of the Tf^A and Tf^{D2} gene products and came to the conclusion that there are three amino acid differences between the two proteins, each substitution occurring within well-separated regions of the primary sequence. This is a most unusual finding, since in most other examples of similar allelic variation, mutations due to a single base change within a gene result in only one amino acid substitution.

III. SUMMARY

The study of transferrin polymorphism within the animal kingdom has revealed an extensive degree of variability at the transferrin gene locus. In most species, where reasonable numbers of animals have been available for study, multiple transferrin alleles have been discovered. This polymorphism has been put to a practical use in a variety of ways, including:

1. The study of interspecies hybridization (e.g., frogs and toads)
2. Providing data to assist in the taxonomic classification of animal species, and the study of their phylogenetic relationships (e.g., snakes, rats, and dogs)
3. Paternity testing (e.g., horses)
4. The study of animal migration patterns (e.g., fishes, birds, and squirrels)

The magnitude of genetic variation observed at the molecular level in natural populations of various animal species has raised the question of how this variation is maintained. The question that is still unresolved concerns the extent to which balancing selection assists in the maintenance of protein polymorphism. One school of thought asserts that variability is maintained mainly by the process of random genetic drift (Kimura)[181] whilst the other believes that almost all polymorphism is maintained by some form of balancing selection (Lewontin).[182] Amongst the many animals in which transferrin polymorphism has been detected, there is evidence that not all the alleles are selectively neutral, and that some might be maintained by the operation of balanced polymorphisms. Examples of the latter include the following: tuna, toad, pigeon, macaque, deer mouse, vole, house mouse, pig, reindeer, and cattle.

REFERENCES

1. **Dessauer, H. C., Fox, W., and Hartwig, Q. L.,** Comparative study of transferrins of amphibia and reptilia using starch-gel electrophoresis and autoradiography, *Comp. Biochem. Physiol.,* 5, 17, 1962.
2. **Palmour, R. M. and Sutton, H. E.,** Vertebrate transferrins. Molecular weights, chemical compositions, and iron-binding studies, *Biochemistry,* 10, 4026, 1971.
3. **van Eijk, H. G., van Dijk, J. P., van Noort, W. L., Leijnse, B., and Moonfort, C. H.,** Isolation and analysis of transferrin from different species, *Scand. J. Haematol.,* 9, 267, 1972.
4. **Hudson, B. G., Ohno, M., Brockway, W. J., and Castellino, F. J.,** Chemical and physical properties of serum transferrins from several species, *Biochemistry,* 12, 1047, 1973.
5. **Graham, I. and Williams, J.,** A comparison of glycopeptides from the transferrins of several species, *Biochem. J.,* 145, 263, 1975.
6. **Jarritt, P. H.,** The effect of iron on sedimentation-velocity and gel filtration behaviour of transferrin from several species, *Biochem. Biophys. Acta,* 453, 332, 1976.
7. **Princiotto, J. V.,** Differences between human and rabbit transferrins, *Biochem. Biophys. Acta,* 539, 81, 1978.
8. **Regoeczi, E. and Hatton, M. W. C.,** Transferrin catabolism in mammalian species of different body sizes, *Am. J. Physiol.,* 238, 306, 1980.
9. **Lim, B. C., Peters, T., and Morgan, E. H.,** Iron-binding properties and amino acid compositions of marsupial transferrins: comparison with eutherian mammals and other vertebrates, *Comp. Biochem. Physiol. A,* 89, 559, 1988.

10. **Bobak, P., Stratil, A., and Valenta, M.**, A comparison of molecular weights of transferrins of various vertebrates, *Comp. Biochem. Physiol. B*, 79, 113, 1984.

11. **Welch, S. and Skinner, A.**, A comparison of the structure and properties of human, rat and rabbit transferrin, *Comp. Biochem. Physiol. B*, 93, 417, 1989.

12. **Lim, B. C. and Morgan, E. H.**, Transferrin-receptor interaction and its significance to protein evolution, Proc. Int. Conf. Prot. Iron Metab. 7th Villeneuve D'Ascq., France, 1985, 13.

13. **Welch, S.**, A comparison of the structure and properties of serum transferrin from 17 animal species, *Comp. Biochem. Physiol. B*, 97, 417, 1990.

14. **Penhallow, R. C., Mason, A. B., and Woodworth, R. C.**, Electrophoretic characterisation of human, equine and bovine transferrins, *Comp. Biochem. Physiol. B*, 98, 41, 1991.

15. **Martin, A. W., Huebers, E., Huebers, H., Webb, J., and Finch, C. A.**, A monosited transferrin from a representative deuterostome: the ascidan *Pyura stolonifera* (sub phylum Urochordate), *Blood*, 64, 1047, 1984.

16. **Mao, S-H. and Dessauer, H. C.**, Selectively neutral mutations, transferrins and the evolution of natricine snakes, *Comp. Biochem. Physiol. A*, 40, 669, 1971.

17. **Prager, E. M., Wilson, A. C., Osuga, D. T., and Feeney, R. E.**, Evolution of flightless land birds on southern continents: transferrin comparison shows monophyletic origin of ratites, *J. Mol. Evol.*, 8, 283, 1976.

18. **Ho, C. Y.**, Penguin evolution. Protein comparisons demonstrate relationship to flying aquatic birds, *J. Mol. Evol.*, 8, 271, 1976.

19. **Prager, E. M., Brush, A. H., Nolan, R. A., Nakanishi, M., and Wilson, A. C.**, Slow evolution of transferrin and albumin in birds according to micro-complement fixation analysis, *J. Mol. Evol.*, 3, 243, 1974.

20. **Ashton, G. C.**, Serum protein differences in cattle by starch gel electrophoresis, *Nature*, 180, 917, 1957.

21. **Smithies, O.**, Variations in human serum β-globulins, *Nature*, 180, 1482, 1957.

22. **Ashton, G. C.**, Polymorphism in the β-globulins of sheep, *Nature*, 181, 849, 1958.

23. **Ashton, G. C. and McDougall, E. I.**, β-Globulin polymorphism in cattle, sheep and goats, *Nature*, 182, 945, 1958.

24. **Turner, R. J. and Jamieson, A.**, Transferrin in fishes, *Anim. Genet.*, 18(Suppl. 1), 70, 1987.

25. **Creysell, R., Richard, G. B., and Silberzahu, P.**, Transferrin variants in carp serum, *Nature*, 212, 5068, 1966.

26. **Valenta, M. and Kalal, L.**, Polymorphism of serum transferrin in the carp and the tench, *J. Univ. Agr. Prague Ser. B*, p 93, 1968.

27. **Reichenbach-Klinke, H. H.**, Investigation of the serum polymorphism of trout and carp, in *Genetics and Mutagenisis in Fish*, J. H. Schroder, Ed., Springer-Verlag, Berlin, 1973, 315.

28. **Klose, J., Wolf, U., Hitzeroth, H., and Ritter, H.**, Polyploidization in the fish family Cyprinidae. Duplication of the gene loci coding for lactate dehydrogenase and 6-phosphogluconate dehydrogenase, *Humangenetik*, 7, 245, 1969.

29. **Valenta, M., Stratil, A., Slechtova, V., Kalal, L., and Slechta, V.**, Polymorphism of transferrin in carp (*Cyprinus carpio* L.): genetic determination, isolation, and partial characterisation, *Biochem. Genet.*, 14, 27, 1976.

30. **McKensie, J. A. and Martin, C.**, Transferrin polymorphism in blueback herring *Alosa aestivalis* (Mitchell), *Can. J. Zoology*, 53, 1479, 1975.

31. **DeLigny, W.**, Polymorphism of serum transferrin in Plaice, Proc. 11th Europ. Conf. Anim. Blood Groups and Biochem. Polymorphisms, Warsaw, 1968, 527.

32. **Moller, D.**, Genetic differences between cod groups in the Lofoten area, *Nature*, 212, 824, 1966.

33. **Fujino, K. and Kang, T.**, Transferrin groups of tunas, *Genetics*, 59, 79, 1968.

34. **Russell, H. A. and Jeffrey, J. E.**, Serum transferrin polymorphism in grey trout, *Cynoscion regalis*, from the lower Rappahannock river, *Esturaries*, 2, 269, 1979.

35. **Teixiera, A. S., Raposo, J. C. P., and Jamieson, A.,** Transferrin variation in jaraquis, *Semaprochilodus taeniurus* and *S. insignis,* in the Amazon region, *Anim. Genet.,* 21, 419, 1990.

36. **Hitron, J. W.,** Serum transferrin phenotypes in striped bass, *Morone saxatilis* from the Hudson river, *Chesapeake Sci.,* 15, 246, 1974.

37. **Tsuyuki, H., Roberts, E., and Best, E. A.,** Serum transferrin systems and haemoglobin of the Pacific halibut (*Hippoglossus stenolepsis*), *J. Fish. Res. Board Can.,* 26, 2351, 1969.

38. **Jeffrey, J. E.,** Distribution of serum transferrin in spot, *Leiostomus xanthurus, Anim. Blood Groups Biochem. Genet.,* 12, 139, 1981.

39. **Johnson, A. G. and Beardsley, A. J.,** Biochemical polymorphism of starry flounder, *Platichthys stelatus,* from northwestern and northeastern Pacific ocean, *Anim. Blood Groups Biochem. Genet.,* 6, 9, 1975.

40. **Mangaly, G. and Jamieson, A.,** Genetic tags applied to the European hake, *Anim. Blood Groups Biochem. Genet.,* 10, 39, 1979.

41. **Child, A. R., Burnell, N. P., and Wilkins, N. P.,** The existence of two races of Atlantic salmon (*Salmon salar* L.) in British Isles, *J. Fish Biol.,* 8, 35, 1976.

42. **Monostory, Z., Nagy, A. M., Gervai, J., and Csanyi, V.,** Polymorphism and inheritance of serum esterases and β-globulins in the paradise fish (*Macropodus opercularis*; Anabantidae), *Anim. Blood Groups Biochem. Genet.,* 15, 1, 1984.

43. **Guttman, S.,** Transferrin and haemoglobin polymorphism, hybridization and introgression in two African toads, *Bufo regularis* and *Bufo rangeri, Comp. Biochem. Physiol.,* 23, 871, 1967.

44. **Guttman, S.,** Blood proteins, in *Evolution in the Genus* Bufo, W. F. Blair, Ed., University of Texas Press, Austin, 1972, 265.

45. **Guttman, S. I. and Wilson, K. G.,** Genetic variation in the Genus *Bufo.* An extreme degree of transferrin and albumin polymorphism in a population of the American toad (*Bufo americanus*), *Biochem. Genet.,* 8, 329, 1973.

46. **Gartside, D. F. and Watson, G. F.,** Inheritance in progeny of *in vitro* crosses involving the tree frog *Littoria ewingi* (Anura: Hylidae), *Comp. Biochem. Physiol. B,* 53, 431, 1976.

47. **Dunlap, D. G.,** Linkage analysis of the transferrin, albumin, and haemoglobin in leopard frogs, *J. Hered.,* 73, 247, 1982.

48. **Platz, J. E.,** Sympatric interaction between two forms of leopard frogs (*Rana pipiens* complex) in Texas, *Copeia,* 1972, 232, 1972.

49. **Dessauer, H. C. and Nevo, E.,** Geographic variation of blood and liver proteins in cricket frogs, *Biochem. Genet.,* 3, 171, 1969.

50. **Gorman, G. C. and Dessauer, H. C.,** The relationships of *Anolis* of the *Roquet* species group (Sauria: Iguanidiae) — electrophoretic comparison of blood proteins, *Comp. Biochem. Physiol.,* 19, 845, 1966.

51. **Ogden, A. L., Morton, J. R., Gilmour, D. G., and McDermid, E. M.,** Inherited variants in the transferrins and conalbumins of the chicken, *Nature,* 195, 1026, 1962.

52. **Stratil, A.,** A contribution towards the study of transferrins and conalbumins of the domestic fowl, in *Polymorphismes Biochimiques des Animaux. Proc. 10th Europ. Conf. Anim. Blood Groups and Biochem. Polymorphisms,* Institut National de la Recherche Agronomique, Paris, 1966, 241.

53. **Crozier, G.,** Polymorphismes biochimiques de la poule domestique. Analyse genetique des proteines du blanc d'oeuf chez des poules de races francaises et etrangeres, *Ann. Biol. Anim. Biochim. Biophys.,* 6, 379, 1966.

54. **Baker, C. M. A.,** Molecular genetics of avian proteins. Chemical and genetic polymorphism of conalbumin and transferrin in a number of species, *Comp. Biochem. Physiol.,* 20, 949, 1967.

55. **Stratil, A.,** Transferrin and albumin loci in chickens, *Gallus gallus* L., *Comp. Biochem. Physiol.,* 24, 113, 1968.

56. **Williams, J.,** A comparison of conalbumin and transferrin in the domestic fowl, *Biochem. J.,* 83, 355, 1962.
57. **Kimura, M., Ito, S., Morishima, Y., and Isogai, I.,** Conalbumin electrophoretic pattern of the quail *Coturnix coturnix japonica, Jpn. J. Genet.,* 52, 251, 1977.
58. **Ito, S., Asano, H., Hanai, H., Ishikawa, K., Kimura, M., and Isogai, I.,** Genetic control and population survey of transferrin in the Japanese quail, *Anim. Blood Groups Biochem. Genet.,* 12, 145, 1981.
59. **Baker, C. M. A. and Hanson, H. C.,** Molecular genetics of avian proteins. Evolutionary implications of blood proteins of eleven species of geese, *Comp. Biochem. Physiol.,* 17, 997, 1966.
60. **Valenta, M. and Stratil, A.,** Polymorphism of transferrin and conalbumin in the domestic goose (*Anser anser*), *Anim. Blood Groups Biochem. Genet.,* 9, 129, 1978.
61. **Milne, H. and Robertson, F. W.,** Polymorphisms in egg albumen protein and behaviour in the eider duck, *Nature,* 205, 367, 1965.
62. **Mueller, J. O., Smithies, O., and Irwin, M. R.,** Transferrin variation in Columbidae, *Genetics,* 47, 1385, 1962.
63. **Ferguson, A.,** Geographic and species variation in transferrin and ovotransferrin polymorphism in the Columbidae, *Comp. Biochem. Physiol. B,* 38, 477, 1971.
64. **Desborough, S. and Irwin, M. R.,** Additional variation in serum proteins in Columbidae, *Physiol. Zool.,* 39, 66, 1966.
65. **Frelinger, J. A.,** The maintenance of transferrin polymorphism in pigeons, *Proc. Natl. Acad. Sci. U.S.A.,* 69, 326, 1972.
66. **Frelinger, J. A.,** Maternally derived transferrin in pigeon squabs, *Science,* 171, 1260, 1971.
67. **Brown, R. V. and Sharp, H. B.,** Association of transferrin and glutathione in pigeons, *Anim. Blood Groups Biochem. Genet.,* 1, 113, 1970.
68. **Frelinger, J. A.,** Chemical basis of transferrin polymorphism in pigeons, *Anim. Blood Groups Biochem. Genet.,* 4, 35, 1973.
69. **Baker, C. M. A. and Manwell, C.,** Molecular genetics of avian proteins. Egg white proteins of the migratory quail — new concepts of "hybrid vigour", *Comp. Biochem. Physiol.,* 23, 21, 1967.
70. **Stratil, A. and Valenta, M.,** Protein polymorphism of egg white and yolk in geese and ducks, *Folia Biol. (Prague),* 12, 307, 1966.
71. **Ferguson, A.,** An Electrophoretic Study of the Blood and Egg White Proteins of Some Columbidae, Ph.D. thesis, Queen's University, Belfast, 1969.
72. **Buettner-Janusch, J.,** Evolution of serum protein polymorphisms, *Annu. Rev. Genet.,* 4, 47, 1970.
73. **Nute, P. E. and Buettner-Janusch, J.,** Genetics of polymorphic transferrins in the genus *Lemur, Folia Primatol.,* 10, 181, 1969.
74. **Shimaoka, T.,** Genetic variations in albumin and transferrin as species markers in plasma of Callithricidae, *Jikken Dobutsu,* 33, 105, 1984.
75. **Buettner-Janusch, J.,** Haemoglobin and transferrin of baboons, *Folia Primatol.,* 1, 73, 1963.
76. **Lai, L. Y. C.,** Transferrin in *Macaca irus, Folia Primatol.,* 17, 193, 1972.
77. **Nute, P. E. and Buettner-Janusch, J.,** Serum transferrins of Pongidae: *Pan, Pongo,* and *Hylobates, Folia Primatol.,* 8, 282, 1968.
78. **Goodman, M., Wisecup, W. G., Reynolds, H. H., and Kratochuil, C. H.,** Transferrin polymorphism and population differences in the genetic variability of chimpanzees, *Nature,* 187, 1035, 1960.
79. **Goodman, M. and Poulik, E.,** Serum transferrins of the genus *Macaca*: species distribution of nineteen phenotypes, *Nature,* 191, 1407, 1961.
80. **Goodman, M. and Poulik, E.,** Effects of speciation on serum proteins in the genus *Macaca* with special reference to the polymorphic state of transferrin, *Nature,* 190, 171, 1961.

81. **Devor, E. J.**, Genetic variation of transferrin alleles of rhesus macaques, *Macaca mullata*, *Am. J. Phys. Anthropol.*, 48, 165, 1978.

82. **Brown, R. V., Goodman, M., and Gavan, J. A.**, Glutathione and transferrin in rhesus monkey, *Anim. Blood Groups Biochem. Genet.*, 1, 189, 1970.

83. **Smith, D. G. and Small, M. F.**, Selection and the transferrin polymorphism in monkeys (*Macaca mulatta*), *Folia Primatol.*, 37, 127, 1982.

84. **Goodman, M., Kulkarni, A., Poulik, E., and Reklys, E.**, Species and geographic differences in the transferrin polymorphism of Macaques, *Science*, 147, 884, 1965.

85. **Buettner-Janusch, J.**, Distribution of transferrin phenotypes in selected troops of Kenya baboons, *Am. J. Phys. Anthropol.*, 33, 303, 1970.

86. **Buettner-Janusch, J.**, Genetic studies of serum transferrins of free-ranging rhesus macaques, *Am. J. Phys. Anthropol.*, 41, 217, 1974.

87. **Boyer, S. H. and Young, W. J.**, β-Globulin polymorphism in chimpanzees, *Nature*, 187, 1035, 1960.

88. **Goodman, M., McBride, R., Poulik, E., and Reklys, E.**, Serum transferrins in the Orange Park chimpanzee colony classified by the Boyer and Young scheme, *Nature*, 197, 259, 1963.

89. **Goodman, M. and Riopelle, A. J.**, Inheritance of serum transferrins in chimpanzees, *Nature*, 197, 261, 1963.

90. **Petras, M. L.**, Studies of natural populations of Mus. Biochemical polymorphisms and their bearing on breeding structure, *Evolution*, 21, 259, 1967.

91. **Selander, R. K. and Yang, S. Y.**, Protein polymorphism in wild populations, *Genetics*, 61, s54, 1969.

92. **Ashton, G. C. and Braden, A. W. H.**, Serum β-globulin polymorphism in mice, *Aust. J. Biol. Sci.*, 14, 248, 1961.

93. **Cohen, B. L. and Shreffler, D. C.**, A revised nomenclature for the mouse transferrin locus, *Genet. Res.*, 2, 306, 1961.

94. **Ashton, G. C. and Dennis, M. N.**, Selection at the transferrin locus in mice, *Genetics*, 67, 253, 1971.

95. **Bernstein, S. E.**, Hereditary hypotransferrinemia with hemosiderosis, a murine disorder resembling human atransferrinemia, *J. Lab. Clin. Med.*, 110, 690, 1987.

96. **Huggenvik, J. I., Craven, C. M., Idzerda, R. L., Berstein, S., Kaplan, J., and McKnight, G. S.**, A splicing defect in the mouse transferrin gene leads to congenital atransferrinemia, *Blood*, 74, 482, 1989.

97. **Moriwaki, K., Tsuchiya, K., and Yosida, T. H.**, Genetic polymorphism in the serum transferrin of *Rattus rattus*, *Genetics*, 63, 193, 1969.

98. **Moriwaki, K., Kato, H., Imai, H., Tsuchiya, K., and Yosida, T.**, Geographical distribution of twelve transferrin alleles in black rats of Asia and Oceania, *Genetics*, 79, 295, 1975.

99. **Rasmussen, D. I. and Koehn, R. K.**, Serum transferrin polymorphism in the deer mouse, *Genetics*, 54, 1353, 1966.

100. **Griswold, K. E. and Dawson, W. D.**, Transferrin and haptoglobin inheritance in *Peromyscus*, *J. Hered.*, 62, 339, 1971.

101. **Canham, R. P., Birdsall, D. A., and Cameron, D. G.**, Disturbed segregation at the transferrin locus of the deer mouse, *Genet. Res.*, 16, 355, 1970.

102. **Ootsu, K., Matsumoto, T., and Hiroano, T.**, An electrophoretic polymorphism in the serum transferrins of *Praomys (Mastomys) natalensis*, *Biochem. Genet.*, 14, 687, 1976.

103. **Nadler, C. F.**, The serum proteins and transferrins of the ground squirrel subgenus *Spermophilus*, *Comp. Biochem. Physiol.*, 27, 487, 1968.

104. **Nadler, C. F. and Youngman, P. M.**, Further studies of transferrins of the artic ground squirrel *Spermophilus undulatus*, *Comp. Biochem. Physiol.*, 36, 81, 1970.

105. **Nadler, C. F., Voronstov, N. N., Hoffman, R. S., Formichova, I. I., and Nadler, C., Jr.**, Zoogeography of transferrins in artic and long-tailed ground squirrel populations, *Comp. Biochem. Physiol. B*, 44, 33, 1973.

106. **Nadler, C. F., Sukernik, R. I., Hoffman, R. S., Vorontsov, N. N., Nadler, C. F., Jr., and Fomichova, I. I.,** Evolution in ground squirrels. Transferrins in holartic populations of *Spermophilus, Comp. Biochem. Physiol. A,* 47, 663, 1974.

107. **Maurer, F. W.,** Heritability of the plasma transferrin protein in three species of *Microtus, Nature,* 215, 95, 1967.

108. **Tamarin, R. H. and Krebs, C. J.,** *Microtus* population biology. Genetic changes at the transferrin locus in fluctuating populations of two vole species, *Evolution,* 23, 183, 1969.

109. **Gaines, M. S., Myers, J. H., and Krebs, C. J.,** Experimental analysis of relative fitness in transferrin genotypes of *Microtus achrogaster, Evolution,* 25, 443, 1971.

110. **Tamarin, R. H. and Krebs, C. J.,** Selection at the transferrin locus in cropped vole populations, *Heredity,* 30, 53, 1973.

111. **Gilman-Sachs, A. and Hanley, W. C.,** Enzymes and other proteins in serum and other tissues: rabbit, in *Inbred and Genetically Defined Strains of Laboratory Animals,* Vol. 3, Part 2, C. A. Wright and D. D. Katz, Eds., Federation for Experimental Biology, MD, 1979, 578.

112. **Binette, J. P., MacNair, M. B., and Calkins, E.,** Fractionation and characterisation of normal rabbit plasma proteins, *Biochem. J.,* 94, 143, 1965.

113. **Skow, L. C., Fox, R. R., and Womack, J. E.,** Inherited enzyme variation among JAX strains of domestic rabbits, *J. Hered.,* 69, 165, 1978.

114. **Zaragoza, P., Arana, A., and Amorena, B.,** Relationship between rabbit transferrin electrophoretic patterns and plasma iron concentrations, *Anim. Genet.,* 18, 1987.

115. **Arana, A., Zaragoza, P., Rodellar, C., and Amorena, B.,** Evidence for transferrin polymorphism in Spanish wild rabbits, *Anim. Genet.,* 18, 125, 1987.

116. **Ferrand, N., Carvahlo, G., and Amorim, A.,** Transferrin (Tf) polymorphism in wild rabbit, *Oryctolagus cuniculus, Anim. Genet.,* 19, 295, 1988.

117. **Bernoco, D., Sartore, G., and Bona, C.,** Studie preliminari sul polymorfismo biochimico nel cane, *Atti Soc. Ital. Sci. Vet.,* 20, 343, 1966.

118. **Braend, M.,** Serum transferrins of dogs, Proc. 10th Europ. Conf. Anim. Blood Groups and Biochem. Polymorphisms, 1966, 319.

119. **Stevens, R. W. C. and Townsley, M. E.,** Canine serum transferrins, *J. Hered.,* 61, 71, 1970.

120. **Juneja, R. K., Christensen, K., Andresen, E., and Gahne, B.,** Frequencies of transferrin types in various breeds of domestic dogs, *Anim. Blood Groups Biochem. Genet.,* 12, 79, 1981.

121. **Simonsen, V.,** Electrophoretic studies on the blood proteins of domestic dogs and other Canidae, *Hereditas,* 82, 7, 1976.

122. **Fisher, R. A., Putt, W., and Hackel, E.,** An investigation of the products of 53 gene loci in three species of wild Canidae: *Canis lupus, Canis latrans,* and *Canis familiaris, Biochem. Genet.,* 14, 963, 1976.

123. **Braend, M. and Roed, K. H.,** Polymorphism of transferrin and esterase in Alaskan wolves: evidence of close molecular homology with the dog, *Anim. Genet.,* 18, 143, 1987.

124. **Allan, J., Putt, W., and Fisher, R. A.,** An investigation of the products of 23 gene loci in the domestic cat, *Felis catus, Anim. Blood Groups Biochem. Genet.,* 12, 95, 1981.

125. **Balbierz, H. and Nikolajczuk, M.,** Further immunogenetic investigations of breeding foxes, Proc. 10th Europ. Conf. Anim. Blood Groups Biochem. Polymorph., Budapest, 1972, 673.

126. **Juneja, R. K., Niini, T., Lohi, O., Larsen, B., and Gahne, B.,** Genetic polymorphism of plasma B-glycoprotein and transferrin in arctic and silver foxes, *Anim. Genet.,* 19, 237, 1988.

127. **McDermid, E. M. and Bonner, W. N.,** Red cell and serum protein systems of grey seals and harbour seals, *Comp. Biochem. Physiol. B,* 50, 97, 1975.

128. **Kerley, G. I. H.,** Electrophoretic transferrin variation in fur seals (*Arctocephalus* spp) at Marion Island, *Comp. Biochem. Physiol. B,* 92, 361, 1989.

129. **Braend, M. and Stormont, C.,** Studies on hemoglobin and transferrin types of horses, *Nord. Veterinaermed.,* 16, 31, 1964.

130. **Cothran, E. G., Henney, P. J., and King, J. A.,** Inheritance of the equine Tf F3 allele, *Anim. Genet.,* 22, 187, 1991.

131. **Putt, W. and Whitehouse, D. B.,** Genetics of four plasma protein loci in *Equus prze-walskii*: new alleles at the prealbumin, postalbumin and transferrin loci, *Anim. Blood Groups Biochem. Genet.,* 14, 7, 1983.

132. **Stratil, A., Tomasek, V., Bobak, P., and Glasnak, V.,** Heterogeneity of horse trans-ferrin: the role of the carbohydrate moiety, *Anim. Blood Groups Biochem. Genet.,* 15, 89, 1984.

133. **Schmid, D. O. and Braend, M.,** Further evidence for a silent allele in the transferrin locus of the horse, *Anim. Genet.,* 21, 423, 1990.

134. **Ashton, G. C. and McDougall, E. I.,** β-Globulin polymorphism in cattle, sheep and goats, *Nature,* 182, 945, 1958.

135. **Watanabe, S., Nozawa, K., and Suzuki, S.,** Studies on the transferrin of goats. 1. Typing of transferrin of goat serum by starch gel electrophoresis, *Proc. Jpn. Acad.,* 41, 326, 1965.

136. **Watanabe, S. and Suzuki, S.,** Studies on the transferrin of goats. 2. Inheritance mode of serum transferrin types, *Proc. Jpn. Acad.,* 42, 178, 1965.

137. **Watanabe, S. and Suzuki, S.,** Studies on the transferrins of goats. 3. Evidence for a third transferrin allele, *Anim. Blood Groups Biochem. Genet.,* 4, 23, 1973.

138. **Tucker, E. M. and Clarke, S. W.,** Comparative aspects of biochemical polymorphism in the blood of Caprinae species and their hybrids, *Anim. Genet.,* 11, 163, 1980.

139. **Wang, S., Foote, W. C., and Bunch, T. D.,** Transferrin and haemoglobin polymorphism in domesticated goats in the USA, *Anim. Genet.,* 21, 91, 1990.

140. **Ashton, G. C.,** Polymorphism in the β-globulins of sheep, *Nature,* 181, 849, 1958.

141. **Ashton, G. C.,** Further β-globulin phenotypes in sheep, *Nature,* 182, 1101, 1958.

142. **Ashton, G. C. and Ferguson, K. A.,** Serum transferrins in merino sheep, *Genet. Res. Camb.,* 4, 240, 1963.

143. **Stormont, C., Suzuki, Y., Bradford, G. E., and King, P.,** A survey of hemoglobins, transferrins and certain red cell antigens in nine breeds of sheep, *Genetics,* 60, 363, 1968.

144. **Stratil, A.,** Two new sheep transferrin variants and the effect of neuraminidase, *Anim. Blood Groups Biochem. Genet.,* 4, 153, 1973.

145. **Collis, S. C. and Millson, G. C.,** Transferrin polymorphism in Herdwick sheep, *Anim. Blood Groups Biochem. Genet.,* 6, 117, 1975.

146. **Archibald, A. L. and Webster, J.,** A new transferrin allele in sheep, *Anim. Genet.,* 17, 191, 1986.

147. **Erhardt, G.,** Transferrin variants in sheep: separation and characterisation by polyacryl-amide gel electrophoresis and isoelectric focusing, *Anim. Genet.,* 17, 343, 1986.

148. **Nadler, C. F., Woolf, A., and Harris, K. E.,** The transferrins and hemoglobins of bighorn sheep (*Ovis canadensis*), dall sheep (*Ovis dalli*) and mouflon (*Ovis musimon*), *Comp. Biochem. Physiol. B,* 40, 567, 1971.

149. **Lay, D. M., Nadler, C. F., and Hassinger, J. D.,** The transferrins and hemoglobins of wild Iranian sheep (*Ovis linnaeus*), *Comp. Biochem. Physiol. B,* 40, 567, 1971.

150. **Ashton, G. C.,** Thread protein and β-globulin polymorphism in the serum proteins of pigs, *Nature,* 186, 991, 1960.

151. **Kristjansson, F. K.,** Inheritance of a serum protein in swine, *Science,* 131, 1681, 1960.

152. **Schroffel, J.,** New genetic variants of transferrins and haptoglobins in pigs, *Nature,* 210, 1274, 1966.

153. **Baker, L. N.,** New allele in the transferrin system of pigs, Tf[E] Ames, an apparent mutation, *Vox Sang.,* 14, 446, 1968.

154. **Skladanowski, E., Zurkowski, M., Wiatroszak, I., and Filipiak, W.,** Polymorphism of the serum proteins of wild pigs, *Anim. Blood Groups Biochem. Genet.,* 10, 151, 1979.

155. **Palovics, A., Fesus, L., and Osvath, L.,** Tf I transferrin variant in domestic pig, *Anim. Blood Groups Biochem. Genet.,* 13, 61, 1982.

156. **Stratil, A., Glasnak, V., Skladanowski, E., Fesus, L., and Palovics, A.,** A comparison of the fastest moving transferrin variants of the pig, *Anim. Blood Groups Biochem. Genet.,* 13, 59, 1982.

157. **Tanaka, K., Oishi, T., Kurosawa, Y., and Suzuki, S.,** Genetic relationship among several pig populations in East Asia analysed by blood groups and serum protein polymorphisms, *Anim. Blood Groups Biochem. Genet.,* 14, 191, 1983.

158. **Kurosawa, Y. and Tanaka, K.,** Electrophoretic variants of serum transferrin in wild pig populations of Japan, *Anim. Genet.,* 19, 31, 1988.

159. **Kristjansson, F. K.,** Transferrin types and reproductive performance in the pig, *J. Reprod. Fertil.,* 8, 311, 1964.

160. **Lowe, V. P. W. and McDougall, E. I.,** Serum β-globulin types in red deer and other species, and their stability in the presence of bacteria, *Nature,* 192, 983, 1962.

161. **Stratil, A., Glasnak, V., Bobak, P., Cizowa, D., Gabrisova, A., and Kalab, P.,** Variation of some serum proteins in red deer, *Cervus elaphus, Anim. Genet.,* 21, 285, 1990.

162. **Herzog, S.,** Genetic polymorphism of transferrin in fallow deer, *Cervus dama, Anim. Genet.,* 20, 421, 1989.

163. **Shubin, P. N. and Ionova, T. A.,** Genetic interrelation between domestic and wild reindeer, *Rangifer tarandus,* Biologischeskie Problemy Severa (9th Simpozium) Ch. II, Syktyvkar, 1981.

164. **Roed, K. H.,** Genetic differences at the transferrin locus in Norwegian semi-domestic and wild reindeer (*Rangifer tarandus*), *Hereditas,* 102, 199, 1985.

165. **Zhurkevich, N. M. and Fomicheva, I. I.,** Genetic polymorphism of transferrins of blood serum in reindeer (*Rangifer tarandus*) indigenous to northeastern Siberia, *Genetika,* 12, 56, 1976.

166. **Roed, K. H.,** Transferrin variation and body size in reindeer, *Rangifer tarandus, Hereditas,* 106, 67, 1987.

167. **Masina, L.,** Serum albumin and transferrin variants in Italian water buffalo (*Bos bubalis*), *Experimentia,* 27, 587, 1971.

168. **Granciu, I., Duica, S., Curea, I., and Mivolan, E.,** Blood group and biochemical polymorphism studies in *Bos bubalis, Anim. Blood Groups Biochem. Genet.,* 4, 11, 1973.

169. **Amano, T., Nakikawa, T., and Suzuki, S.,** Genetic differences between swamp and river buffaloes in electrophoretic variants of albumin and transferrin, *Proc. Jpn. Acad. B,* 56, 463, 1980.

170. **Makaveyew, T.,** Albumin, transferrin, amylase and blood groups in Bulgarian water buffalo, *Proc. XIth Eur. Conf. Anim. Blood Groups Biochem. Polymorph.,* Warsaw, 1970, 236.

171. **Ashton, G. C.,** Serum protein differences in cattle by starch gel electrophoresis, *Nature,* 180, 917, 1957.

172. **Hickman, C. G. and Smithies, O.,** Polymorphism of β-globulin in cattle, *Proc. Genet. Soc. Can.,* 2, 39, 1957.

173. **Ashton, G. C.,** Genetics of β-globulin polymorphism in British cattle, *Nature,* 182, 370, 1958.

174. **Tsuji, S., Fukishima, T., Shiomi, M., and Abe, T.,** A new serum transferrin phenotype observed in Japanese Black cattle, *Anim. Blood Groups Biochem. Genet.,* 12, 299, 1981.

175. **Ashton, G. C.,** β-Globulin polymorphism and early foetal mortality in cattle, *Nature,* 183, 404, 1959.

176. **Stratil, A. and Spooner, R. L.,** Isolation and properties of individual components of cattle transferrin: the role of sialic acid, *Biochem. Genet.,* 5, 347, 1971.

177. **Richardson, N. E., Buttress, N., Feinstein, A., Stratil, A., and Spooner, R. L.,** Structural studies on individual components of bovine transferrin, *Biochem. J.,* 135, 87, 1973.

178. **Hatton, M. W. C., Regoeczi, E., Wong, K-L., and Kraay, G. J.,** Bovine serum transferrin phenotypes AA, D_1D_1, D_2D_2, and EE: their carbohydrate compositions and electrophoretic multiplicity, *Biochem. Genet.*, 15, 621, 1977.

179. **Maeda, K., McKensie, H. A., and Shaw, D. C.,** Nature of the heterogeneity within genetic variants of bovine serum transferrin, *Anim. Blood Groups Biochem. Genet.*, 11, 63, 1980.

180. **Maeda, K., McKensie, H. A., and Shaw, D. C.,** Comparison of bovine serum transferrin A and D_2. Amino acid residue differences, *Anim. Blood Groups Biochem. Genet.*, 15, 299, 1984.

181. **Kimura, M.,** The neutral theory of molecular evolution, in *Evolution of Genes and Proteins*, M. Nei, and R. K. Kohn, Eds., Sinauer Associates, Sunderland, MA, 1983, 208.

182. **Lewontin, R. C.,** *The Genetic Basis of Evolutionary Change*, Columbia University Press, New York, 1974.

Chapter 10

HUMAN TRANSFERRIN — SELECTED CLINICAL AND PATHOLOGICAL ASPECTS

I. INTRODUCTION

Virtually all of the iron present in human plasma (80 to 180 μg/L, 14 to 32 μM/L) is bound to transferrin, as shown by the near completeness of iron removal from plasma when transferrin is precipitated by specific antibodies. Under normal circumstances, the only other iron found in plasma is that associated with the traces of haemoglobin and lactoferrin usually present. Whilst most red cell destruction occurs within the spleen, a small amount of intravascular haemolysis is not unusual, and when this occurs, the haemoglobin released from the red cells is rapidly complexed with the plasma protein haptoglobin, thus preventing iron loss via the kidneys. The plasma iron in the form of the haemoglobin-haptoglobin complex rarely exceeds 5 μg/100 mL. The only other significant contribution to the plasma iron pool is the molecule of lactoferrin, derived mainly from granulocytes. Lactoferrin is rapidly catabolised and is present in the plasma (1 to 3.5 mg/L) in very much smaller amounts than transferrin (2500 to 4000 mg/L), such that its contribution to the total plasma iron rarely exceeds 0.2 μg/100 mL.

Circumstances where significant amounts of iron appear in the plasma, not bound to transferrin, include iron poisoning and the chronic iron overload associated with such conditions as thalassaemia and idiopathic haemochromatosis. In the latter examples, it is the appearance of ferritin in the plasma that accounts for much of the increase in plasma iron. Ferritin is normally present in the plasma at very low levels, requiring sensitive immunoassay techniques in order to be measured accurately. Increased amounts of ferritin in the plasma usually indicate an increase in the iron stores of the body. When these stores become overloaded, such as in haemochromatosis, plasma levels of ferritin rise dramatically. Since each molecule of ferritin contains as many as 4500 atoms of iron, compared with the maximum of two iron atoms bound to transferrin, the spillage of even small quantities of ferritin into the plasma results in a large rise in the level of plasma iron. Occasionally, iron-containing tissue ferritin appears in the plasma, even when the body iron stores are within the normal range. Circumstances where this occurs include liver disease, leukaemia, and certain other neoplastic disorders where ferritin is released from diseased or damaged tissues.

With these few exceptions in mind, and since most body tissues are dependent upon transferrin for their iron supplies, in a healthy individual plasma iron is assumed to be synonymous with transferrin-bound iron. The clinical assessment of plasma iron status usually involves two measurements. The first of these is the determination of the amount of iron in the plasma (PI), and the second is a measurement of how much iron would be present if the total iron-binding capacity (TIBC) of the plasma was fully saturated. From these two results, two further values can be calculated. First, by subtracting the PI from the TIBC, the unsaturated iron-binding capacity (UIBC) is obtained. Second, and of much more use as a parameter for evaluating plasma iron supply, transferrin saturation (percent) can be calculated: PI/TIBC × 100.

It is not the intention of this chapter to give anything other than a very brief account of either how these measurements are made or their clinical relevance. These subjects are dealt with extensively in most standard textbooks of haematology or clinical chemistry, and have recently been reviewed by Huebers and Finch.[1]

The most commonly employed methods for the measurement of plasma iron involve the acidification of the plasma to liberate iron from transferrin, precipitation of the proteins to minimise turbidity, and finally the addition of a colour-producing iron chelator. Such colorimetric methods are not always entirely specific for iron, and as much as 5% of the colour developed may be due to the presence of copper. Even in normal subjects, plasma iron levels frequently show a significant diurnal variation, with the highest levels being seen in the morning and the lowest in the evening. The cause of the diurnal variation has yet to be fully elucidated, but there is some evidence that it is associated with changes in the amount of iron released by the reticulo-endothelial cells following red cell destruction. The increase in bilirubin levels associated with the diurnal rise in plasma iron certainly supports this hypothesis. Since in adults, less than 5% of the iron passing through the plasma each day comes from dietary absorption, it is not surprising to find that neither meals nor short periods of fasting have any significant effect on the level of plasma iron. Where random fluctuations of plasma iron do occur, the causes have yet to be determined. For example, strenuous physical activity is often followed by an increase of plasma iron by as much as 10%, whereas sleep deprivation is associated with a marked decrease.

Until recently, the measurement of the TIBC was most commonly carried out by adding a large excess of iron to a sample of plasma, in order to ensure that the transferrin was fully saturated with iron. The unbound iron is then removed using magnesium carbonate, and finally the iron content of the plasma is determined using a standard colorimetric procedure, as for the PI. In the last few years, because of the inherent problems associated with this procedure (failure to fully saturate the transferrin with inorganic iron, and failure to remove all of the excess iron), this method has begun to be replaced by direct measurements of plasma transferrin using immunological techniques. On the assumption that nearly all of the plasma iron is bound to transferrin, and knowing that each molecule of transferrin when fully iron saturated carries two atoms of iron, it is possible to calculate TIBC from a knowledge of the transferrin concentration.

Once PI and TIBC are known, transferrin iron saturation can be calculated. Because of the direct relationship between saturation and diferric iron, and also because of the greater capacity for diferric transferrin to deliver iron to tissues, transferrin saturation is the most useful and relevant biological expression of iron supply. The value is usually found to be in the region of 30%, evidence that transferrin is capable of carrying a lot more iron than is normally present in plasma. Since transferrin concentrations do not fluctuate throughout the day, the normal saturation cycles between 40% in the early morning and

20% at night, due principally to the diurnal variation of plasma iron concentration. A transferrin iron saturation of 16% or more is considered to be adequate for the maintenance of basal erythropoiesis in adults.[2] Many of the pathological changes in plasma iron concentrations and transferrin saturation can be explained on the basis of alterations either in the iron supplied to the plasma, or in the iron removed from the plasma by the tissue transferrin receptors. For example, hypoferraemia resulting from the exhaustion of tissue iron reserves, coupled with inadequate dietary intake, results in a decrease of both the PI and the transferrin saturation. Conversely, increases in the PI and transferrin saturation follow a large oral dose of iron or an episode of acute red cell haemolysis. In many such pathological examples, the changes in PI concentration are paralleled by changes in transferrin iron saturation in the same direction, but this is not always the case. There is a second element in the equation, and this is the concentration of plasma transferrin itself. Independent changes may occur in either transferrin concentration or PI, the former usually relating to transferrin synthesis and the latter to changes in either plasma iron supply or utilisation. If there is an acute change in PI concentration and the level of plasma transferrin remains constant, then the transferrin saturation will alter accordingly, and in a predictable direction. However, it is well known that many factors can affect the level of transferrin in the plasma, either by regulating the expression of the transferrin gene (iron, hormones, nutritional state) or by increasing the rate of loss of transferrin from the blood (kidney damage). When the concentration of plasma transferrin is altered as a result of the operation of one of these factors, this can have a direct effect on both the level of PI and the degree of transferrin saturation, but not necessarily in the same direction. For example, when transferrin levels fall dramatically, as occurs in renal loss, the PI concentration will decrease, but the iron saturation of the small amount of transferrin remaining in the plasma may well be found to have increased.

Huebers and Finch[1] have reviewed many of the factors that either directly or indirectly can result in alterations in the level of PI, the concentration of plasma transferrin, and the degree of transferrin saturation. Some of the more commonly encountered examples are summarised in Table 1.

The clinical applications of human transferrin estimations that have been briefly described so far have principally been concerned with the evaluation of iron status, and disorders that disturb iron homeostasis. It has, however, become increasingly apparent over the last 20 years that the presence of transferrin, not only in plasma, but also in other biological fluids, its structural variability (particularly the microheterogeneity resulting from different numbers of sialic acid residues), its ability to bind elements other than iron, its ability to cross membranes (particularly when these become leaky as a result of damage), and its capacity to bind to specific cell membrane receptors, are all properties that can be exploited in many different fields of human pathology. As a result, even a brief inspection of the medical literature reveals that these and other properties of the molecule have been successfully applied

TABLE 1

**Pathological Conditions and Other Factors Affecting Plasma Iron,
Plasma Transferrin, and Transferrin Saturation**

Increase	Decrease
Plasma Iron	
Oral iron — therapeutic accidental	Iron deficiency
Ineffective erythropoiesis	Blood loss
Acute haemolytic anaemia	Pregnancy
Aplastic anaemia	Lactation
Idiopathic haemochromatosis	Inflammation
Liver disease	Hypotransferrinaemia
Nontransferrin iron (ferritin)	Physical activity
Sleep deprivation	Kidney damage (renal loss of transferrin)
Plasma Transferrin	
Iron deficiency	Congenital atransferrinaemia
Pregnancy	Liver damage
Steroid hormones (oestrogen)	Dietary protein deficiency
	Inflammation and infection
	Iron overload — haemochromatosis
	Neoplasm
	Kidney damage (renal loss of transferrin)
Transferrin Saturation	
Iron overload	Iron deficiency
Aplastic anaemia	Inflammation and infection
Haemolytic anaemia	
Ineffective erythropoiesis	
Kidney damage (renal loss of transferrin)	

in a wide range of clinical contexts, ranging from the assessment of nutritional status or the measurement of vascular permeability, to the localisation of tumours or the delivery of drugs and other chemotherapeutic agents to cancer cells. In the remaining sections of this chapter, selected examples of these diverse applications will be briefly described and discussed in order to demonstrate the wide range of areas in which the rich and varied chemical and physical properties of human transferrin have been successfully exploited.

II. HUMAN TRANSFERRIN — A SELECTION OF CLINICAL APPLICATIONS (OTHER THAN AS AN INDEX OF IRON STATUS)

A. INFECTION AND HOST RESISTANCE

Although the primary function of transferrin is considered to be as a carrier and supplier of iron to host tissues, it may also have an important role to play as an antibacterial agent.[1] In fact, it is as a direct result of the ability of plasma transferrin to retard bacterial growth that the molecule was first discovered nearly 50 years ago. Virtually all microorganisms require iron in order to multiply, and since plasma transferrin is rarely more than about 35% saturated with iron, the remaining high-affinity binding sites can act as scavengers of free iron in extracellular fluids, thereby withholding this vital element from the invading microorganisms. Bacterial growth is inhibited in the presence of unsaturated transferrin, but resumes when the transferrrin is fully saturated with iron.[3] Not only has it been proposed that transferrin constitutes an important defence against bacterial invasion, but it has also been speculated that iron deficiency may strengthen this defence by increasing the proportion of unsaturated transferrin.

Certainly, many of the clinical reports in the early 1970s, particularly those from Africa, supported a relationship between unsaturated transferrin and resistance to infection[1] — lower incidences of bacterial infection and malarial attacks amongst those individuals with chronic iron deficiency. Whilst this significant advantage of iron deficiency may be relevant in some parts of the world, there is no evidence that in developed countries such an advantage exists.[1]

Until recently, the explanation for the acute hypoferraemia that invariably occurs within a few hours of onset of infection was provided by the "RES block" hypothesis. This model envisaged a withholding of iron release from the cells of the reticulo-endothelial system (RES), possibly attributable to the action of chemical messengers (? interleukin-2). However, Sawatzki has challenged this explanation and has provided evidence suggesting that the primary cause of the acute postinfection hypoferraemia is the release of lactoferrin from granulocytes. Lactoferrin, being a molecule with a much higher affinity for iron than transferrin, captures the iron from transferrin, and then the iron-lactoferrin complex becomes rapidly cleared from the blood by the liver. Whichever of these two theories one accepts, the net effect is the same — a reduction in PI concentration following infection, thereby producing an iron-deplete environment helping to suppress further bacterial multiplication.

In order to deprive invading pathogens of iron, humans have evolved a complex mechanism involving the cooperation between cells (granulocytes) and iron-binding proteins (transferrin and lactoferrin). In the meantime, the pathogens themselves have not been idle, since they have evolved a battery of mechanisms in order to obtain their iron in this hostile environment (high-affinity iron siderophores and cell membrane receptors for transferrin and lactoferrin).

B. PROTEIN MALNUTRITION

In the field of human nutrition there has been a continuing interest in finding biochemical indices that accurately reflect nutritional status. These are required in order to identify cases of early undernutrition in situations where anthropometric measurements may be unreliable, and also to provide an index which allows the clinician to estimate the severity and prognosis for recovery from the more severe forms of malnutrition. Whilst plasma albumin concentrations are invariably reduced in severe cases of kwashiorkor (protein malnutrition), they are frequently in the normal range in cases of both marasmus (protein-energy malnutrition) and marginal malnutrition.

In an extensive survey carried out by Reeds and Laditan[5] amongst a large group of children in Nigeria, plasma transferrin and plasma albumin concentrations were measured, as well as the usual anthropometric indices. It was discovered that plasma transferrin provided a far better index of the severity of malnutrition than did plasma albumin, since transferrin concentrations are reduced in kwashiorkor and marasmus, with the level being far lower in the former group. In addition, there was found to be a significant correlation between plasma transferrin concentrations and the deficits in length-for-age and weight-for-age measurements, particularly amongst the group of marginally undernourished children. Resulting from these findings, Reeds and Laditan have suggested that plasma transferrin provides a very useful index not only for estimating the severity of malnutrition, but also for the likely prognosis for recovery.

C. MATERNAL NUTRITION AND INFANT BIRTH WEIGHT

In a study of pregnant mothers and their newborn infants, the maternal plasma transferrin concentration at 24 weeks of gestation has been found to have a significant correlation with infant birth weight.[6] Maternal undernutrition, reflected by the low plasma transferrin level, clearly affects the outcome of the pregnancy. On the other hand, data from this same survey showed that there was no correlation between infant birth weight and the maternal concentrations of plasma albumin.

D. SIALOTRANSFERRINS AND ALCOHOL ABUSE

The molecule of human transferrin contains two complex-type glycan chains, each of which have been shown to be capable of exhibiting a wide range of structural variability.[7] Biantennary, triantennary, and tetraantennary branched structures have been shown to exist, and the variability is further compounded by the presence or absence of a residue of sialic acid at the end of each branch. As a result, nine different electrophoretically distinguishable isoforms of transferrin can be present at any one time in human plasma — ranging from molecules totally lacking sialic acid residues (asialotransferrin) to those containing the maximum of eight (octasialotransferrin). The various isoforms of human transferrin can be separated by means of isoelectric focussing in the pH range 5 to 6. Transferrins with the least number of sialic acid residues have the highest isoelectric points.[8,9] In normal plasma, the most predominant isoform carries four sialic acid residues (tetrasialotransferrin) and comprises more than 85% of the total. Apart from the penta (7%) and tri (5%) isoforms, the remaining species (zero, one, two, six, seven, and eight sialic acid residues) are normally found in only trace amounts.

During the last 10 years, the human sialotransferrins have attracted a considerable amount of research interest, and although the structural basis for the heterogeneity is now well understood, the physiological significance of the different isoforms has yet to be fully elucidated.[7,10] One fact that has emerged, however, is that the number of sialic acid residues present on a molecule of iron-laden transferrin profoundly influences the route by which the molecule delivers its iron to tissues, particularly the liver. Normally sialylated transferrin (three, four, or five sialic acid residues) binds to the specific transferrin receptor on cell membranes, and then follows the endocytotic route, described in Chapter 7, whereby the transferrin and the iron both evade capture by the intracellular lysosomes. On the other hand, transferrin molecules from which most or all of the sialic acid residues have been removed (asialotransferrins) have a reduced affinity for the normal transferrin receptor. However, these molecules, stripped of their sialic acid residues and with galactose residues exposed at the free ends of the glycan chains, now have a very high affinity for an alternative membrane receptor known as the asialoglycoprotein receptor. On hepatocyte cell membranes in particular, asialoglycoprotein receptors are far more numerous than transferrin receptors. A possible pathological consequence of these two receptor systems has recently been suggested following the discovery that, whereas iron entering hepatocytes via the transferrin receptor system can be rapidly recycled, iron moving into hepatocytes via the asialoglycoprotein receptor becomes deposited within the lysosomes, and is subsequently far less available for recycling.[11,12] This implies that if the proportion of the asialotransferrin isoform in plasma were to increase for any reason, more iron would be deposited in the "slowly mobilised" iron stores of the liver, increasing the likelihood of the development of hepatic siderosis.[13]

The first clear demonstration of an abnormality in the proportional distribution of sialotransferrin isoforms in human plasma came with the discovery by Stibler et al.[14] in 1978 that one or more of the transferrin bands detected by isoelectric focussing was more pronounced in the serum of alcoholics, this being a reflection of an increased concentration of molecules with a low sialic acid content. Subsequent studies by a number of groups[15-21] have confirmed this observation, and have clearly demonstrated that the most consistent abnormality within the plasma of alcoholics is an increase in the proportions of the transferrin isoforms with isoelectric points 5.7, 5.8, and 5.9. These correspond to the molecules of disialo-, monosialo-, and asialotransferrin, respectively. The measurement of sialic acid-depleted transferrin is usually carried out either by means of isoelectric focussing, or by using a recently developed ion-exchange chromatography technique,[17] the latter method being referred to as the carbohydrate-deficient transferrin (CDT) test. The elevated levels of CDT associated with chronic alcohol abuse have been found to return to normal within one month following alcohol withdrawal.[21] Asialo or CDT now appears to provide one of the most sensitive and specific tests for the detection of alcohol abuse.[20,22]

The molecular basis for the increase in asialotransferrin in alcoholic sera has recently been elucidated. During the final stages of the assembly of molecules of transferrin within the liver, the enzyme α-2,3-sialyltransferase of the Golgi membrane system catalyses the addition of sialic acid residues to the ends of the glycan chains. Once the newly synthesised molecules of transferrin have been released into the plasma, each molecule participates in many cycles between the plasma and the cytoplasm of iron-requiring cells. During the course of these cycles, terminal sialic acid residues are very susceptible to being removed, particularly under the influence of a highly active desialylation enzyme present within the liver endothelium.[23] Much of this damage is later repaired when the transferrin molecules encounter the α-2,3-sialyltransferase of the Golgi system during the course of the normal endocytotic cycle. It therefore appears that the degree of sialylation of plasma transferrin is a result of the balance between these two enzyme activities, one of which removes sialic acid residues, whilst the other adds them back again. In chronic alcohol abuse, it has been shown that alcohol stimulates the activity of the desialylation enzyme,[13] whilst at the same time it inhibits the activity of the sialyltransferase.[25] These two pathological responses to alcohol both serve to increase the proportion of asialotransferrin present within the plasma. Since, as has already been discussed, asialotransferrin delivers its iron to liver cells by way of the asialoglycoprotein receptor into the "slow-release" iron pool, the events outlined above appear to offer a reasonable explanation for the high incidence of hepatic siderosis amongst alcoholics.[13]

E. SIALOTRANSFERRINS AND OCCUPATIONAL EXPOSURE TO ORGANIC SOLVENTS

In the same manner that chronic exposure to alcohol has been shown to increase the levels of plasma asialotransferrin, Petren and Vesterberg[25] have recently discovered that workers in the paint industry exposed to a variety of organic solvents (white spirit, xylene, toluene, and ethyl acetate) have significantly elevated levels of the sialic acid-deficient isoforms of transferrin within their plasma. Since the levels were found to have remained well above the normal values even after the workers' holidays, it was concluded that the effects on the liver caused by the organic solvents were similar to those caused by alcohol abuse, but possibly had a more long-term effect.

F. SIALOTRANSFERRINS IN PREGNANCY

During pregnancy, enormous changes in maternal iron metabolism occur. As gestation progresses, and particularly by the stage of the third trimester, the increasing iron demands of the growing foetus have been found to be associated with alterations in both the concentration and chemical structure of the maternal plasma transferrin:[10,26]

1. The concentration of plasma transferrin has doubled.
2. The proportion of transferrin molecules carrying the more highly branched

glycan chains, particularly the triantennary structures, has increased significantly.

3.   The increase in glycan chain branching is associated with an increase in the proportions of the more highly sialylated transferrin isoforms.

De Jong et al.[10] have described a striking correlation between the progressive increase in the more highly sialylated maternal transferrin isoforms and the increase in transplacental iron transport that occurs during pregnancy. Since iron uptake at the maternal side of the placenta is thought to involve an interaction between maternal iron-loaded transferrin and transferrin receptors on the placental syncytiotrophoblast membrane,[27,28] it has been suggested that the increase in branching and sialylation of the maternal transferrin glycans may have a functional significance.[10]

G. SIALOTRANSFERRINS IN CEREBROSPINAL FLUID AND THE DIAGNOSIS OF CSF LEAKAGE

Cerebrospinal fluid (CSF) leakage resulting from a dural tear (skull fracture, tumour, infections, postoperative trauma, etc.), and commonly presenting as otorrhea or rhinorrhea, can be a dangerous and potentially life-threatening occurrence, especially when accompanied by bacterial meningitis.[29] Radiographic procedures have not always been successful in demonstrating small or delayed CSF leaks, and chemical analysis of fluid secretions for the presence of contaminating CSF have, until recently, been notoriously unreliable, especially when these secretions have contained even small amounts of blood. For this reason, a rapid, sensitive, and reliable test for the detection of CSF admixture in a variety of body secretions has been required.

Meurman et al.[30] described a potentially useful method for the detection of CSF leakage following their discovery that CSF contained a unique electrophoretic isoform of transferrin (β_2-transferrin/or the tau-protein) that did not appear to be present in any of the other body fluids tested (serum, nasal secretions, saliva, tears, and lymph). It has now been established that the β_2-transferrin of CSF is equivalent to the sialic acid-deficient isoform asialotransferrin. The microheterogeneity of human transferrin is therefore not just confined to human plasma. CSF contains a significant amount of asialotransferrin, whereas this particular isoform is normally present in only trace amounts in other fluids, including plasma. In a number of recent clinical studies, it has been confirmed that by analysing the pattern of transferrin microheterogeneity within a suspected fluid, and demonstrating the presence of a pronounced asialotransferrin band, the diagnosis of CSF leakage can be made with a high degree of reliability.[29-31]

H. SIALOTRANSFERRIN AS A DIAGNOSTIC MARKER IN CASES OF A RARE INHERITED DISORDER OF GLYCOPROTEIN SYNTHESIS

In 1984, Jaeken et al.[33] described a new genetic syndrome in two identical twins, presenting as a complex array of neurological disorders and multiple serum protein abnormalities. Predominant amongst the plasma protein abnormalities was a significant increase in the concentrations of disialotransferrin and asialotransferrin. A similar disorder has recently been described in seven Swedish children, and given the name disialotransferrin developmental deficiency syndrome.[34] Stibler and Jaeken[35] have reviewed these and similar cases, concluding that they are examples of a rare inherited disorder affecting the synthesis of plasma glycoproteins. Since transferrin is one of the most abundant members of this group of proteins, Stibler and Jaeken have attempted to discover the abnormality associated with the structure of the plasma transferrin from these patients in the hope that this might provide the key to an understanding of the molecular basis of this rare inherited condition. All the patients were found to have about a tenfold increase in the concentration of the carbohydrate-deficient isoforms of plasma transferrin. Further chemical analysis revealed that the carbohydrate deficiency was not confined just to the sialic acid residues. In addition, the content of galactose and *N*-acetyl galactosamine was found to be significantly reduced. From these results Stibler concluded that the disorder affected a number of the Golgi system glycosyl transferase enzymes, resulting in the production of shortened versions of the glycan chains, missing the sugars that normally comprise the terminal three residues of each chain — sialic acid, galactose, and *N*-acetyl galactosamine. Measurement of the plasma asialotransferrin appears to provide a simple diagnostic test for this rare systemic hereditary syndrome.

I. URINARY TRANSFERRIN AND THE EARLY DIAGNOSIS OF DIABETIC NEPHROPATHY

As an early manifestation of the glomerular basement membrane damage associated with diabetes, the appearance of plasma albumin in the urine has usually been assumed to provide a sufficiently sensitive and specific test in order to predict the subsequent development of clinically overt diabetic nephropathy. Recent experimental results, however, indicate that the presence of plasma transferrin in the urine (microtransferrinuria) is an even more sensitive indicator of early glomerular damage than microalbuminuria.[36,37] Since the molecular radius of transferrin (4.0 nm) is larger than albumin (3.6 nm), it is difficult to imagine how a gradual enlargement of the glomerular basement membrane pores would lead to the appearance of transferrin in the urine before the appearance of albumin. If size is not the deciding factor, then possibly the difference in net charge between the two proteins may be significant, transferrin being less anionic than albumin. Despite the absence of experimental evidence necessary to provide a rational explanation for selective escape of transferrin in advance of albumin, Bernard et al.[38] have recently confirmed that amongst a group of 176 diabetics, many more of the patients showed signs of microtransferrinuria than microalbuminuria, this being particularly noticeable in those patients with Type 1 (insulin-dependent) diabetes. Furthermore, these observations were reproduced experimentally in streptozotocin-induced diabetic rats, the animals showing a higher relative increase in the urinary excretion of transferrin than of albumin.

J. URINARY TRANSFERRIN — A MARKER FOR PROSTATIC CANCER

The prostate is the urologic organ most often affected by benign or malignant neoplasms. Several tumour markers, such as acid phosphatase, alkaline phosphatase, and lactate dehydrogenase, are traditionally measured in the plasma in order to monitor the extent of tumour progression and the presence of metastases in prostate carcinoma patients. However, many of these markers have been criticised for their lack of sensitivity and specificity.[39] Prostatic fluid, which is in direct contact with the prostate epithelium, contains high levels of transferrin. Since the fluid can enter the urine directly via the urethra, proteins originally present in the fluid and finding their way into the urine represent potentially useful markers for diseases affecting the prostate epithelium.

Fernandez et al.[39] compared the concentration of urinary transferrin in a control group (0.38 mg/L) with that from a group of patients with benign prostatic hyperplasia (1.5 mg/L) and prostatic cancer (13.7 mg/L). Since the highest levels were found amongst the patients at the more advanced stages of the disease, it appears that urinary transferrin could provide a useful additional marker for adenocarcinoma of the prostate epithelium.

K. SEMINAL PLASMA TRANSFERRIN AND FERTILITY

Seminal plasma contains high levels of transferrin,[40] this being necessary to satisfy the iron demands of the developing spermatocytes. The essential role of transferrin-bound iron in the process of spermatogenesis is supported by the presence of transferrin receptors on human spermatocytes and spermatids.[41] Since the architecture of the seminiferous tubules creates an effective blood-testis barrier, most of the transferrin found in seminal plasma originates from the secretions of the Sertoli cells of the testis, and not the blood plasma.[42] Sertoli cells respond to many of the hormones that regulate spermatogenesis (FSH, testosterone), and transferrin alone comprises as much as 5% of the total protein secreted by these cells into the seminal plasma.[43]

Because of the vital role played by the Sertoli cells in providing the nutrient environment essential for the proper development of sperm, there has been a considerable amount of research carried out during the last 10 years in order to find reliable markers of the functional activity of these cells. In 1982, Holmes et al.[44] demonstrated a positive correlation between sperm density and the level of seminal plasma transferrin. These early results indicated that abnormalities in Sertoli cell function, leading to a reduced secretion of transferrin, had a direct effect on male fertility. These observations have been subsequently confirmed by many independent reports.[45-51] The concentration of seminal plasma transferrin is considerably lower in subjects with azoospermia or oligospermia, and the transferrin level correlates well with sperm count, sperm motility, and the ability of the sperm to fertilize human oocytes *in vitro,* providing an early and specific marker of Sertoli cell function.

L. GLYCOSYLATED PLASMA TRANSFERRIN AND SHORT-TERM DIABETIC CONTROL

The chronic hyperglycaemia associated with uncontrolled diabetes results in an accentuation of the nonenzymic glycosylation of many body proteins.[52] This particular type of posttranslational protein glycosylation, as distinct from that involved in the formation of the glycan chains of glycoproteins, occurs in two steps, neither of which requires the presence of an enzyme. The initial step, which is both rapid and reversible, involves the formation of an aldimine link (Schiff base) between the aldehyde group of a glucose molecule and an amino group on the protein. Subsequently, an Amadori rearrangement forms a stable and irreversible ketoamine link. The glycosylation of proteins such as collagen, capillary and glomerular basement membrane proteins, myelin, and lens crystallin, is thought to account for many of the clinical complications that are frequently associated with poor diabetic control — peripheral neuropathy, kidney damage, and blindness. In addition to these examples of structural proteins, posttranslational glycosylation also affects many of the soluble proteins in cells and tissue fluids, including, for example, red cell haemoglobin. The levels of glycosylated haemoglobins are raised in chronic hyperglycaemia, and correlate closely with the average blood glucose levels over the previous 6 to 8 weeks.[53-55] Since the process of non-enzyme-catalysed glycosylation is irreversible, and the life-span of the red cell is 120 days, measurements of glycosylated haemoglobin levels are routinely used in order to assess the long-term diabetic control in patients.

As a means of obtaining a retrospective estimate of the time-averaged blood glucose level experienced by a diabetic patient over shorter time periods (2 to 8 days), glycosylated haemoglobin is not a particularly sensitive index. On the other hand, measuring the extent of posttranslational glycosylation of plasma transferrin (half-life 7 to 9 days) does appear to provide a reliable marker of short-term glycaemic control.[56]

M. PLASMA TRANSFERRIN AND THE ASSESSMENT OF VASCULAR PERMEABILITY, PARTICULARLY WITHIN THE LUNGS

For many years, radioiodinated plasma albumin has been a standard procedure used in clinical and experimental investigations of abnormal capillary permeability. The recent development of the technique of positron emission tomography (PET) has led to the possibility of studying the effects of tissue damage-induced changes in vascular permeability *in situ*. Iron, indium, and gallium are metals known to complex tightly with plasma transferrin, and iron-52, indium-110, and gallium-68 are all positron-emitting radionuclides that can be produced and used in PET studies. They have the additional advantage of short half-lives (8 hours, 66 minutes, and 68 minutes, respectively). Otsuki et al.[57] have recently demonstrated that whereas the iron-transferrin complex (exclusively) and the gallium-transferrin complex (preferentially) are removed from the circulation via the cell membrane transferrin receptor, the indium-transferrin complex has a very low affinity for the receptor, and its escape from the circulation provides a convenient macromolecular tracer to estimate vascular permeability and vessel pore size in tumours and systemic tissues. This follows an earlier report by Mintun et al.[58] suggesting the potential usefulness of the gallium-68 transferrin complex in PET studies for the assessment of increased pulmonary vascular permeability in adult respiratory distress syndrome.[58]

In the absence of PET, increased vascular permeability following acute lung injury can be monitored using the radioactive indium-113-transferrin complex.[59,60]

N. TRANSFERRIN AND THE LOCALISATION OF TUMOURS

Transferrin receptors are found in abundance on the cell membranes of cancerous tissues and malignant cell lines,[61] evidence of the increased iron demands of these rapidly dividing cells. Transferrin receptors of cancerous tissues have been actively investigated as potential tools for both the diagnosis and treatment of malignancies.

Gallium-67 citrate localises in a wide variety of soft-tissue tumours and has been used for over 20 years as a diagnostic imaging agent in clinical nuclear medicine.[62] The mechanism by which administered gallium is transported to, and accumulated by, malignant cells is now well understood. The administration of trace amounts of radioactive gallium is rapidly followed by the binding of the gallium to plasma transferrin. This in turn transports the gallium to cells and tissues, whereupon the radioactive isotope is taken into cells via the membrane transferrin receptor. It is the enhanced expression of transferrin receptors on malignant cells that explains why gallium-67 has proved to be such a useful imaging agent for the diagnosis of soft-tissue tumours.

O. TRANSFERRIN AS A VEHICLE FOR THE DELIVERY OF DRUGS AND OTHER CHEMOTHERAPEUTIC AGENTS

The presence of large numbers of transferrin receptors on tumour cells has provided a target upon which to focus potential therapeutic agents for the purpose of suppressing cell proliferation. Two alternative approaches have recently been investigated. The first of these has been the use of monoclonal antibodies against the transferrin receptor, either as a means of blocking iron-transferrin uptake (and thereby inhibiting cell growth and division), or as a vehicle for the delivery of cytotoxic agents (in the form of receptor antibody-drug conjugates) to tumour cells. Although many *in vitro* experiments have shown promising results using this approach,[61] its application in the clinical field is likely to be of limited value, since the monoclonal antibodies, often of mouse origin, will be recognised by the patients as foreign proteins, against which an immune response will be mounted.

A more promising technique has been the use of homologous transferrin to deliver cytotoxic agents to the tumour cells via their membrane receptors.

One of the first successful demonstrations of this method was reported by Kohgo et al.[61] in 1985. Human diferric transferrin was complexed with neocarzinostatin, a polypeptide antibiotic that is cytotoxic to human leukaemia and other cancer cells. *In vitro* experiments demonstrated that the transferrin-antibiotic conjugate was far more effective in bringing about the death of cultured cancer cells than was the free antibiotic alone. Even more encouraging was the demonstration of the effectiveness of the conjugate in suppressing tumour growth *in vivo*.

Since this first report, further successful applications of therapeutic regimes in which transferrin has been used to deliver drugs to tumour cells have been reported. These include the treatment of human leukaemia with a transferrin-adriamycin conjugate,[64] breast cancer and liver cancer with transferrin-platinum complexes,[65,66] and human lymphomas with gallium salts that subsequently become bound to human plasma transferrin.[67] The subject of drug targetting using transferrin as a delivery vehicle has been reviewed by Faulk.[68]

P. TRANSFERRIN AS A VEHICLE FOR THE INTRODUCTION OF FOREIGN DNA INTO EUKARYOTIC CELLS

Most current gene-transfer methods (retroviral vectors, microinjection, calcium phosphate precipitation), whilst functioning well with adherent cells of established cell lines in culture, have met with limited success when similar transfection procedures have been attempted on primary, nonadherent eukaryotic cells. In addition, many of the reagents that have been used to enhance DNA uptake have proved to have serious cytotoxic side effects. It is only recently that alternative protocols employing electroporation or DEAE-dextran have met with some degree of success.

A novel approach for the introduction of DNA into eukaryotic cells using transferrin as the vehicle, and receptor-mediated uptake as the port of entry, has recently been reported.[69,70] Transferrin alone has little or no affinity for DNA. However, if the transferrin is first conjugated with a large polycation such as protamine or polylysine, the resulting conjugate binds double-stranded DNA by means of electrostatic attraction. Incubation of recipient cells with the transferrin-polycation-DNA complex results in the uptake of the DNA via the membrane transferrin receptors. The successful transfer and subsequent expression of plasmid DNA by eukaryotic cells is further enhanced if the cells have been previously treated with iron-chelating agents in order to increase the numbers of membrane transferrin receptors. DNA molecules as large as 14,000 bp have been successfully transferred into cells using this new method, a technique which the authors have called "transferrinfection".[69,70]

Q. TRANSFERRIN, ALUMINIUM TOXICITY, AND ALZHEIMER'S DISEASE

Aluminium has yet to be shown to have an essential role to play in human metabolism. However, the accumulation of excessive amounts of this element within the body, coupled with its slow release from tissues (half-life 45 days), is thought to be responsible for many of the well-known toxic effects of aluminium. A wide variety of human cells and tissues are susceptible to aluminium poisoning, including the brain,[71] red cells,[72] bone,[73] joints,[74] and muscles.[75]

Although aluminium is present in very low amounts in most foods, there are certain dietary components known to contain high concentrations of aluminium. These include soya bean, tea, and any manufactured cakes to which aluminium silicates have been added in the form of baking powder. Fortunately, the capacity of the intestinal tract to absorb aluminium is extremely low, such that it has been calculated that the length of time it would take a human to accumulate, via a normal diet, levels of aluminium within the brain likely to induce even the mildest form of encephalopathy, is in the region of 150 years. Consequently, those people at greatest risk of accumulating toxic levels of aluminium within their bodies before the end of a normal life-span include:

1. Individuals with impaired renal function, including premature neonates, in which the ability to eliminate aluminium from the body via the kidneys is severely reduced.
2. People exposed to high levels of aluminium within an industrial environment.
3. Patients who inadvertently receive aluminium by a route that bypasses the normal barrier of the gastrointestinal tract. This includes particularly those patients who receive maintenance dialysis because of their non-functioning kidneys. The acquisition of aluminium from the dialysis fluid is thought to account for the increased incidence of microcytic anaemia, osteomalacia, and encephalopathy amongst this group.[77]
4. People who ingest large amounts of aluminium, for example, the widespread consumption of antacid preparations based on aluminium hydroxide. The ingestion of antacids coupled with reduced renal function (in old age) leads to an elevation of serum aluminium levels and the accumulation of toxic levels of aluminium within bones.[78]

Of the three main groups of clinical disorders in which aluminium toxicity has been implicated, microcytic anaemia, osteomalacia, and encephalopathy, it is the last of these, particularly the association between aluminium and Alzheimer's disease, that has received considerable attention in recent years. Alzheimer's disease is an insidious and ultimately fatal form of dementia affecting as many as 1% of the population. Although the precise cause is not yet known, both genetic and environmental factors are thought to be involved. There have been many reports suggesting an association between aluminium and Alzheimer's disease. These have included: the increased levels of aluminium in the affected parts of the brain of Alzheimer patients;[79–86] a geographical relationship between the incidence of Alzheimer's disease and the concentration of aluminium in the drinking water;[87] and the similarities of the neurochemical, neuropathological, and cerebral disturbances exhibited by dialysis patients and people with Alzheimer's disease.[88]

Whether plasma transferrin plays a significant role in the accumulation of aluminium within the brain is a question that has yet to be fully resolved. Plasma normally contains very low levels of aluminium (2 to 8 ng/mL). Whilst the vast majority of this aluminium is found complexed to the vacant metal-binding sites of transferrin, a small proportion is bound to plasma albumin, and the remainder is associated with low-molecular-weight chelators, principally citrate.[89,90] At least two mechanisms have been suggested to account for the uptake of aluminium across the blood-brain barrier into the brain. One logical possibility is that aluminium follows the same route as iron — bound to the transferrin in plasma, taken up by the endothelial cells of the blood-brain barrier by receptor-mediated endocytosis, and finally transferred to the transferrin present in the CSF. An alternative suggestion, which does not directly involve plasma transferrin, is that the aluminium-citrate complex in the plasma plays an essential role in the process of intracellular accumulation, and hence the toxicity, of aluminium.[90,91] Evidence supporting this second route has recently been reported by Farrar et al.[92] Plasma from patients with Alzheimer's disease has been found to contain a much higher proportion of the aluminium associated with low-molecular-weight complexes (citrate) than with transferrin. From these results it has been suggested that the plasma transferrin of Alzheimer's patients has unusual metal-binding properties. The degree of iron saturation of the transferrin was found to be significantly increased (60%), whereas the ability of the transferrin to bind aluminium was considerably reduced. Since, as a result, a greater proportion of the aluminium was bound to citrate, it was suggested that in the form of the citrate complex more aluminium entered the brain, thereby causing the neurotoxicity seen in Alzheimer's disease. The implication of these preliminary findings is that a defective form of transferrin (genetic?) in Alzheimer's patients, because of its reduced affinity for aluminium, results in more of the metal being present in the plasma in the form of a low-molecular-weight citrate complex, which in turn leads to an increased uptake of aluminium by the brain.

R. CIRCULATING TRANSFERRIN RECEPTORS IN HUMAN PLASMA

The final example of a possible clinical application of human transferrin concerns not the transferrin molecule itself, but rather the membrane receptor for transferrin and its presence in biological fluids. There is now abundant evidence that the number of transferrin receptors on the membrane of a cell controls its rate of iron uptake from circulating transferrin. Increased numbers of membrane receptors have been described in a wide variety of haematological disorders[93,94] and on the malignant cells of many tumours.[95]

In 1985, Kohgo et al.[61] discovered the presence of human transferrin receptors circulating within the blood plasma. The molecular weight of this soluble form of the receptor was found to be 180,000, which is the same size as the receptor dimer normally associated with cell membranes. From these results it appeared that complete receptor molecules could be shed from cell membranes into the plasma. This initial observation has been confirmed in many subsequent reports.[96-101] By using a sensitive enzyme-linked immunoassay procedure, plasma transferrin-receptor concentrations have been measured in a number of clinical disorders, and the results compared with those of normal healthy individuals.[102,103] The level of circulating transferrin receptors has been found to be significantly reduced in aplastic anaemia, polycythemia, and posttransplant aplasia, whereas it has been found to be sharply elevated in patients with haemolytic anaemia, iron-deficiency anaemia, sickle cell anaemia, myeloproliferative disorders, and chronic lymphocytic leukaemia. From these preliminary observations it has been suggested that plasma transferrin-receptor levels could be a useful clinical index of bone marrow proliferative activity, as well as an indicator of disease progression in a variety of malignant and nonmalignant disorders.[102,103]

REFERENCES

1. **Huebers, H. A. and Finch, C. A.,** The physiology of transferrin and transferrin receptors, *Physiol. Rev.,* 67, 520, 1987.
2. **Bainton, D. F. and Finch, C. A.,** The diagnosis of iron deficiency anaemia, *Am. J. Med.,* 37, 62, 1964.
3. **Weinberg, E. G.,** Iron withholding: a defence against infection and neoplasia, *Physiol. Rev.,* 64, 65, 1984.
4. **Sawatzki, G.,** The role of iron binding proteins in bacterial infections, in *Iron Transport in Microbes, Plants and Animals,* G. Winkelmann, D. Van der Helm, and J. B. Neilands, Eds., VCH Publishers, Weinheim, West Germany, 1987, chap. 25.
5. **Reeds, P. J. and Laditan, A. A. O.,** Serum albumin and transferrin in protein-energy malnutrition. Their use in the assessment of marginal undernutrition and the prognosis of severe undernutrition, *Br. J. Nutr.,* 36, 255, 1976.
6. **Maletnlema, T. N. and Eddy, T. P.,** Serum transferrin of pregnant mothers related to birth weight of their infants, *Br. Med. J.,* 3, 386, 1972.
7. **De Jong, G. and Van Eijk, H. G.,** Functional properties of the carbohydrate moiety of human transferrin, *Int. J. Biochem.,* 21, 253, 1989.
8. **Van Eijk, H. G., Van Noort, W. L., Dubelaar, M. L., and Van der Heul, C.,** The microheterogeneity of human transferrins in biological fluids, *Clin. Chim. Acta,* 132, 167, 1983.
9. **Van Eijk, H. G., Van Noort, W. L., Kroos, M. J., and Van der Heul, C.,** The heterogeneity of human transferrin and transferrin preparations in isoelectric focussing gels, *Clin. Chim. Acta,* 121, 2009, 1982.
10. **De Jong, G., Van Dijk, J. P., and Van Eijk, H. G.,** The biology of transferrin, *Clin. Chim. Acta,* 190, 1, 1990.
11. **Tavassoli, M.,** The role of liver endothelium in the transfer of iron from transferrin to hepatocytes, *Ann. N.Y. Acad. Sci.,* 528, 83, 1988.
12. **Irie, S. and Tavassoli, M.,** Transferrin-mediated cellular iron uptake, *Am. J. Med. Sci.,* 292, 103, 1987.

13. **Mihas, A. A. and Tavassoli, M.**, The effect of ethanol on the uptake, binding, and desialylation of transferrin by rat liver endothelium: implications in the pathogenesis of alcohol-associated hepatic siderosis, *Am. J. Med. Sci.*, 301, 299, 1991.

14. **Stibler, H., Allgulander, C., Borg, S., and Kjellin, K. G.**, Abnormal micro-heterogeneity of transferrin in serum and cerebrospinal fluid in alcoholism, *Acta Med. Scand.*, 205, 49, 1978.

15. **Stibler, H. and Borg, S.**, Evidence of a reduced sialic acid content in serum transferrin in male alcoholics, *Alcoholism Clin. Exp. Res.*, 5, 545, 1981.

16. **Vesterberg, O., Petren, S., and Schmidt, D.**, Increased concentrations of a transferrin variant after alcohol abuse, *Clin. Chim. Acta*, 141, 33, 1984.

17. **Stibler, H., Borg, S., and Joustra, M.**, Micro anion exchange chromatography of carbohydrate-deficient transferrin in serum in relation to alcohol consumption, *Alcoholism Clin. Exp. Res.*, 10, 535, 1986.

18. **Storey, E. L., Mack, U., Anderson, G. J., Powell, L. W., and Halliday, J. W.**, Desialylated transferrin as a serological marker of chronic excessive alcohol ingestion, *Lancet*, 1292, June 1987.

19. **Petren, S. and Vesterberg, O.**, Concentration differences in isoforms of transferrin in blood from alcoholics during abuse and abstinence, *Clin. Chim. Acta*, 175, 183, 1988.

20. **Behrens, U. J., Worner, T. M., Braly, L. F., Schaffner, F., and Lieber, C. S.**, Carbohydrate-deficient transferrin, a marker for chronic alcohol consumption in different ethnic populations, *Alcoholism Clin. Exp. Res.*, 12, 427, 1988.

21. **Behrens, U. J., Worner, T. M., and Lieber, C. S.**, Changes in carbohydrate-deficient transferrin levels after alcohol withdrawal, *Alcoholism Clin. Exp. Res.*, 12, 539, 1988.

22. **Schellenberg, F., Benard, J. Y., Goff, A. M., and Weill, J.**, Evaluation of carbohydrate-deficient transferrin compared with Tf index and other markers of alcohol abuse, *Alcoholism Clin. Exp. Res.*, 13, 605, 1989.

23. **Irie, S. and Tavassoli, M.**, Desialylation of transferrin by liver endothelium is selective for its triantennary chains, *Biochem. J.*, 263, 491, 1989.

24. **Malagolini, N., Dall'Orio, F., Serafini-Cessi, F., and Cessi, C.**, Effect of acute and chronic ethanol administration on rat liver α 2,3 sialyltransferase activity responsible for sialylation of serum transferrin, *Alcoholism Clin. Exp. Res.*, 13, 649, 1989.

25. **Petren, S. and Vesterberg, O.**, Studies of transferrin in serum of workers exposed to organic solvents, *Br. J. Ind. Med.*, 44, 566, 1987.

26. **Leger, D., Campion, B., Decottignies, J., Montreuil, J., and Spik, G.**, Physiological significance of the marked increased branching of the glycans of human serum transferrin during pregnancy, *Biochem. J.*, 257, 231, 1989.

27. **Booth, A. G. and Wilson, M. J.**, Human placental coated vesicles containing receptor-bound transferrin, *Biochem. J.*, 196, 355, 1981.

28. **Pearse, B. M. F.**, Coated vesicles from human placenta carry ferritin, transferrin and immunoglobulin G, *Proc. Natl. Acad. Sci. U.S.A.*, 79, 451, 1982.

29. **Oberscher, G.**, Cerebrospinal fluid otorrhea — new trends in diagnosis, *Am. J. Otology*, 9, 102, 1988.

30. **Meurman, O. H., Irjala, K., and Suonpaa, J.**, A new method for the identification of cerebrospinal fluid leakage, *Acta Otolaryngol.*, 87, 366, 1979.

31. **Reisinger, P. W. M. and Hochstraber, K.**, The diagnosis of CSF fistulae on the basis of detection of β_2-transferrin by polyacrylamide gel electrophoresis and immunoblotting, *J. Clin. Chem. Clin. Biochem.*, 27, 169, 1989.

32. **Rouah, E., Rogers, B. B., and Buffone, G. J.**, Transferrin analysis by immunofixation as an aid in the diagnosis of cerebrospinal fluid otorrhea, *Arch. Pathol. Lab. Med.*, 111, 756, 1987.

33. **Jaeken, J., Van Eijk, H. G., Van der Heul, C., Corbeel, L., Eeckels, R., and Eggremont, E.**, Sialic acid-deficient serum and CSF transferrin in a newly recognised genetic syndrome, *Clin. Chim. Acta*, 144, 245, 1984.

34. **Kristiansson, B., Andersson, M., Tonnby, B., and Hagberg, B.,** The disialotransferrin developmental deficiency (DDD) syndrome, *Arch. Dis. Child.,* 64, 71, 1989.

35. **Stibler, H. and Jaeken, J.,** Carbohydrate deficient serum transferrin in a new systemic hereditary syndrome, *Arch. Dis. Child.,* 65, 107, 1990.

36. **Martin, P., Walton, C., Chapman, C., Bodansky, H. J., and Stickland, M. H.,** Increased urinary excretion of transferrin in children with Type 1 diabetes mellitus, *Diab. Med.,* 7, 35, 1990.

37. **Cheung, C. K., Cockram, C. S., Yeung, V. T. F., and Swaminathan, R.,** Urinary excretion of transferrin by non-insulin dependent diabetics: a marker for early complications?, *Clin. Chem.,* 35, 1672, 1989.

38. **Bernard, A. M., Ouled Amor, A. A., Goemaere-Vanneste, J., Antoine, J. L., Lauwerys, R. R., Lambert, A., and Vandeleene, B.,** Microtransferrinuria is a more sensitive indicator of early glomerular damage in diabetes than microalbuminuria, *Clin. Chem.,* 34, 1920, 1988.

39. **Fernandez, C., Rifai, N., Wenger, A. S., Mickey, D. D., and Silverman, L. M.,** A preliminary study of urinary transferrin as a marker for prostatic cancer, *Clin. Chim. Acta,* 161, 335, 1986.

40. **Tauber, P. F., Zaneveld, L. J. D., Propping, D., and Schumacher, G. F. B.,** Components of human split ejaculates. Spermatozoa, fructose, immunoglobulins, albumin, lactoferrin, transferrin, and other plasma proteins, *J. Reprod. Fertil.,* 43, 249, 1975.

41. **Vanelli, B. G., Orlando, C., Barni, T., Natali, A., and Baldoni, G. C.,** Immuno-staining of transferrin and transferrin receptors in human seminiferous tubules, *Fertil. Steril.,* 45, 536, 1986.

42. **Skinner, M. K. and Griswold, M. D.,** Sertoli cells synthesise and secrete transferrin-like protein, *J. Biol. Chem.,* 255, 9523, 1980.

43. **Wilson, R. M. and Griswold, M. D.,** Secreted proteins from rat Sertoli cells, *Exp. Cell Res.,* 123, 127, 1979.

44. **Holmes, S. D., Lipshultz, L. I., and Smith, R. G.,** Transferrin and gonadal dysfunction in man, *Fertil. Steril.,* 38, 600, 1982.

45. **Sueldo, C., Marrs, R. P., Berger, T., Kletzky, O. A., and O'Brien, T. J.,** Correlation of semen transferrin concentration and sperm fertilizing capacity, *Am. J. Obstet. Gynecol.,* 150, 528, 1984.

46. **Chan, S. Y. W., Loh, T. T., Wang, C., and Lawrence, C. H.,** Seminal plasma transferrin and seminiferous tubular dysfunction, *Fertil. Steril.,* 45, 687, 1986.

47. **Foresta, C., Manoni, F., Businaro, V., Donadel, C., Indino, M., and Scandellari, C.,** Possible significance of transferrin levels in seminal plasma of fertile and infertile men, *J. Androl.,* 7, 77, 1986.

48. **Orlanda, C., Caldani, A. L., Barni, T., Wood, W. G., Strasburger, C., Natali, A., Maver, A., Forti, G., and Serio, I.,** Ceruloplasmin and transferrin in human seminal plasma: are they an index of seminiferous tubular function?, *Fertil. Steril.,* 43, 290, 1985.

49. **Canale, D., Voliani, S., Izzo, P. L., Esposito, G., Giorgi, P. M., Ferdeghini, M., Meschini, P., and Menchini-Fabris, G. F.,** Human seminal transferrin: correlation with seminal and hormonal parameters, *Andrologia,* 20, 379, 1988.

50. **Mallea, L., Mas, J., Padron, R. S., and Diaz, J. W.,** Transferrin in seminal plasma of fertile and infertile men, *Andrologia,* 20, 15, 1988.

51. **Ber, A., Vardinon, N., Yogev, L., Yavetz, H., Hommonai, Z. T., Yust, I., and Paz, G.,** Transferrin in seminal plasma and in serum of men: its correlation with sperm quality and hormonal status, *Hum. Reprod.,* 5, 294, 1990.

52. **Brownlee, M. and Cerami, A.,** The biochemistry of the complications of diabetes, *Annu. Rev. Biochem.,* 50, 385, 1981.

53. **Bunn, H. F.,** Evaluation of glycosylated hemoglobin in diabetic patients, *Diabetes,* 30, 613, 1981.

54. **Goldstein, D. E., Parker, M., England, J. D., England, J. E., Weidmeyer, H., Rawlings, S. S., Hess, R., Little, R. R., Simonds, J. F., and Breyfogle, R. P.,** Clinical application of glycosylated hemoglobin measurements, *Diabetes,* 31, 70, 1982.

55. **McDonald, J. M. and Davis, J. E.,** Glycosylated hemoglobins and diabetes mellitus, *Hum. Pathol.,* 10, 279, 1979.

56. **Kemp, S. F., Creech, R. H., and Horn, T. R.,** Glycosylated albumin and transferrin: short-term markers of blood glucose control, *J. Paediatr.,* 105, 394, 1984.

57. **Otsuki, H., Brunetti, A., Owens, E. S., Finn, R. D., and Blasberg, R. G.,** Comparison of iron-59, indium-111, and gallium-69 transferrin as a macromolecular tracer of vascular permeability and the transferrin receptor, *J. Nucl. Med.,* 30, 1676, 1989.

58. **Mintun, M. A., Dennis, D. R., Welch, M. J., Mathias, C. J., and Schuster, D. P.,** Measurement of pulmonary vascular permeability with PET and gallium-68 transferrin, *J. Nucl. Med.,* 28, 1704, 1987.

59. **Hultkvist, U. and Bjellin, L.,** The indium-113m-transferrin complex as an indicator of serotonin-induced vascular changes in the golden hamster lung, *Int. J. Microcirc. Clin. Exp.,* 6, 333, 1987.

60. **Wetterberg, T., Svensjo, E., Larsson, A., Sigurdsson, G., Wagnerm, Z., and Willen, H.,** Acute lung injury monitored with radiolabelled transferrin and lung volume measurements, *Acta Anaesth. Scand.,* 33, 359, 1989.

61. **Kohgo, Y., Niitsu, Y., Nishisato, T., Urushizaki, Y., Kondo, H., Fukushima, M., Tsushima, N., and Urushizaki, I.,** Transferrin receptors of tumour cells: potential tools for diagnosis and treatment of malignancies, in *Proteins of Iron Storage and Transport,* G. Spik, J. Montreuil, R. R. Crichton, and J. Mazurier, Eds., Elsevier, Amsterdam, 1985, 155.

62. **Vallabhajosula, S. R., Harwig, J. F., Siemsen, J. K., and Wolf, W.,** Radiogallium localisation in tumours: blood binding and transport and the role of transferrin, *J. Nucl. Med.,* 21, 650, 1980.

63. **Trowbridge, I. S. and Domingo, D. L.,** Anti-transferrin receptor monoclonal antibody and toxin-antibody conjugates affect growth of human tumour cells, *Nature,* 294, 171, 1981.

64. **Faulk, W. P.,** Preliminary clinical study of transferrin-adriamycin conjugate for drug delivery to acute leukaemia patients, *Mol. Biother.,* 2, 57, 1990.

65. **Eillott, R. L., Stjerholm, R., and Elliott, M.,** Preliminary evaluation of platinum transferrin (MPTC-63) as a potential nontoxic treatment for breast cancer, *Cancer Det. Prev.,* 12, 469, 1988.

66. **Hamada, Y.,** Experimental studies on the treatment of hepatocellular carcinoma with cis-platinum transferrin complex, *Hokkaido Igaku Zasshi,* 63, 864, 1988.

67. **Warrell, R. P., Coonley, C. J., Strauss, D. J., and Young, C. W.,** Treatment of patients with advanced malignant lymphoma using gallium nitrate administered as a seven day continuous infusion, *Cancer,* 51, 1982, 1983.

68. **Faulk, W. P.,** Recent advances in cancer research: drug targetting without the use of monoclonal antibodies, *Am. J. Reprod. Immunol.,* 21, 151, 1989.

69. **Zenke, M., Steilein, P., Wagner, E., Cotten, M., Beug, H., and Birnstiel, M. L.,** Receptor-mediated endocytosis of transferrin-polycation conjugates: an efficient way to introduce DNA into hematopoietic cells, *Proc. Natl. Acad. Sci. U.S.A.,* 87, 3655, 1990.

70. **Cotten, M., Langle-Rouault, F., Kirlappos, H., Wagner, E., Mechtler, K., Zenke, M., Beug, H., and Birnstiel, M. L.,** Transferrin-polycation-mediated introduction of DNA into human leukemic cells: stimulation by agents that affect the survival of transfected DNA or modulate transferrin receptor levels, *Proc. Natl. Acad. Sci. U.S.A.,* 87, 4033, 1990.

71. **Boegman, R. J. and Bates, L. A.,** Neurotoxicity of aluminium, *Can. J. Phys. Pharm.,* 62, 1010, 1984.

72. **McGonigle, R. J. S. and Parsons, V.,** Aluminium-induced anaemia in haemodialysis patients, *Nephron,* 39, 1, 1985.

73. **Ott, S. M., Maloney, N. A., Coburn, J. W., Alfrey, A. C., and Sherard, D. J.,** The prevalence of bone aluminium deposition in renal osteodystrophy and its relation to the response to calcitrol therapy, *N. Eng. J. Med.,* 307, 709, 1982.

74. **Netter, P., Kessler, M., Gancher, A., Gillet, P., Delons, S., Burnel, D., Benoit, J., and Got, C.,** Aluminium and dialysis arthropathy, *Lancet,* 1, 886, 1988.

75. **Gittleman, H. J.,** *Aluminium and Health: a Critical Review,* Marcel Dekker, New York, 1989.

76. **Ganrot, P. O.,** Metabolism and possible health effects of aluminium, *Environ. Health Perspect.,* 65, 363, 1986.

77. **Wills, M. R. and Savory, J.,** Aluminium poisoning: dialysis encephalopathy, osteomalacia, and anaemia, *Lancet,* 2, 29, 1983.

78. **Davie, M. W. J., Worsfold, M., Sharp, C. A., Perks, J., and Day, J. P.,** Evaluation of serum osteocalcin associated with mobilisation of bone aluminium by desferrioxamine, *Bone,* 10, 478, 1989.

79. **Crapper, D. R., Krishman, S. S., and Dalton, A. J.,** Brain aluminium distribution in Alzheimer's disease and experimental neurofibrillary degeneration, *Science,* 180, 511, 1973.

80. **Crapper, D. R., Krishman, S. S., and Quittkat, S.,** Aluminium, neurofibrillary degeneration and Alzheimer's disease, *Brain,* 99, 67, 1976.

81. **Perl, D. P. and Brody, A. R.,** Alzheimer's disease: X-ray spectrometric evidence of aluminium accumulation in neurofibrillary tangel-bearing neurons, *Science,* 208, 297, 1980.

82. **Perl, D. P.,** Relationship of aluminium to Alzheimer's disease, *Environ. Health Perspect.,* 63, 149, 1985.

83. **Candy, J. M., Oakley, A. E., Klinowsky, J., Carpenter, T. A., Perry, R. H., Atack, J. R., Perry, E. K., Blessed, G., Fairbairn, A., and Edwardson, J. A.,** Aluminosilicates and senile plaque formation in Alzheimer's disease, *Lancet,* 1, 354, 1986.

84. **Ward, N. I. and Mason, J. A.,** Neutron activational analysis techniques for identifying elemental status in Alzheimer's disease, in *Modern Trends in Activational Analysis,* Copenhagen, 1986, 925.

85. **Shore, D. and Wyatt, R. J.,** Aluminium and Alzheimer's disease, *J. Nerv. Ment. Dis.,* 171, 553, 1983.

86. **Kellett, J. M., Taylor, A., and Oram, J. J.,** Aluminosilicates and Alzheimer's disease, *Lancet,* 1, 683, 1986.

87. **Martyn, C. N., Osmond, C., Edwardson, J. A., Barker, D. J. P., Harris, E. C., and Lacey, R. F.,** Geographical relationship between Alzheimer's disease and aluminium in drinking water, *Lancet,* 1, 59, 1989.

88. **Scholtz, C. L., Swash, M., Gray, A., Kogeoros, J., and Marsh, F.,** Neurofibrillary neuronal degeneration in dialysis dementia: a feature of aluminium toxicity, *Clin. Neuropathol.,* 6, 93, 1987.

89. **Trapp, G. A.,** Plasma aluminium is bound to transferrin, *Life Sci.,* 33, 311, 1983.

90. **Van Ginkel, M. F., Van der Voet, G. B., Van Eijk, H. G., and Wolff, F. A.,** Aluminium binding to serum constituents: a role for transferrin and for citrate, *J. Clin. Chem. Clin. Biochem.,* 28, 459, 1990.

91. **Farrar, G., Morton, A. P., and Blair, J. A.,** The intestinal speciation of gallium: possible models to describe the bioavailability of aluminium, in *Trace Element Analytical Chemistry in Medicine and Biology,* Vol. 5, P. Bratter and P. Schramel, Eds., Walter de Gruyter, Berlin, 1988, 343.

92. **Farrar, G., Altmann, P., Welch, S., Wychrij, O., Ghose, B., Lejeune, J., Corbett, J., Prasher, V., and Blair, J. A.,** Defective gallium-transferrin binding in Alzheimer's disease and Down's syndrome: possible mechanism for accumulation of aluminium in brain, *Lancet,* 335, 747, 1990.

93. **Matu, K., Nishimura, J., Ideguchi, H., Umemura, T., and Ibayashi, H.,** Erythroblast transferrin receptors and transferrin kinetics in iron deficiency and various anaemias, *Am. J. Hematol.,* 25, 155, 1987.

94. **Barnett, D., Wilson, G. A., Lawrence, A. C., and Buckley, G. A.,** Transferrin receptor expression in the leukaemias and lymphoproliferative disorders, *Clin. Lab. Haematol.,* 9, 361, 1987.

95. **Sutherland, R., Delia, D., Schnieder, C., Newman, R., Kemshead, J., and Greaves, M.,** Ubiquitous cell-surface glycoprotein on tumour cells is proliferation-associated receptor for transferrin, *Proc. Natl. Acad. Sci. U.S.A.,* 78, 4515, 1981.

96. **Kohgo, Y., Nishisato, T., Kondo, H., Tsushima, N., Niitsu, Y., and Urushizaki, I.,** Circulating transferrin receptor in human serum, *Br. J. Haematol.,* 64, 277, 1986.

97. **Kohgo, Y., Niitsu, Y., and Kondo, H.,** Serum transferrin receptor as a new index of erythropoiesis, *Blood,* 70, 1955, 1987.

98. **Kohgo, Y., Niitsu, Y., Nishisato, T., Kato, J., Sasaki, K., Tsushima, N., Hirayama, M., Kondo, H., and Urushizaki, I.,** Externalisation of transferrin receptor in established cell lines, *Cell. Biol. Int. Rep.,* 11, 871, 1987.

99. **Kohgo, Y., Niitsu, Y., and Nishisato, T.,** Quantitation and characterisation of serum transferrin receptor in patients with anaemias and polycythemias, *Jpn. J. Med.,* 27, 64, 1988.

100. **Beguin, Y., Heubers, H. A., Josephson, B., and Finch, C. A.,** Transferrin receptors in rat plasma, *Proc. Natl. Acad. Sci. U.S.A.,* 85, 637, 1988.

101. **Heubers, H. A., Beguin, Y., Pootrakul, P., Einsphar, D., and Finch, C. A.,** Intact transferrin receptors in human plasma and their relation to erythropoiesis, *Blood,* 75, 102, 1990.

102. **Flowers, C. A., Skikne, B. S., Covell, A. M., and Cook, J. D.,** The clinical measurement of serum transferrin receptor, *J. Lab. Clin. Med.,* 114, 368, 1989.

103. **Klemow, D., Einsphar, D., Brown, T., Flowers, C. H., and Skikne, B. S.,** Serum transferrin receptor measurements in hematologic malignancies, *Am. J. Hematol.,* 34, 193, 1990.

INDEX

R

Rabbit, transferrin polymorphism in, 236
Radioimmunoassay, of transferrin plasma
levels, 66
Rare earth ions, see Lanthanides
Rat, transferrin polymorphism in, 234
Receptor-mediated endocytosis, 164,
178–181
Red blood cells, release of iron in, 37
Redox-mediated plasma membrane model,
181
Relativity, Special Theory of, 7
Reptilia, transferrin polymorphism in,
229–230
Respiratory complex III, iron-sulphur
protein component of, 11
Reticulocytes
diferric transferrin binding to, 170
iron uptake mechanism in, 102
receptor-mediated uptake of transferrin-
bound iron by, 179
transferrin-iron cycle in, 176
transferrin receptors of, 167, 169
Reticuloendothelial system (RES), iron
turnover in, 37
Reticuloendothelial system block
hypothesis, 258
Rhizobacteria, symbiotic relationship of
with crop plants, 19
Ribonucleotide reductase, 12
Rieske's protein, 11
Rodents, transferrin polymorphism in,
234–236
Rough endoplasmic reticulum (RER)
insertion of polypeptide chain into, 168
transferrin gene in, 140–143
Rubredoxins, 11

S

Samarium, 122
Scandium, binding of to transferrin, 116
Sciatin, 153
Seal, transferrin polymorphism in, 237–238
Seminal plasma transferrin, fertility and,
264
Seminiferous tubules
architecture of, 264
transferrin receptors in, 163
Serine residue-24, phosphorylation of, 169
Sertoli cells

markers of function of, 264
transferrin in, 44, 56
transferrin receptors in, 163
transferrin synthesis in, 149–150
Serum transferrin, 44
amino acid composition of, 70–71,
72–74
disulphide bridges of, 79–80
functions of, 49–50
glycan chains in, 80–81
iron binding and, 81–98
iron release and, 99–102
physical and chemical properties of,
69–81
plasma concentration and electrophoretic
mobility of, 65–69
potential heterogeneity of, 67–69
primary sequence of, 75
primary structure of, 71–74
purification of, 69
secondary structure of, 74–76
size, shape, and quaternary structure of,
69–71
tertiary structure of, 76–79
Sheep, transferrin polymorphism in, 239
Shen Nung, and iron as cure for anaemia,
26
Shigella dysenteriae, growth inhibition of,
44–45
Sialic acid residues, number of in
transferrins, 259
Sialotransferrin
and alcohol abuse, 259–261
in cerebrospinal fluid, diagnosis of CSF
leakage and, 262
as diagnostic marker in rare glycoprotein
synthesis inherited disorder,
262–263
and occupational exposure to organic
solvents, 261
in pregnancy, 261–262
Sialyltransferase, 261
Sickle cell anaemia, and structurally
abnormal haemoglobin, 188
Siderite, 3
Siderophilins
amino acid sequences of, 74
ancestor of, 137
characteristics of, 42–44
comparison of structures, functions, and
properties of, 47–56
crystallographic data on, 76–77